Clinical Exercise Testing *and* Prescription

Theory and Application

Edited by

Scott O. Roberts
Robert A. Robergs
Peter Hanson

CRC Press
Boca Raton Boston London New York Washington, D.C.

Acquiring Editor: Marsha Baker
Project Editor: Debbie Didier
Cover Design: Dawn Boyd
PrePress: John Gandour

Library of Congress Cataloging-in-Publication Data

Clinical exercise testing and prescription : theory and application /
   edited by, Scott O. Roberts, Robert A. Robergs, Peter Hanson.
        p.   cm.
     Includes bibliographical references and index.
     ISBN 0-8493-4593-6
     1. Exercise therapy.   2. Exercise tests.   I. Roberts, Scott O.
   II. Robergs, Robert A.   III. Hanson, Peter (Peter G.)
     [DNLM: 1. Exercise Therapy--methods.   2. Exercise Test--methods.
   WB 541 C641 1997]
   RM725.C585   1997
   615.8'2--dc20
   DNLM/DLC
   for Library of Congress   96-24940
                                                                                                CIP

No claim to original U.S. Government works
International Standard Book Number 0-8493-4593-6
Library of Congress Card Number 96-24940
Printed in the United States of America   2 3 4 5 6 7 8 9 0
Printed on acid-free paper

The Editors

Scott Owen Roberts, Ph.D., is an Assistant Professor in the Department of Health, Physical Education, and Recreation at Texas Tech University, Lubbock, Texas.

Dr. Roberts obtained a B.S. in Physical Education from California State University, Chico, in 1986; an M.S. in Exercise Physiology from California State University, Sacramento, in 1988; and a Ph.D. in Exercise Physiology from the University of New Mexico in 1995.

Dr. Roberts' research interests include the role of ergogenic aids in sports, the effects of exercise in prepubescent children, and the role of exercise in the treatment and prevention of chronic diseases. Dr. Roberts has had numerous original scientific articles, trade articles, chapters, and books published. His most recent publications include serving as a section editor for *Exercise Management for Persons With Chronic Diseases and Disabilities,* Champaign, IL: Human Kinetics; and co-author of *Exercise Physiology: Exercise Performance and Clinical Applications,* St. Louis, MO: Mosby.

Dr. Roberts is a member of The American College of Sports Medicine, The Texas Chapter of the American College of Sports Medicine, The American Heart Association, The American Association of Cardiovascular and Pulmonary Rehabilitation, and The Texas Chapter of The American Association of Cardiovascular and Pulmonary Rehabilitation. He serves on a variety of committees for all of these organizations. He is a fellow of the American Association of Cardiovascular and Pulmonary Rehabilitation and a certified Exercise Program Director through the American College of Sportsmedicine.

Robert A. Robergs, Ph.D., is an Associate Professor of Exercise Physiology and Biochemistry and Director of the Center For Exercise and Applied Human Physiology at the University of New Mexico.

Dr. Robergs obtained a B.Ed Degree in Physical Education at Victoria University, Melbourne, Australia, in 1982. After teaching Physical Education in high school for three years, he began a Master's Degree in Exercise Physiology at The University of Western Australia, Perth. After being accepted into the Sports Science and Cardiac Rehabilitation Program under Paul Ribisl of Wake Forest University in the fall of 1985, he travelled to the United States and completed this degree in 1987. He then worked with David Costill at Ball State University for his Ph.D. in Bioenergetics. After graduating in 1990, achieving recognition on the Dean's List For Academic Excellence, Dr. Robergs accepted his present position at the University of New Mexico.

Dr. Robergs has a rapidly growing publication record in a diverse number of topics, including altitude physiology, muscle biochemistry, substrate use during exercise, the effects of exercise on the autonomic nervous system, applications of magnetic resonance to understanding muscle biochemistry during exercise, and exercise nutrition. He is primary author, along with Scott Roberts, of a graduate text on exercise physiology, a member of the American College of Sports Medicine, and a certified Exercise Test Technologist.

Peter Hanson, M.S., M.D., is a Professor of Medicine (Cardiology) and codirector of the Preventive Cardiology Program at the University of Wisconsin Clinical Science Center, Madison, WI.

Dr. Hanson obtained an M.S. degree in Physiology from the University of Illinois in 1962. He completed medical school at the University of New Mexico in Albuquerque, graduating with honors in 1971. He completed his medical residency training and served as a research fellow at the Cardiovascular Research Institute at the University of California, San Francisco.

Dr. Hanson's clinical and research interests have focused on clinical exercise physiology, baroreflex control of the circulation, and exercise training in a variety of patient populations, including patients with hypertension, ischemic heart disease, advanced heart failure, and postheart transplantation. His publication record includes over 100 original research articles, review papers, and chapters.

Dr. Hanson is a member of the American Physiological Society, a fellow of the American College of Sports Medicine, and a fellow of the American Heart Association Council on Circulation. He serves as an editorial reviewer for a number of journals including *Circulation, American Journal of Cardiology, Medicine and Science in Exercise and Sports, Journal of the American Medical Association, Archives of Internal Medicine, Journal of Applied Physiology, and American Journal of Hypertension.*

Contributors

Thomas Chick, M.D.
Department of Pulmonary Medicine
Matagorda General Hospital
Bay City, Texas

Thomas D. Fahey, Ed.D.
Exercise Physiology Laboratory
California State University
Chico, California

Robert G. Holly
Department of Exercise Science
University of California
Davis, California

Carolyn I. Johns, M.S., C.A.N.P.
Department of Cardiology
Lovelace Medical Center
Albuquerque, New Mexico

Miqdad Khan, M.D.
Blodgett Medical Center
Grand Rapids, Michigan

Karen E. Krstich, M.A.
Internal Medicine
University of California
Sacramento, California

Larry C. Kuo, M.D.
Department of Cardiology
Lovelace Medical Center
Albuquerque, New Mexico

Arthur S. Leon, M.D., M.S.
Division of Kinesiology
University of Minnesota
Minneapolis, Minnesota

David Lombard, M.S.
Psychology Department
Virginia Tech
Blacksburg, Virginia

Steven C. Port, M.D.
Cardiovascular Associates
Milwaukee, Wisconsin

Mark Richardson, Ph.D.
College of Education
University of Alabama
Tuscaloosa, Alabama

Robert A. Robergs, Ph.D.
Center for Exercise and Applied Human
    Physiology
University of New Mexico
Albuquerque, New Mexico

Scott O. Roberts, Ph.D.
Exercise and Sport Sciences
Texas Technological University
Lubbock, Texas

George Salem, Ph.D.
Department of Biokinesiology and Physical
    Therapy
University of Southern California
Los Angeles, California

Roy J. Shephard, M.D., Ph.D.
School of Physical and Health Education
University of Toronto
Toronto, Ontario, Canada
and
Health Studies Programme
Brock University
St. Catherines, Ontario, Canada

Douglas R. Southard, Ph.D., M.P.H., P.A.-C.
Department of Human Nutrition, Foods, and
  Exercise
Virginia Tech
Blacksburg, Virginia

Ray W. Squires, Ph.D.
Director, Cardiovascular Health Clinic
Associate Professor of Medicine
Division of Cardiovascular Diseases and Internal
  Medicine
Mayo Clinic and Foundation
Rochester, Minnesota

Jack E. Turman, Jr., Ph.D., P.T.
Department of Biokinesiology and Physical
  Therapy
University of Southern California
Los Angeles, California

Steven Ung, M.D.
Department of Cardiology
Lovelace Medical Center
Albuquerque, New Mexico

Contents

Clinical Exercise Testing *and* Prescription

Theory and Application

Chapter 1

Overview of Clinical Exercise Physiology

Robert A. Robergs

CONTENTS

I. INTRODUCTION

The stresses of exercise vary relative to the type, intensity, and duration of exercise, the environmental conditions, and also the health status of the individual. These multifactorial determinants of the physiological responses to exercise make a concise review of the physiology of exercise a daunting task. Nevertheless, as exercise training is becoming increasingly accepted in clinical treatment, rehabilitation, and preventative functions of the medical community, the need to appreciate the demands of exercise and its role in the promotion of health is paramount. This chapter will provide a concise review of the components of the science of exercise physiology that are involved in the clinical applications of exercise.

II. CLINICAL APPLICATIONS OF EXERCISE

Exercise is used in clinical settings for diagnostic, rehabilitative, and preventative purposes. In each application, there are fundamental principles that need to be understood concerning the quantification of exercise intensity and the interactions among exercise intensity, muscle energy metabolism, and systems physiology.

A. QUANTIFYING EXERCISE INTENSITY

Exercise intensity can be expressed relative to the mechanical energy generated by the exercise (e.g., watts or kilocalories generated from cycle ergometry) or to the energy expended by the individual during the exercise. The former expression requires knowledge of ergometry and energy conversions, while the latter example requires knowledge of indirect gas analysis calorimetry.

Table 1 Conversion Factors for the Different Units of Work, Power, Force, Pressure, and Mass

WORK	kJ	kcal	ft lb	kgm			
1 kJ	1.0	0.2388	737	1786.9			
1 kcal	4.1868	1.0	3,086	426.4			
1 ft lb	0.000077	0.000324	1.0	0.1383			
1 kgm	0.000560	0.002345	723	1.0			
POWER	**Horsepower**	**kgm · min⁻¹**	**ft lb · min⁻¹**	**watt**	**kcal · min⁻¹**	**kJ · min⁻¹**	
1 Horsepower	1.0	4564.0	33,000.0	745.7	10.694	44.743	
1 kgm · min⁻¹	0.000219	1.0	7.233	0.16345	0.00234	0.0098068	
1 ft lb · min⁻¹	0.00003	0.1383	1.0	0.0226	0.000324	0.0013562	
1 watt	0.001314	6.118	44.236	1.0	0.014335	0.060	
1 kcal · min⁻¹	0.0936	426.78	3,086.0	69.697	1.0	4.186	
1 kJ · min⁻¹	0.02235	101.97	737.30	16.667	0.2389	1.0	
FORCE	**lb**	**kg**	**N**				
lb	1.0	0.4545	0.04635				
kilogram (kg)	2.2	1.0	0.10197				
Newton (N)	19.614	9.807	1.0				
PRESSURE	**mmHg**	**kPa**	**torr**	**mbar**			
mmHg	1.0	0.1333	1.0	0.7502			
kPa	7.501	1.0	7.501	5.6272			
torr	1.0	0.1333	1.0	0.7502			
mbar	1.333	0.1777	1.333	1.0			
MASS	**ounce**	**gram**	**pound**	**kg**			
ounce	1.0	28.35	0.0625	0.028			
gram	0.0353	1.0	0.0022	0.001			
pound	16.129	454	1.0	0.454			
kg	35.714	1000	2.2	1.0			

Note: For these conversion tables, the conversion factors represent how many units listed down the page equal the units listed across the page. For example, 1 kJ equals 0.2388 kcal and 1786.9 kgm.

1. Energy, Work, Power, and the Science of Ergometry

The science of ergometry concerns the measurement of work. Work (W) is accomplished during the application of force against gravity (F) over a distance (D) and, hence, is expressed as $W = F \times D$. As movement of the body is based on lever systems of the musculoskeletal system, often performed against gravity, ergometry also has application to human movement. A device that can be used to measure work is called an ergometer, and a commonly used ergometer during exercise is the stationary cycle, or *cycle ergometer.*

Table 1 provides conversions of different scientific units. The internationally recognized unit of work is the joule, and the recognized unit of power (W/Time) is joules per second (J/s) or J/min.[5] These units are extremely small, so they are usually expressed in increments of 1000 (kJ). Despite the joule being the internationally recognized unit of work and energy, the units of kilogram meters (kgm) and kgm/min and Watts are routinely used as units for work and power, respectively. An understanding of the relationships among kilojoules, Watts, and kilocalories is advantageous for the understanding of research finding from internationally circulated journals (see References 4 and 8).

The distinction between work and power is important during exercise. Almost any individual can perform a given amount of work if given enough time. However, not all individuals can perform a similar quantity of work in a given time interval. Consequently, during ergometry, exercise intensity is quantified in units of power, which enables comparisons to be made within and between individuals. Individuals who can sustain high power outputs during prolonged exercise without becoming fatigued have high cardiorespiratory endurance fitness. Conversely, individuals who can generate high maximal power values during very short bursts of exercise have high muscle power and would be suited to sprint and other intense short-term exercise.

The development of the cycle ergometer enabled the calculation of work and power during cycle exercise. A modern example of a cycle ergometer, and the principles that it uses to quantify work and power, is illustrated in Figure 1.

The application of friction via a belt around the front flywheel is quantified by the force required to move a pendulum attached to the belt. The distance moved by the pendulum is calibrated and generally

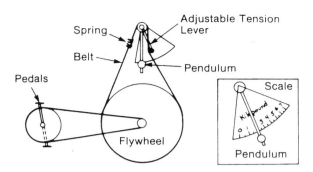

Figure 1 Externally braked cycle ergometers apply load to a flywheel by means of a friction belt. The frictional resistance from the belt is calibrated by applying known weights and adjusting the pendulum meter to read appropriate weight increments. The application of a given exercise intensity using externally braked cycle ergometers requires a constant cadence. In contrast, cycle ergometers that are electronically braked do not need to be ridden at a constant cadence, as the resistance is computer controlled to accommodate alterations in cadence (the exact tolerance for changes in cadence is not unlimited and is specified by the cycle manufacturer — usually between 40 and 120 rpm). (From Fox, Bowers, and Foss, *The Physiological Basis of Physical Education and Athletics*, 4th ed., 1988. With permission.)

labeled in 0.5-kg units on a scale fixed behind the pendulum. A person pedaling the bike will spin the front flywheel, and the product of the distance traversed by the circumference of the flywheel and the frictional force applied to the belt is equal to work, expressed as kilogram meters (kgm). The Body Guard™ and Monark™ ergometers traverse 6 m per crank revolution.

For a Monark ergometer, work and power can be calculated as follows:

$$\text{WORK} = \text{cadence (r/min)} \times \text{load (kg)} \times 6 \text{ (m)} \times \text{duration (min)}$$

For example, a person riding at 60 r/min at 3 kg load for 30 min will perform work equal to

$$\text{Work (kgm)} = 60 \times 3 \times 6 \times 30$$
$$= 32,400$$

and

$$\text{Power (kgm/min)} = 32,400/30$$
$$= 1080$$

$$\text{Power (Watts)} = 1080/6.118$$
$$= 176.5$$

$$\text{Power (kcal/min)} = 1080/426.4$$
$$= 2.5$$

$$\text{Power (kJ/min)} = 2.5 \times 4.1868$$
$$= 10.5$$

The Monark ergometer is an example of an externally loaded ergometer. A cycle ergometer more commonly used in research and clinical settings is the *constant load ergometer*. The constant load ergometer has an electronic resistance mechanism that applies resistance to the flywheel that varies with cadence. At increasing cadence, the resistance decreases so that the power output and exercise intensity remain constant. Consequently, the constant load ergometer allows cadence to vary without affecting work and power.

Another type of cycle ergometer is the isokinetic ergometer. This cycle provides the user with the option to set a given cadence, and the force applied to the pedals and crankshaft during cycling is measured. The work and power generated is computed by the computer integration that accompanies the equipment. Similar ergometers exist for rowing.

The treadmill is not really an ergometer. During level-grade walking or running, there is minimal force applied against gravity, which precludes calculations of work and power. However, when the treadmill is used for either running or walking up a grade, body weight can be used as the force against gravity, and the vertical distance traversed is used for the distance component of the work equation.

By definition, any exercise mode that does not allow for the measurement of mechanical power is not an ergometer. Such exercise equipment would be exemplified by the many forms of home and gymnasium exercise equipment: stair climbing, Nordic track skiing, recumbent cycling, rowing, etc. For these exercise equipment and exercise performed outdoors without stationary ergometry equipment, exercise intensity must be quantified by the metabolic energy expenditure that is derived from the principles of *calorimetry.*

2. Indirect Calorimetry and Oxygen Consumption

Based on the first law of thermodynamics, *energy is neither created nor destroyed,* the forms and relative amounts of energy released during the chemical reactions of the body are relatively constant. As heat is one such form of energy, the heat released from chemical reactions is relatively constant. Thus, during exercise, when the net sum of all reactions (metabolism) is increased, *the increase in metabolic heat production is proportional to the increase in exercise intensity.*

The science of calorimetry concerns the measurement of heat production by the body. Calorimetry can either be direct, involving the measurement of heat released by the body, or indirect, calculating the heat production by the body based on other measurements. Direct calorimetry is invalid when trying to measure heat production during exercise. The body stores heat, thereby reducing available heat release to the environment. In addition, the frictional heat generated by exercise further complicates the issue. The most valid and reliable means of computing energy expenditure during exercise is to measure expired gas volumes and concentrations and to calculate oxygen consumption and carbon dioxide production. Based on these calculations, and known energy equivalents for oxygen consumption at given carbon dioxide production rates, a very accurate estimation of energy expenditure can be calculated.

To understand why this can occur, we have to once again apply the first law of thermodynamics. The combustion of either carbohydrate or lipid to carbon dioxide and water will yield the same total energy release, regardless of how the molecules are catabolized.

glucose

$$C_6H_{12}O_6 + 6CO_2 \longrightarrow 6CO_2 + 6H_2O + ENERGY$$
$$VCO_2/VO_2 = 1.0$$

palmitate

$$C_{16}H_{32}O_2 + 23O_2 \longrightarrow 16CO_2 + 146H_2O + ENERGY$$
$$VCO_2/VO_2 = 0.69$$

As heat release in the body for these reactions represents a given proportion of total energy release, knowing the amount of oxygen required to combust substrates in metabolism provides a means to quantify heat production, as well as total energy release (expenditure). Also, as there are differences in carbon dioxide production between carbohydrate and lipid catabolism, the ratio of carbon dioxide production to oxygen consumption (respiratory quotient, or RQ) can be used to reflect different proportions of carbohydrate and lipid substrates used in metabolism. Based on research that dates back to the late 1800s and early 1900s, the specific contribution of fat and carbohydrate for given values of RQ has been determined, as have the energy expenditure values relative to the amount of oxygen consumed[7] (Table 2). In 1928, Lusk[7] corrected these values to remove contributions from amino acid catabolism, and computations of energy expenditure are now easily completed using the "non-protein" data in Table 3 when oxygen consumption, carbon dioxide production, and, of course, RQ are known. These values are only valid to use when exercise is performed under steady state conditions and during nutritional conditions characterized by ample carbohydrate stores so that minimal amino acid oxidation is occurring.

Table 2 Heat Release[†] and Caloric Equivalents for Oxygen[†] for the Main Macronutrients of Catabolism

Food	Rubner's[a] kcal/g	kcal/g Bomb Cal	kcal/g Body	RQ	kcal/LO$_2$
Mixed CHO	**4.1**	**4.1**	**4.0**	**1.0**	**5.05**
Glycogen		4.2		1.0	5.05
Glucose		3.7		1.0	4.98
Fructose		3.7		1.0	5.00
Glycerol		4.3		0.86	5.06
Mixed FAT	**9.3**	**9.3**	**8.9**	**0.70**	**4.73**
Palmitate (C 16:0)		9.3		0.70	4.65
Stearate (C 18:0)		9.5		0.69	4.65
Triacylglycerol (C 18:0)		9.6		0.70	4.67
Medium chain length Triacylglycerols		8.4		0.74	4.69
Mixed PROTEIN	**4.1**	**5.7**	**4.3**	**0.81**	**4.46**
Alanine		4.4		0.83	4.62
Aspartate		2.69		1.17	4.60
Glutamate		3.58		1.0	4.58
Isoleucine		6.89		0.73	4.64
ALCOHOL		**7.1**	**7.0**	**0.82**	**4.86**
MIXED DIET				**0.84**	**4.83**

Note: Bomb Cal = Bomb calorimetry data; Body = data calculated from body catabolism; RQ = respiratory quotient; CHO = carbohydrate.

[a] See Lusk.[7]

3. The Measurement and Applied Meaning of VO$_2$max

The ability to measure oxygen consumption (VO$_2$) during many different types of exercise, where an ergometer cannot be used, not only provides a means to calculate energy expenditure, but also provides information of exercise intensity. For a given submaximal exercise intensity, VO$_2$ is remarkably similar between individuals (Figure 2). Differences in VO$_2$ that do exist between individuals are small and result from differences in mechanics, which influences the mechanical efficiency during exercise, which in turn alters the actual intensity of the exercise.

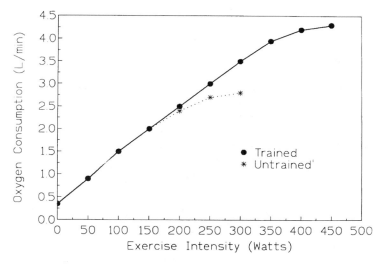

Figure 2 As exercise intensity increases, so does VO$_2$. This linear increase only applies over a range of intensities, between rest and near VO$_2$max. During submaximal exercise, individuals have a similar VO$_2$ for a given intensity. However, the more endurance trained the individual, the higher will be the intensity at VO$_2$max.

Table 3 Caloric Equivalents for the Range of Nonprotein Respiratory Quotient (RQ) Values

RQ	kcal/lO$_2$	%CHO	kcal/lO$_2$ CHO	%Fat	kcal/lO$_2$ Fat
1.00	5.047	100.00	5.047	0.0	0.000
0.99	5.035	96.80	4.874	3.18	0.160
0.98	5.022	93.60	4.701	6.37	0.230
0.97	5.010	90.40	4.529	9.58	0.480
0.96	4.998	87.20	4.358	12.80	0.640
0.95	4.985	84.00	4.187	16.00	0.798
0.94	4.973	80.70	4.013	19.30	0.960
0.93	4.961	77.40	3.840	22.60	1.121
0.92	4.948	74.10	3.666	25.90	1.281
0.91	4.936	70.80	3.495	29.20	1.441
0.90	4.924	67.50	3.324	32.50	1.600
0.89	4.911	64.20	3.153	35.80	1.758
0.88	4.899	60.80	2.979	39.20	1.920
0.87	4.887	57.50	2.810	42.50	2.077
0.86	4.875	54.10	2.637	45.90	2.238
0.85	4.862	50.70	2.465	49.30	2.397
0.84	4.850	47.20	2.289	52.80	2.561
0.83	4.838	43.80	2.119	56.20	2.719
0.82	4.825	40.30	1.944	59.70	2.880
0.81	4.813	36.90	1.776	63.10	3.037
0.80	4.801	33.40	1.603	66.60	3.197
0.79	4.788	29.90	1.432	70.10	3.356
0.78	4.776	26.30	1.256	73.70	3.520
0.77	4.764	22.30	1.062	77.20	3.678
0.76	4.751	19.20	0.912	80.80	3.839
0.75	4.739	15.60	0.739	84.40	4.000
0.74	4.727	12.00	0.567	88.00	4.160
0.73	4.714	8.40	0.396	91.60	4.318
0.72	4.702	4.76	0.224	95.20	4.476
0.71	4.690	1.10	0.052	98.90	4.638
0.707	4.686	0.0	0.000	100.00	4.686

Note: To convert kcal to kJ, multiply by 4.184.

Based on data from Lusk.[7]

Caloric values from each of carbohydrate and fat are also listed for each RQ value.

As indicated in Figure 2, VO$_2$ increases linearly with increases in exercise intensity, until the maximal rate of VO$_2$ is achieved (VO$_2$max). VO$_2$ then plateaus, or in some individuals may decrease (overshoot phenomenon). The measure of VO$_2$max has been interpreted as the best index of cardiorespiratory endurance[1,2] and is also used to standardize exercise intensities among individuals of different cardio-respiratory fitness. For example, exercise at 50% VO$_2$max for two individuals with very different VO$_2$max values is assumed to be of a similar relative intensity, demanding similar metabolic and endocrinological changes and similar relative changes in ventilatory and cardiovascular responses.

III. METABOLIC AND SYSTEMS PHYSIOLOGY RESPONSES DURING EXERCISE AND FOLLOWING TRAINING

The scope of the acute adaptation of the body to exercise is presented in Table 4. As previously mentioned, the magnitude of these responses will be determined by extraneous variables, such as the absolute and relative exercise intensity, fitness, health status, medications, age, and even gender.

The transition of the body from rest to exercise stimulates neuromuscular responses that cause muscle contraction. Muscle contraction alters the cellular equilibrium of metabolism, resulting in the increased

Table 4 Multiple Components of the Response of the Body during Exercise

Skeletal Muscle

↓ creatine phosphate[a]
↑ glycogenolysis[a]
↑ glycolysis[a]
↑ glucose uptake
↑ lipolysis[a]
↑ mitochondrial respiration
↑ potassium release
↑ adenosine release
↑ temperature
↓ pH[a]

Cardiovascular

↑ heart rate, stroke volume, and cardiac output
↑ ejection fraction
↓ peripheral vasular resistance[a]
↑ vasodilation of skeletal muscle vasculature
↓ vasodilation (vasoconstriction) to sphlancnic vasculature

Pulmonary

↑ depth and frequency of breathing, and ventilatory volume
↑ dilation of bronchioles
Improved ventilation-perfusion of the lung
Respiratory compensation for metabolic acidosis[a]

Endocrinological

↑ catecholamine release[a]
↑ growth hormone release
↑ cortisol release[a]
↑ glucagon release[a]
↓ insulin release
↑ ADH release[a]
↑ aldosterone[a]

Thermoregulatory

↑ cutaneous blood flow
↑ sweat rate[a]

[a] Dependent on exercise intensity and/or duration.

rate of many reactions, the activation and inhibition of specific enzymes which also affect reaction rates, and indirectly stimulates the local regulation of blood flow. Additional immediate responses also exist, such as the neural stimulation of an increased heart rate and cardiac output and the increased depth and rate of breathing. The clinical application of exercise requires the practitioner to understand normal acute responses to exercise and to interpret the functional significance of deviations from normality. An understanding of the chronic effects of exercise training is also required for the application of exercise training for rehabilitation and disease prevention (Table 5).

Table 5 Multiple Components of the Chronic Adaptations of the Body to Exercise

Strength/Power	Endurance
Skeletal Muscle	
↑ hypertrophy	↑ hypertrophy
↑ creatine phosphate	↑ mitochondrial density
↑ strength	↑ capillarization
↑ buffering capacity	Glycogen sparing
	↑ glucose uptake capacity
Cardiovascular	
?	↑ maximal cardiac output
	↑ stroke volume
	↑ blood volume
	↑ plasma volume
	↓ resting blood pressure
	↓ resting heart rate
Pulmonary	
↑ buffering capacity	?
Endocrinological	
?	↓ circulating stress hormones
Thermoregulatory	
?	Earlier onset of sweating
	Improved temperature regulation

REFERENCES

1. **Gollnick, P. D., R. B. Armstrong, B. Saltin, C. W. Saubert IV, W. L. Sembrowhich, and R. E. Shepherd.** Effect of training on enzyme activity and fiber composition of human skeletal muscle. *J. Appl. Physiol.* 33(3):312–319, 1972.
2. **Holloszy, R. L. and E. F. Coyle.** Adaptations of skeletal muscle to endurance training and their metabolic consequences. *J. Appl. Physiol.* 56(4):831–838, 1984.
3. **LaFontaine, T. P., B. R. Londeree, and W. K. Spath.** The maximal steady state versus selected running events. *Med. Sci. Sports Exerc.* 13(3):190–192, 1981.
4. **Lippert, H. and H. P. Lehmann.** *SI Units in Medicine. An Introduction to the International System of Units with Conversion Tables and Normal Ranges.* Urban & Schwarzenberg, Baltimore, 1978.
5. **Livesey, G. and M. Elia.** Estimation of energy expenditure, net carbohydrate utilization, and net fat oxidation and synthesis by indirect calorimetry: evaluation of errors with special reference to the detailed composition of fuels. *Am. J. Clin. Nutr.* 47:608–628, 1988.
6. **Luft, U., L. Myhre, and J. Loeppky.** Validity of Haldane calculation for estimating respiratory gas exchange. *J. Appl. Physiol.* 35(4):546–551, 1973.
7. **Lusk, G.** *The Elements of the Science of Nutrition.* 4th ed., W.B. Saunders, Philadelphia, 1928.
8. **Young, D. S.** Implementation of SI units for clinical laboratory data. Style specifications and conversion tables. *Ann. Intern. Med.* 106:114–120, 1987.

Chapter 2

Cardiovascular Function and Adaptation to Exercise

Thomas D. Fahey

CONTENTS

I. INTRODUCTION

Exercise places increased demands on the cardiovascular system. Cardiac output is increased to meet the increased demands of metabolism, temperature regulation, and blood pressure regulation. These demands are often conflicting and contradictory. For example, maintenance of blood pressure is central to cardiovascular regulation.[33] During intense exercise, skin and muscle blood flow must sometimes be compromised so that blood pressure can be maintained.[32,35] Teleologically, the system chooses survival (by maintaining blood pressure) over performance (by compromising muscle and skin blood flow).

Cardiovascular control is elegant and usually very effective. The system is driven by higher neural regulators that receive sensory information from peripheral sensors.[26,33] The heart, while largely neurally controlled, has built-in automaticity that gives it a regulatory redundancy and allows it to respond rapidly to stimuli such as exercise.

II. MAXIMAL OXYGEN CONSUMPTION

$\dot{V}_{O_{2max}}$ is considered to be the best measure of cardiovascular capacity.[9] Many sports medicine experts think of it as the single most important measure of physical fitness. It is defined as the point at which O_2 consumption fails to rise despite an increased exercise intensity or power output. The greater ability of trained people to sustain a high exercise intensity is largely due to a greater $\dot{V}_{O_{2max}}$.

$\dot{V}_{O_{2max}}$ is equal to the product of maximum cardiac output and maximum arteriovenous oxygen difference (Equation 1):

$$\dot{V}_{O_{2max}} = \dot{Q}_{max(a-v)O_{2max}} \qquad (1)$$

where $\dot{V}_{O_{2max}}$ is the maximal rate of O_2 consumption $(1 \cdot min^{-1})$, $\dot{Q}_{max}$ is the maximum cardiac output $(1 \cdot min^{-1})$, and $(a-v)\,O_{2max}$ is the maximum arterial-venous O_2 difference (ml $O_2 \cdot 100$ ml^{-1}). Thus, $\dot{Q}_{max}$ is a function of the maximum rate of oxygen transport and oxygen utilization.[9]

During the transition from rest to maximal exercise, there is a linear increase in $(a-v)\,O_2$. Arterial oxygen partial pressure (Pa_{O_2}) is well maintained in most athletes during exercise.[15] The increase is due to the decrease in venous oxygen partial pressure (Pv_{O_2}). There is only a limited capacity to increase oxygen extraction through endurance training. The venous blood draining the active muscles of both trained and untrained people during maximal exercise contains relatively little oxygen.

To be successful in competition, athletes in sports that require endurance must have a large cardiac output capacity.[8,19] Maximum cardiac output is the product of maximum heart rate (HR) and maximum stroke volume (SV) (Equation 2).

$$\dot{Q}_{max} = \left(HR_{max}\right)\left(SV_{max}\right) \qquad (2)$$

Maximum heart rate is largely determined by heredity and age. It is not appreciably affected by training.[20] Because HR_{max} and $(a-v)\,O_{2max}$ are stable, changes in $\dot{V}_{O_{2max}}$ with training are mostly due to changes in stroke volume.

Stroke volume is affected by hemodynamic and myocardial factors. It is closely linked to venous return of blood to the heart.[13] The ability of the heart to contract with increased force as its chambers are stretched (e.e., preload) is described by the Frank–Starling principle. Factors affecting preload include blood volume, body position, intrathoracic pressure, atrial contribution to ventricular filling, pumping action of skeletal muscle, venous tone, and intrapericardial pressure.[9] These hemodynamic factors can have acute and chronic effects on stroke volume, oxygen transport capacity, and perception of fatigue.[23] For example, during endurance exercise where there is a decrease in blood volume due to dehydration or a decrease in venous tone. There is a compensatory increase in heart rate and an increase in perceived exertion. Increased blood volume resulting from endurance training also causes an increase in stroke volume.

Stroke volume is also affected by myocardial contractility.[26] The contractile force of the myocardium changes in response to circulating catecholamines, the force–frequency relationship of the muscle, sympathetic nerve impulses, intrinsic depression, loss of myocardium, pharmacological depressants, and inotropic agents. Inotropic agents include digitalis, hypoxemia, hypercapnia, and acidosis.[10] Endurance training increases myocardial contractility by increasing Ca^{++}-mypsin ATPase activity.[25] The combination of increased preload and contractility is responsible for the increase in stroke volume that occurs with endurance training. Both of these factors are limited by ventricular volume, which is affected by genetic and environmental factors during growth and development.[6] Stroke volume can be changed to some extent through endurance training.

The oxygen consumption capacity of a muscle varies according to fiber type.[9] The ability of the mitochondria to extract oxygen from blood is approximately three to five times greater in slow-twitch red than in fast-twitch white fibers. Training can double the mitochondrial mass. It is possible for elite endurance athletes to have 10 times the muscle oxygen-extracting capacity in their trained muscles as sedentary people. A high correlation ($r \approx 0.80$) exists between $\dot{V}_{O_{2max}}$ and leg muscle mitochondrial acitivity.[9] Cardiac output and muscle mitochondrial capacities are important determinants of the upper limits of $\dot{V}_{O_{2max}}$.

There is a strong genetic component for $\dot{V}_{O_{2max}}$.[1,6,7] The well-known exercise physiologist Per-Olaf Åstrand has stated that to become an Olympic-level endurance athlete requires choosing parents carefully! Genetic studies typically show less variance in $\dot{V}_{O_{2max}}$ and muscle fiber type between monozygous twins than between dizygous twins.[22] However, these studies also show that training is critical for success. The ability to improve performance in response to an endurance training program depends on genetic factors.

Intense endurance training results in a maximum increase in $\dot{V}_{O_{2max}}$ of approximately 20%.[4,28] However, greater increases are possible if the initial physical fitness of the subject is low. Only certain types of exercise promote the cardiac alterations necessary for increased $\dot{V}_{O_{2max}}$. Maximal stroke volume can be increased in response to a volume overload induced by participation in sports such as running, cycling, and swimming. However, in pressure-overload sports, such as weight lifting, left ventricular wall thickness increases with no increase in left ventricular volume.[32] Changes in $\dot{V}_{O_{2max}}$ and endurance capacity are not the same. Endurance performance can be improved by much more than 20%.[9,28] This is possible by improving mitochondrial density, speed, running economy, and body composition.[27]

A high $\dot{V}_{O_{2max}}$ is a prerequisite to performing at elite levels in endurance events. The evidence for a minimum aerobic capacity requirement is circumstantial:[9]

- All elite endurance athletes have high aerobic capacities. Even though $\dot{V}_{O_{2max}}$ is a poor predictor of performance among athletes at the same level of competition, the variance in maximal aerobic power between them is small.
- Oxygen consumption increases as a function of velocity in all endurance events. Although athletes vary somewhat in their efficiencies, the variance between them is small.

Even though a high $\dot{V}_{O_{2max}}$ is important for achieving superior levels of endurance, it is not the only requirement for success.

Noakes[27,28] has questioned the validity of $\dot{V}_{O_{2max}}$ as a predictor of endurance performance. His reservations are based on these observations:

- Much of the evidence of an oxygen limitation during exercise is circumstantial. Noakes analyzed the data of the classic studies that established $\dot{V}_{O_{2max}}$ as a laboratory benchmark for cardiovascular performance. He found that most subject did not show that $\dot{V}_{O_{2max}}$ leveled off with increasing intensity of exercise at maximum.
- Studies have attempted to show that O_2 transport is limiting by transfusion or O_2 breathing. None of these studies has demonstrated that its subjects reached a plateau in $\dot{V}_{O_{2max}}$ during normal exercise. There was no evidence of an O_2 transport limitation before the experimental intervention.
- In blood-doping studies there is a dissociation between changes in and performance. Performance changes last only a few days while changes in $\dot{V}_{O_{2max}}$ last longer.
- Exercise at extreme altitudes is not limited by high blood lactate levels or by indications of central limitations in cardiac or respiratory function.
- Exhaustion during maximal exercise occurs at a lower oxygen consumption during cycling than during running in the same subjects.
- Blood lactate levels at exhaustion during progressive treadmill exercise testing are lowest in elite athletes.
- Changes in running performance with training occur without equivalent changes in $\dot{V}_{O_{2max}}$.

Noakes's data suggest that a good predictor of endurance performance is peak treadmill velocity. He hypothesized that maximum speed may be related to the capacity of the muscles for high cross-bridge cycling and respiratory adaptations. Respiratory adaptations may make it possible to prevent the onset of exercise-induced dyspnea.

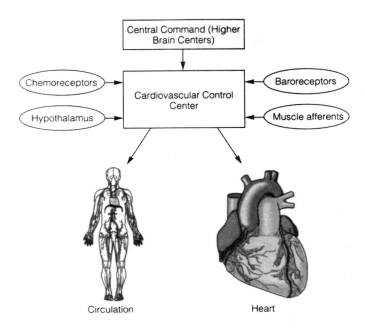

Figure 1   Schematic diagram of CVC.

III. CARDIOVASCULAR CONTROL DURING EXERCISE

The control of blood flow is critical during exercise (Figure 1). Blood must be rapidly directed to working muscles to meet their demands for oxygen and fuels.[21] Blood pressure must be maintained. Uninterrupted blood flow to the heart is needed to ensure blood supply to critical areas such as the central nervous system.[16]

At rest, a large portion of the cardiac output is directed to the spleen, liver, kidneys, brain, and heart.[16] Muscles comprise over 40% of body tissue. Yet, they only receive about 20% of the total blood flow. During exercise the muscles can receive more than 85% of the cardiac output. Circulatory control mechanisms carefully balance their central role of maintaining blood pressure with the increased metabolic demands of exercising muscle.

Peripheral resistance decreases during exercise as a result of increasing blood flow to active muscles.[3,33] To maintain blood pressure, blood vessels are constricted in less-active tissues. Cardiac output is increased. Circulatory controls make it possible to maintain blood pressure, supply blood to important areas, and satisfy metabolic needs of working muscles. The heart and circulation are mainly controlled by higher brain centers (central command) and cardiovascular control areas in the brain stem. Control is also affected by baroreceptors, chemoreceptors, muscle afferents, local tissue metabolism, and circulating hormones.[131]

Regulation of blood pressure and tissue circulation is affected by cardiovascular neural control centers, local tissue metabolic regulation, and muscle afferents.[24,31] Extrinsic neural control is directed toward maintaining blood pressure. Local regulation of blood flow is directed toward meeting tissue metabolic requirements. A close match between cardiac output and muscle blood flow is critical in maintaining blood pressure during exercise. Regulation of the heart and circulation during exercise are closely coupled.

During exercise, various circulatory control mechanisms act to increase or maintain blood pressure. They also supply blood to tissues and cool the body. Unfortunately, the maximum demands of each requirement cannot be met simultaneously. During intense exercise, a limitation is placed on maximum blood flow to active muscle and the skin so blood pressure can be maintained. Neural and hormonal control mechanisms operate to balance the demand for blood to active tissues with the critical requirement of maintaining blood pressure. The cardiovascular control mechanisms (muscle afferents, central command, baroreceptors, chemoreceptors, hypothalamus, hormones) are redundant rather than additive.[5,12,18] If one mechanism is blocked, others will respond.

A. NEURAL CONTROL

Neural control of the heart is integrated into regulation of the cardiovascular system.[24] Mechanisms that regulate arterial blood pressure, blood volume, and the intake of fluid and electrolytes affect the heart and circulation.

Circulatory requirements during exercise easily exceed the ability of the Frank–Starling mechanism to increase cardiac output. Fortunately, the heart is supplied with sympathetic and parasympathetic nerves from the autonomic nervous system.[10,17] These nerves affect the contractile strength of the heart and the heart rate. The sympathetic nerves stimulate the heart. The parasympathetics suppress the heart.

Parasympathetic nerve terminals innervate the sinoatrial (SA) node, the atrial myocardium, the atrioventricular (AV) node, and the ventricular myocardium. Sympathetic stimulation is directed at stimulating heart rate and the force of cardiac contraction. It also increases blood pressure by peripheral vasoconstriction of blood vessels. The sympathetics also allow more blood to pass through the coronary arteries.

Neural control of circulation involves the cerebral cortex (central command), cardiovascular control center, and peripheral afferents. Peripheral afferents include baroreceptors, chemoreceptors, and muscle afferents.[24,30] Neural control mechanisms match vascular conductance (blood flow) with cardiac output. The heart, arteries, arterioles, venules, and veins are sympathetically innervated.

Neural control of circulation involves the cerebral cortex (central command), cardiovascular control center, and peripheral afferents. Peripheral afferents include baroreceptors, chemoreceptors, and muscle afferents.[24,30] Neural control mechanisms match vascular conductance (blood flow) with cardiac output. The heart, arteries, arterioles, venules, and veins are sympathetically innervated. Neural control of circulation arises from a central area of the brain called the subthalamic locomotor region.[31] This area has also been associated with motor unit recruitment and ventilatory control. Central command is responsible for controlling heart rate, arterial blood pressure, and left ventricular contractility.[24] It does this by controlling the level of efferent activity of the sympathetic (cardiovascular control center) and parasympathetic nervous system (vagus nerve). Central command is involved in withdrawal of parasympathetic influences during exercise by its stimulation of the cardioinhibitory center in the medulla.[34]

Central command starts sympathetic activity by directly influencing the cardiovascular control areas.[24] These are located in the reticular formations. During exercise, stimulation of the cardiovascular control center by central command results in circulatory vasoconstriction, increased heart rate, increased strength of contraction by the myocardium, and increased impulse conduction velocity in the heart.

1. Cardiovascular Control Center

The cardiovascular control center (CVC) is a loose connection of nerve cells in the reticular formation of the brain stem, centered mainly in the pons and medulla.[31,36] During exercise, the CVC receives impulses from central command, hypothalamus, baroreceptors, chemoreceptors, and muscle afferents. These inputs determine the level of cardiac output and peripheral resistance. The CVC is also directly affected by the levels of O_2 and CO_2 in blood. Decreased CO_2, which can result during hyperventilation, causes a decrease in blood pressure. Low P_{O_2} stimulates the CVC.

2. Hypothalamus

The hypothalamus lies in the upper part of the brain stem, above the pons.[17,36] It is involved in many physiological processes. These include neuroendocrine control, hunger and satiety, body water control, temperature regulation, and circulatory control. The hypothalamus is particularly active in influencing circulation during temperature challenges from the environment or exercise. The anterior hypothalamus influences the cardiovascular control areas to vasodilate skin vessels in response to increased body temperature. The posterior hypothalamus induces vasoconstriction in response to falling body temperature.

3. Baroreceptors

Baroreceptors influence the CVC.[5] They affect heart rate, cardiac contractility, vascular resistance, and compliance. The baroreceptors are stretch receptors located in the heart, major arteries (particularly in the carotid sinus and aortic bodies), and pulmonary vessels. Atrial baroreceptors stimulate the release of arganine-vasopressin from the pituitary. Baroreceptors are involved in the chronic as well acute regulation of blood pressure.

Baroreceptors work by establishing a blood pressure set point.[31] If pressure increases above the set point, the baroreceptors send impulses to the CVC. This reduces the level of sympathetic activity and causes blood pressure to decrease. When pressure again reaches the set point, activity of the baroreceptors decreases. The reverse is true when blood pressure is below the set point. Impulses from the baroreceptors to the CVC decrease, which causes blood pressure to increase.

At the onset of exercise the baroreceptor set point increases.[31] This causes an immediate increase in heart rate and blood pressure. The baroreflex may be critical in the rapid cardiovascular response that occurs during exercise. Baroreceptor responsiveness has been found to be higher in fit subjects. The baroreceptors have an important effect on active skeletal muscle circulation. Muscle circulation is stimulated to vasodilate when blood pressure increases. This occurs by inhibiting the CVC pressor center. Muscles vasoconstrict when blood pressure begins to fall.

4. Chemoreceptors

Chemoreceptors are located in the aortic and carotid bodies.[17] They respond to decreased P_{O_2}, decreased pH, and increased P_{CO_2} by sending impulses to the pressor area of the CVC. As with the baroreceptors, they establish a set point and work by negative feedback. They increase impulses to the CVC when P_{O_2} or pH is below and P_{CO_2} is above the set point. They decrease impulses when the values go in the other direction.

5. Muscle Afferents

Muscle afferents are classified as Types I, II, III, and IV.[24] Types I and II are highly myelinated nerve fibers that serve as endings for the muscle spindles and Golgi tendon organs.[9] They have no effects on cardiovascular function. Type III and IV afferents are excited by mechanical, thermal, and chemical stimuli. When stimulated, they send signals to the CVC. These signals increase blood pressure by accelerating heart rate. The signals also increase the strength of cardiac contraction and vasoconstrict blood vessels.[38]

Type III afferents are particularly sensitive to stretch and mechanical deformation. They have been called ergoreceptors because they are activated by muscle contraction. During exercise (particularly isometric exercise), they respond more quickly than the Type IV fibers. Type IV fibers are more responsive to chemical stimuli. They respond later than the Type III fibers during exercise. Factors that increase Type IV stimulation of circulation include potassium, decreased pH, and prostaglandins.

Muscle afferents are most active during intense exercise. Increases in metabolism in muscle tend to cause local vasodilation through circulatory metabolic regulation (see discussion of metabolic regulation in this chapter). However, if muscles are allowed to maximally vasodilate, blood pressure would fall. Feedback from muscle afferents limits local muscle vasodilation so blood pressure is maintained.

B. HORMONAL CONTROL MECHANISMS

The release of catecholamines epinephrine and norepinephrine affects the circulation as well as the heart. In the heart, both hormones enhance the effect of the specific sympathetic stimulation. However, they have dissimilar effects on circulatory vasoconstriction.[9] Both hormones stimulate the heart by increasing its rate, force and speed of contraction, speed of conduction, and its irritability. However, while norepinephrine acts to cause peripheral vasoconstriction, epinephrine causes vasodilation.

1. Adrenergic Receptors

Catecholamines interact with specific receptors in vascular smooth muscle membranes to cause vasoconstriction or vasodilation. In muscle vasculature, α-adrenergic receptors cause vasoconstriction when stimulated. β_2 receptors, the most predominant adrenergic receptor type in muscle, cause vasodilation when stimulated.

2. Renin–Angiotensin Mechanism

The renin–angiotensin mechanism is another hormone control system that exerts a relatively acute effect on blood pressure and blood flow.[31] When blood pressure falls, the enzyme renin is released from the kidneys. The production of renin leads to the production of angiotensin II, a potent vasoconstrictor of both arteries and veins. The resulting vasoconstriction causes an increase in peripheral resistance and venous return which raises blood pressure. The system works in only one direction. It acts to raise pressure when it falls too low but has no effect when pressure is too high. There is some evidence that this mechanism plays a role in increasing blood pressure during exercise.

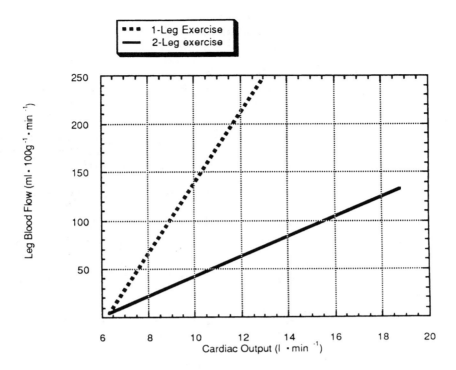

Figure 2 Leg muscle blood flow during one- and two-leg exercise. When an isolated muscle is exercised (i.e., one-leg exercise), muscle blood flow is high. As the mass of exercising muscle increases (i.e., during two-leg exercise), cardiac output capacity limits blood flow available to working muscles. In order to maintain blood pressure, increased sympathetic activity causes vasoconstriction in exercising muscles, which overrides chemical signals within the muscles that normally cause vasodilation of muscle blood vessels. (Adapted from Saltin, B. *Am. J. Cardiol.* 62:30E–35E, 1988.)

The renin–angiotensin system also causes kidneys to retain fluid and salt and thus increases blood volume. This may be its most potent effect on blood pressure. Angiotensin will also have acute (24-h) effects on aldosterone secretion. Aldosterone also increases water and salt retention. Aberrations in this control mechanism are suspected to be related to the development of some types of hypertension.

C. METABOLIC REGULATION OF BLOOD FLOW

Metabolic or local control of blood flow is critical for redirecting blood to active muscles during exercise. It allows local tissues to vasodilate, while less-active tissues are vasoconstricting to maintain blood pressure. At rest, metabolic regulation of blood flow is directed toward maintaining tissue perfusion at a relatively constant rate. During exercise, it is directed toward increasing blood flow to working muscles. Local metabolic regulation of blood flow occurs in response to tissue demands for oxygen and fuels and responses to CO_2, hydrogen ion, and temperature.[9]

Skeletal muscle blood flow is determined by the balance between the metabolic requirements of the muscle with the need to maintain blood pressure. When blood flow is inadequate, vasodilator metabolites accumulate, which stimulates blood flow. Factors that stimulate vasodilation of active blood vessels include low P_{O_2}, high P_{CO_2}, adenosine, low pH, and lactic acid.

Muscle blood flow increases exponentially with metabolism.[33] As oxygen requirements of muscles increase, the arterioles vasodilate to allow more blood flow. At lower levels of metabolism, the precapillary sphincters open and then close. At higher intensities, the vessels tend to stay open. However, as discussed, there is a limit to maximal muscle blood flow (Figure 2).

Sympathetic nervous activity to most tissues, including active muscle, increases with intensity of exercise. It does this so that blood pressure is maintained. At high exercise intensities, skeletal muscle becomes a primary site of vasoconstriction.[33] This is because high muscle blood flow becomes a threat to maintaining blood pressure. While blood flow remains high (60 to 70 ml $\cdot$ 100 g muscle $\cdot$ min^{-1}), it is well short of the maximum flow capacity of the muscle.

D. SUMMARY

Cardiovascular control is aimed at maintaining blood pressure. Local circulatory control can override central command (to a point) so local tissue requirements are met. The following control mechanisms occur during exercise to meet the demands of maintaining blood pressure, satisfying local tissue demands, and cooling the body:

- **Exercise begins: central command stimulates the CVC to begin cardiovascular responses.** These responses include increased heart rate, increased strength of cardiac contraction, and vasoconstriction. The CVC works in coordination with central nervous system centers that control motor unit recruitment and breathing.
- **Vagus tone decreased.** This removes parasympathetic inhibition on the heart which increases blood pressure.
- **Muscle pump facilitates venous return of blood to the heart.** Large muscles activated during exercise, as well as cyclical changes in intrathoracic pressure caused by increased breathing, help push blood toward the heart.
- **Baroreceptor set point raised.** This results in stimulation of the CVC to stimulate cardiovascular activity. Activity includes increased heart rate, increased strength of cardiac contraction, and circulatory vasoconstriction.
- **The hypothalamus is stimulated by increased temperature,** which results in stimulation of the CVC.
- **Type III muscle afferents are stimulated by muscle contraction** and stretch (particularly during isometric exercise). This stimulates the CVC to increase cardiovascular activity.
- **Release of catecholamines from adrenals** results in stimulation of the heart and vasodilation in muscle blood vessels. It also has widespread effects on metabolism.
- **Sympathetic stimulation results in vasoconstriction** in tissues such as the spleen, kidneys, gastrointestinal tract, and inactive muscles. Vasoconstriction in the veins is particularly important for maintaining venous return of blood to the heart.
- **Local changes in metabolism stimulate metabolic regulation of blood flow.** This results in vasodilation in active muscle.
- **As the intensity of exercise increases, activity of Type III and IV muscle afferents increases.** This causes vasoconstriction in active muscle. During exercise using many large muscle groups, maximum blood flow is limited so blood pressure is maintained. Even so, at rest, skeletal muscle receives approximately 20% of cardiac output. During maximal exercise, this value increases to 85%.
- **As exercise progresses, signals from central command, the CVC, hypothalamus, baroreceptors, chemoreceptors, and muscle afferents are balanced.** Cardiac output and circulatory conductance are balanced to maintain blood pressure.

IV. CARDIOVASCULAR RESPONSES TO EXERCISE

The heart and circulation respond to the requirements of metabolism during exercise by increasing blood flow to active areas. Blood flow to less critical areas is decreased. The principal cardiovascular responses to exercise include

- Increased cardiac output. This occurs by increasing heart rate and stroke volume. Increased cardiac output enhances oxygen and substrate delivery to active skeletal muscle and the heart. It also speeds removal of CO_2 and metabolites.
- Increased skin blood flow to help remove heat.
- Decreased blood flow to the kidneys, resulting in diminished urinary output.
- Decreased visceral blood flow, resulting in reduced activity in the gastrointestinal tract.
- Maintenance or slight increase in brain blood flow.
- Increased blood flow to the coronary arteries of the heart.
- Increased muscle blood flow. Maximum muscle blood flow is limited by the need to maintain blood pressure. Active muscle will vasoconstrict at high rates of blood flow if blood pressure cannot be maintained.

output.

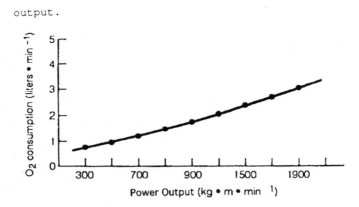

Figure 3   Oxygen consumption increases as a function of power output.

The cardiovascular responses to physical activity depend on the type and intensity of exercise. Dynamic exercise requiring a large muscle mass causes the largest response from the cardiovascular system. Large increases occur in cardiac output, heart rate, and systolic blood pressure. There is little change in diastolic blood pressure. Strength exercises cause marked increases in systolic, diastolic, and mean blood pressure. There are more-moderate increases in heart rate and cardiac output.

A. OXYGEN CONSUMPTION

Oxygen consumption is proportional to the intensity of exercise[9] (Figure 3). It is determined by the rate at which oxygen is transported to the tissues, the oxygen-carrying capacity of blood.

During exercise in which the intensity gradually increases from rest to maximal intensity, stroke volume increases during the early phase of exercise. Heart rate and (a-v) O_2 increase almost linearly with exercise intensity. Cardiac output and (a-v) O_2 each account for about 50% of the increase in oxygen consumption during submaximal exercise. Cardiac output (mainly heart rate) plays a more important role in increasing oxygen consumption as the intensity of exercise approaches maximum. At maximum exercise, it accounts for approximately 75% of the increased oxygen uptake above rest.

The (a-v) O_2 difference and cardiac output are related. The (a-v) O_2 difference is not solely dependent on the capacity of mitochondria to use oxygen. It also depends on the rate of diffusion of oxygen from the blood into the cell. Factors such as blood flow, the oxyhemoglobin dissociation curve, hemoglobin, and myoglobin also affect (a-v) O_2 difference.

Oxygen-carrying capacity of blood is approximately 18 to 20 ml $O_2 \cdot$ ml^{-1} in most healthy people living at sea level.[9,17] Because of their higher hemoglobin content, males have a higher oxygen-carrying capacity than females.

Oxygen consumption increases with exercise intensity. In some subjects it plateaus near maximum effort. As discussed, the highest achievable level of oxygen consumption is called $\dot{V}_{O_{2max}}$. In some people, after $\dot{V}_{O_{2max}}$ is reached, further increases in exercise intensity do not lead to a further increase in oxygen consumption.

B. HEART RATE

Heart rate is the most important factor increasing cardiac output during exercise. In dynamic exercise, heart rate increases with exercise intensity and oxygen consumption. It levels off at $\dot{V}_{O_{2max}}$. Typically, heart rate will increase from about 70 beats/min at rest to 180 to 200 beats/min at maximal exercise.[9] Exercise and maximum heart rates are affected by fitness, age, and gender.

During a constant level of submaximal exercise, heart rate increases and then levels off as the oxygen requirements of the activity have been satisfied. As exercise intensity increases, it takes longer for heart rate to level off. At high exercise intensities, heart rate may not level off. During prolonged exercise, heart rate increases steadily at the same work rate. This phenomenon is called cardiovascular drift. Cardiovascular drift results from decreased stroke volume. The heart rate must increase to maintain cardiac output and blood pressure at the same level. It is caused by a diminished capacity of the circulation to return blood to the heart (i.e., decreased venous return). Decreased venous return may be due to

d plasma volume caused by filtration of fluid from the blood or sweating. It may also be due
    sed sympathetic tone.
    At rest and during low-intensity exercise, heart rate may be elevated above normal. Causes include
anxiety, dehydration, high ambient temperature, altitude, or digestion. "Resting heart rates" of over 90
to 130 beats/min are not unusual before anxiety-producing events such as treadmill testing and sports
competitions.[17]

Heart rates are lower during strength exercises such as weight lifting than during endurance exercise
such as running. During strength exercises, the heart rate increases according to the percentage of
maximum voluntary contraction. A dynamic lift, such as a clean and jerk, using heavy weights, will
increase the heart rate more than a one-arm biceps curl using minimum resistance.

At the same power output, heart rate is higher during upper-body exercise than lower-body exercise.
Upper-body exercise also results in higher $\dot{V}_{O_2}$, mean arterial pressure, and total peripheral resistance.
The higher circulatory load in upper-body exercise results from the use of a smaller muscle mass,
increased intrathoracic pressure, and a less-effective muscle pump. Near maximal contraction using
smaller muscle mass restricts blood flow. All three factors decrease venous return of blood to the heart.

Heart rate can be valuable in writing an exercise prescription. By measuring the heart rate during or
immediately after exercise, the metabolic cost of the activity can be estimated. Exercise heart rate can
provide a good estimate of cardiac load. Heart rate is used in combination with systolic blood pressure
to get an index called the rate–pressure product (RPP). RPP is heart rate × systolic blood pressure. RPP
provides a rough index for coronary blood flow myocardial oxygen consumption.[9]

C. STROKE VOLUME

Stroke volume incrases during exercise in the upright posture. Stroke volume increases steadily until
about 25 to 50% of maximum then tends to level off. Echocardiography measurements suggest that in
some subjects stroke volume decreases as exercise intensity increases toward maximum. After 50%
intensity is achieved, stroke volume decreases toward resting levels.[11,15] This finding is controversial and
has not been found by all investigators. Heart rate is responsible for increasing cardiac output at higher
intensities of exercise. Athletes have a higher exercise cardiac output because they have a higher stroke
volume.

The effects of upright and supine postures: Stroke volume increases during upright exercise. It
does not change from rest to exercise when the subject is supine. At rest, stroke volume is higher in the
supine than in the upright posture. Studies using radionuclide angiography have shown that left ventricular end-diastolic volume (EDV) increases during upright exercise.[31] It is unchanged during supine
exercise. EDV is the amount of blood in the left ventricle during the resting or diastolic portion of the
cardiac cycle. Ejection fraction increases during upright exercise because of an increased cardiac contractility. Ejection fraction is the percent of EDV pumped from the heart with each cardiac contraction.
When exercise intensity is the same, stroke volume is equal in the supine and erect postures.

Stroke volume is perhaps the most important factor determining individual differences in $\dot{V}_{O_{2max}}$. This
is readily apparent when comparing the components of cardiac output of a sedentary man with those of
a champion cross-country skier. Both men have maximum heart rates of 185 beats/min. Yet, the maximum
cardiac output of the untrained man is 16.6 l · min⁻¹. The skier has 32 l · min⁻¹. The maximum stroke
volumes of the skier and sedentary man were 173 and 90 ml, respectively.[9]

D. ARTERIOVENOUS OXYGEN DIFFERENCE

Arteriovenous oxygen difference increases with exercise intensity. The resting value of about 5.6 vol% (ml
$O_2 \cdot dl^{-1}$) is increased to about 16 vol% at maximal exercise. There is always some oxygenated blood returning
to the heart even at exhaustive levels of exercise. This is because some blood continues to flow through
metabolically less-active tissues. These tissues do not fully extract the oxygen from the blood. However,
oxygen extraction approaches 100% when (a-v) O_2 is measured across a maximally exercising muscle.

E. BLOOD PRESSURE

It is very important that blood pressure increases during exercise. Blood flow must be maintained to
critical areas such as the heart and brain.[29] The requirements of working muscles and skin must also be
met. Blood pressure is a function of cardiac output and peripheral resestance (Equation 3).

$$\text{Blood pressure (mmHg)} = Q \cdot TPR \tag{3}$$

where Q = cardiac output (1 · min⁻¹) and TPR = total peripheral resistance (dyn s · cm⁻⁵). Peripheral resistance decreases during exercise. Vasoconstriction in nonexercising tissue is not enough to compensate for the vasodilation in active muscles. Blood pressure does not fall during exercise; it increases. Cardiac output increases greatly during exercise, which more than compensates for the fall in peripheral resistance. For example, in a fit 20-year-old male, cardiac output will increase from about 5 l at rest to approximately 20 l during maximal exercise. Even though peripheral resistance may fall by almost 300% during exercise, systolic blood pressure increases.

Systolic blood pressure rises steadily during exercise. It increases from about 120 mmHg at rest to 180 mmHg or more during maximal exercise. It follows the same general trend as heart rate. The increase in exercise blood pressure varies between people. Maximum systolic pressure may be as little as 150 to more than 250 mmHg in a normal person. The mean arterial pressure increases from about 90 mmHg at rest to about 155 mmHg at maximal exercise. Mean arterial blood (MAP) pressure is described in Equation 4

$$MAP = 1/3 \text{ (systolic blood pressure – diastolic blood pressure)} + \text{diastolic blood pressure} \quad (4)$$

Failure to increase systolic and mean arterial blood pressures during exercise suggests heart failure. A fall in pressure near the end of an exercise test is particularly dangerous. Falling blood pressure during exercise is an absolute reason for stopping an exercise-tolerance test.

There is debate about the maximum safe systolic pressure during exercise. Some experts do not become concerned about systolic blood pressures above even 250 mmHg. Others suggest terminating exercise tests when systolic blood pressure exceeds 220 mmHg. The characteristics of the subject are important. A high systolic pressure is very significant in a hypertensive patient. It is probably meaningless in a world-class endurance athlete. During exercise, systolic blood pressure increases with cardiac output. Endurance athletes have extremely high cardiac output capacities. Their systolic blood pressures will naturally be higher. Systolic blood pressures greater than 450 mmHg have been reported in weight lifters during exercise with no ill effects.

High systolic pressure during exercise in untrained people is a matter of concern. The combination of a high heart rate and systolic blood pressure suggests a high oxygen consumption by the heart. In fact, the RPP is an excellent predictor of myocardial load.[31] As discussed, the RPP is systolic blood pressure times heart rate. If a person has heart disease, extreme levels of systolic blood pressure could easily result in myocardial hypoxemia. This is insufficient supply of oxygen to the heart.

Diastolic pressure changes little during exercise in normal people. Typically, there is either no change or a slight decrease of less than 10 mmHg during exercise. There is also a small decrease during recovery of less than 4 mmHg. A significant increase in diastolic pressure (>15 mmHg or above 110 mmHg) is associated with a greater prevalence of coronary artery disease.[9]

F. BLOOD FLOW

During exercise, blood is redistributed from inactive to active tissues. Critical areas such as the brain and heart are spared the vasoconstriction that occurs in other areas.[29,35] A progressive increase in the sympathetic vasomotor activity occurs with increasing severity of exercise. Even active skeletal muscle is not spared some vasoconstriction during intense exercise.[33] Maintenance of blood pressure takes precedence over delivering maximum blood flow to active muscle.

Resting blood flow to the spleen and kidneys is about 2.8 l · min⁻¹. It is reduced to about 500 ml during maximal exercise.[9] The marked reduction in blood flow to these areas is caused by sympathetic stimulation and circulating catecholamines. Sympathetic enervation is particularly strong in these tissues. In the kidneys, the reduction in blood flow during exercise is accompanied by postexercise proteinuria, hemoglobinuria, and myoglobinuria. These terms mean increased protein, hemoglobin, and myoglobin in the urine, respectively. Urine changes are probably due to decreased plasma volume during exercise. Other causes include increased permeability of the glomeruli and partial inhibition of reabsorption in the kidney tubules.[31]

Skin blood flow increases during submaximal exercise. It decreases to resting values during maximal exercise when muscle blood flow is highest. Relative skin blood flow, as a percentage of cardiac output, changes very little during exercise. Peripheral perfusion of skin blood vessels during exercise contributes to cardiovascular drift and to fatigue during endurance exercise. This is particularly true when exercising in the heat.

The coronary arteries have a large capacity for increasing blood flow.[2] Coronary blood flow increases with intensity during exercise. It increases from about 260 ml · min^{-1} at rest to 900 ml · min^{-1} at maximal exercise. This large coronary reserve is extremely important. It provides adequate blood flow even in the face of significant coronary artery disease. Coronary blood flow is not thought to limit oxygen transport capacity in people without coronary artery disease. Increases in coronary blood flow occur mainly by metabolic regulation and mainly during diastole. Severe coronary artery disease which impedes blood flow will interfere with metabolic regulatory control of blood flow. It may cause coronary ischemia.

Warm-up before endurance exercise is important in facilitating the increase in coronary blood flow during the early stages of exercise. Electrocardiographic (ECG) changes have occurred in healthy people subjected to sudden strenuous exercise. These changes included ST segment depression, which may indicate coronary ischemia. ECG changes with sudden exercise are usually benign is healthy people. They could be very dangerous in people with heart disease.

V. SUMMARY

The cardiovascular system has a large capacity for blood flow during exercise. Circulatory regulation balances the needs of tissues for oxygen and nutrients with the more important function of regulating blood pressure. Maximal oxygen consumption is considered the best measure of cardiovascular capacity.[4] However, many researchers have questioned its value as the *sine qua non* of endurance capacity — the relationship between maximal performance and $V_{O_{2max}}$ break down under a variety of circumstances. During exercise, circulatory regulators do a good job of carefully balancing blood pressure regulation with peripheral tissue requirements.

REFERENCES

1. **Adams, T. D., F. G. Yanowitz, A. G. Fisher, J. D. Ridges, A. G. Nelson, et al.** Heritability of cardiac size: an echocardiographic study of monozygotic and dizygotic twins. *Circulation* 71:39–44, 1985.
2. **Altman, J. D., J. Kinn, D. J. Duncker, and R. J. Bache.** Effect of inhibition of nitric oxide formation on coronary blood flow during exercise in the dog. *Cardiovasc. Res.* 28:119–124, 1994.
3. **Andersen, P.** Capillary density in skeletal muscle of man. *Acta Physiol. Scand.* 95:203–205, 1975.
4. **Åstrand, P. O.** *Experimental Studies of Physical Work Capacity in Relation to Sex and Age.* Copenhagen: Munksgaard, 1952.
5. **Barney, J. A., T. R. J. Ebert, L. Groban, P. A. Farrell, C. V. Hughes, and J. J. Smith.** Carotid baroreflex responsiveness in high-fit and sedentary young men. *J. Appl. Physiol.* 65:2190–2194, 1988.
6. **Bielen, E., R. Fagard, and A. Amery.** Inheritance of heart structure and physical exercise capacity: a study of left ventricular structure and exercise capacity in 7-year-old twins. *Eur. Heart J.* 11:7–16, 1990.
7. **Bouchard, C., F. T. Dionne, J. A. Simoneau, and M. R. Boulay.** Genetics of aerobic and anaerobic performances. In: *Exercise and Sport Sciences Reviews,* J. O. Holloszy (Ed.), Baltimore: Williams and Wilkins, 1992, pp. 27–58.
8. **Brodal, P., F. Ingjer, and L. Hermansen.** Capillary supply of skeletal muscle fibres in untrained and endurance trained men. *Am. J. Physiol.* 232:H705–712, 1977.
9. **Brooks, G. A., T. D. Fahey, and T. White.** *Exercise Physiology: Human Bioenergetics and its Applications.* Mountain View, CA: Mayfield Publishing Co., 1995 (3rd edition).
10. **Brunwald, E.** *Heart Disease: A Textbook of Cardiovascular Medicine.* Philadelphia: W. B. Saunders, 1992.
11. **Concu, A.** Stroke volume: acute and chronic effects of exercise. In: Fahey, T. D. (Ed.), *Encyclopedia of Sports Medicine and Exercise Physiology.* New York: Garland Publishing Co., 1995.
12. **Connolly, R. J.** Flow patterns in the capillary bed of rat skeletal muscle at rest and after repetitive tetanic contraction. In: *Microcirculation,* Grayson, J. and W. Zingg (Eds.), New York: Plenum Press, 1976.
13. **Convertino, V. A., G. W. Mack, and E. R. Nadel.** Elevated central venous pressure: a consequence of exercise training-induced hypervolemia? *Am. J. Physiol. (Reg. Integr. Comp. Physiol.)* 29:R273–R277, 1991.
14. **Dempsey, J. A., P. Hanson, and K. Henderson.** Exercise-induced arterial hypoxemia in healthy humans at sealevel. *J. Physiol.* (London) 355:161–175, 1984.
15. **Ginzton, L. E., R. Conant, M. Brizendine, and M. M. Laks,** Effect of long-term high intensity aerobic training on left ventricular volume during maximal upright exercise. *J. Am. Coll. Cardiol.* 14:364–371, 1989.
16. **Green, J. F.** *Fundamental Cardiovascular and Pulmonary Physiology.* Philadelphia: Lea & Febiger, 1987.
17. **Guyton, A.** *Textbook of Medical Physiology.* Philadelphia: W. B. Saunders, 1986.
18. **Honig, C. R., C. L. Odoroff, and J. L. Frierson.** Active and passive capillary control in red muscle at rest and in exercise. *Am. J. Physiol.* 243:H196–H206, 1982.
19. **Ingjer, F.** Maximal aerobic power related to the capillary supply of the quadriceps femoris muscle in man. *Acta Physiol. Scand.* 104:238–240, 1978.

20. **Katona, P. G., M. McLean, D. H. Dighton, and A. Guz.** Sympathetic and parasympathetic cardiac control in athletes and nonathletes at rest. *J. Appl. Physiol. Respir., Environ. Exercise Physiol.* 52:1652–1657, 1982.
21. **Kjellmer, I.** Effect of exercise on the vascular bed of skeletal muscle. *Acta Physiol. Scand.* 62:18–30, 1964.
22. **Klissouras, V.** Prediction of athletic performance: Genetic considerations. *Can. J. Sport Sci.* 1:195–200, 1976.
23. **Mellander, S. and B. Johansson,** Control of resistance, exchange, and capacitance vessels in the peripheral circulation. *Pharmacol. Rev.* 20:117–196, 1968.
24. **Mitchell, J. H. and R. F. Schmidt.** Cardiovascular reflex control by afferent fibers from skeletal muscle receptors. In: *Handbook of Physiology. The Cardiovascular System. Peripheral Circulation and Organ Blood Flow.* Bethesda, MD: American Physiological Society, 1983, pp. 623–658.
25. **Morris, G. S., R. R. Roy, T. P. Martin, and K. M. Baldwin.** The effect of weight lifting exercise on cardiac myosin isoenzyme distribution. *Med. Sci. Sports Exercise* 2:S29, 1990.
26. **Musch, T. I., G. H. Haidet, G. A. Ordway, J. C. Longhurst, and J. H. Mitchell.** Training effects on regional blood flow response to maximal exercise in foxhounds. *J. Appl. Physiol.* 62:1724–1732, 1987.
27. **Noakes, T. D.** *Lore of Running* (3rd edition). Champaign, IL: Leisure Press, 1991.
28. **Noakes, T. D.** Implications of exercise testing for prediction of athletic performance: a contemporary perspective. *Med. Sci. Sports Exercise* 20:319–330, 1988.
29. **Rogers, H. B., T. Schroeder, N. H. Secher, and J. H. Mitchell.** Cerebral blood flow during static exercise in humans. *J. Appl. Physiol.* 68:2358–2361, 1990.
30. **Rowell, L. B. and D. S. O'Leary.** Reflex control of the circulation during exercise: chemoreflexes and mechanoreflexes. *J. Appl. Physiol.* 69:407–418, 1990.
31. **Rowell, L. B.** *Human Circulatory Regulation During Physical Stress.* London: Oxford University Press, 1986.
32. **Sagiv, M., R. Metrany, N. Fisher, E. Z. Fisman, and J. J. Kellermann.** Comparison of hemodynamic and left ventricular responses to increased after-load in healthy males and females. *Int. J. Sports Med.* 12:41–45, 1991.
33. **Saltin, B.** Capacity of blood flow delivery to exercising skeletal muscle in humans. *Am. J. Cardiol.* 62:30E–35E, 1988.
34. **Smith, M. L., D. L. Hudson, H. M. Graitzer, and P. B. Raven.** Exercise training bradycardia: the role of autonomic balance. *Med. Sci. Sports Exercise* 21:40–44, 1989.
35. **Thomas, S. N., T. Schroeder, N. H. Secher, and J. H. Mitchell.** Cerebral blood flow during submaximal and maximal dynamic exercise in man. *J. Appl. Physiol.* 67:744:748, 1989.
36. **Vander, A., J. Sherman, and D. Luciano.** *Human Physiology.* New York: McGraw Hill, 1975, pp. 228–282.
37. **Vigorito, C., L. DeCaprio, S. Poto, S. Maione, and M. Charello.** Protective role of collaterals in patients with coronary artery disease. *Int. J. Cardiol.* 3:401–415, 1983.
38. **Walgenbach-Telford, S.** Arterial baroreflex and cardiopulmonary mechanoreflex function during exercise. In: *Reflex Control of the Circulation.* Gilmore, J. P. and I. H. Zucker (Eds.), Caldwell, NJ: Telford, 1990.

Chapter **3**

Pulmonary Function and Adaptation to Exercise

Robert A. Robergs

CONTENTS

0-8493-4593-6/97/$0.00+$.50

I. INTRODUCTION

During exercise, the contracting muscles consume oxygen to fuel mitochondrial respiration and produce carbon dioxide. The lungs function to provide a means for oxygen to be transferred between atmospheric air and the blood and for the majority of metabolically produced carbon dioxide to be removed from the body. As carbon dioxide content in blood influences blood acid–base balance, the lungs are also important for regulating blood pH. As one progresses from rest to intense exercise the volumes of air inhaled and exhaled by the lungs may increase from 6 to 160 l/min, with larger values possible for individuals who are larger and more endurance trained. These large and rapid changes in lung function require intricate and sensitive control systems that optimize the ability of the lung to continue to exchange gases between the blood and alveolar air and to retain normal blood pH. For a diverse range of exercise intensities, exercise actually improves lung function. However, moderate-to-extreme altitude and intense exercise in highly endurance-trained individuals may tax the abilities of the lung to maintain optimal function.

II. BASIC ANATOMY OF THE LUNG AND PULMONARY CIRCULATION

Air is directed to and from the lungs by the *trachea,* which is a long tube supported by cartilage that extends from the larynx to the diverging bronchi and bronchioles of the lungs. The trachea and each of the left and right *bronchi* have circumferentially layered smooth muscle and are structurally supported by numerous C-shaped rings of cartilage. Collectively, the mouth and nasal passages, trachea, bronchi and *bronchioles* compose the *conducting zone* of the lungs, whereas the *respiratory bronchioles, alveoli ducts,* and *aveoli,* which are the sites of gas exchange and responsible for the largest lung gas volumes, are referred to as the *respiratory zone* of the lung. During the divergence from the conducting to the respiratory zones of the lung there is a large increase in the cross-sectional area of the airways (Figure 1). This change results in the largest air flow velocities in the upper regions of the conducting zone and in a decrease in air flow velocity toward the respiratory zone. In addition, the greatest air flow resistance occurs in the upper levels of the conducting zone, which is regulated by neurally and hormonally induced vasodilation of the smooth muscle surrounding the trachea, bronchi, and bronchioles.

The respiratory zone of the lung is the location of lung inflation and, as the category name suggests, is the site of *respiration* or gas exchange. The average diameter of an alveolus is approximately 0.25 mm, the average membrane thickness of the respiratory structures is 0.5 μm, and there are approximately 300 million respiratory bronchioles that diverge into numerous alveoli within the two lungs.[54] The alveoli and respiratory bronchioles are connected by openings or holes in their membranes, termed *pores of Kohn.* Originally, it was believed that these holes allowed air to flow from one alveolus to another; however, recent research has shown that the pores are normally filled with fluid and are responsible for the distribution of water and surfactant throughout the respiratory zone.[2] Collectively, the respiratory bronchioles and alveoli make up a surface area of approximately 70 m².

Blood from the heart is pumped through the pulmonary arteries to the lungs, and blood is directed back to the left side of the heart via the pulmonary veins. The circulation of blood to and through the lung is termed the *pulmonary circulation,* and is a low-pressure circuit having a resting normal blood pressure of 25/8 mmHg compared with the normal systemic blood pressure of 120/80 mmHg. A dense capillary bed surrounds the structures of the respiratory zone, providing almost as much surface area of blood as that of the respiratory membranes.

III. LUNG VOLUMES AND CAPACITIES

The conducting zone of the lung is often referred to as the *anatomical dead space,* as it does not have a respiratory function. The anatomical dead space comprises an average volume of 150 ml, although this value will vary in a positive relationship with body size.

The remaining volumes of the lung (Figure 2) are subdivisions of the total lung capacity and essentially comprise the *residual volume* and *vital capacity.* The vital capacity is the maximal volume of air that can be exhaled from the lungs, and, as it is measured during the forced expiration following a maximal inspiratory effort, it can be divided into inspiratory and expiratory components using the method of *spirometry.* Normal resting breathing involves the inspiration and expiration of 500 ml of air, termed the *tidal volume,* and it is the product of the tidal volume and breathing frequency that determines the volume of *ventilation.*

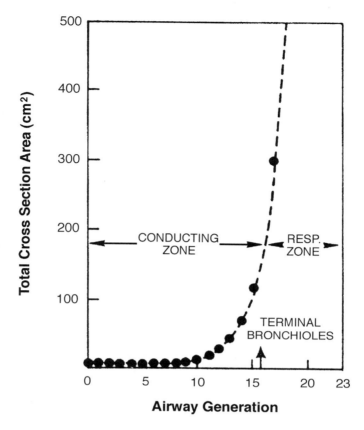

Figure 1 The progression along the lungs from the conducting to respiratory zones involves tremendous divergences, resulting in an exponential increase in the cross-sectional area of the lung. The greatest cross-sectional area corresponds to the alveoli, which are the main locations for gas exchange. (From West, *Respiratory Physiology*, 3rd ed., 1990. With permission.)

IV. VENTILATION

The term *ventilation* is synonomous with the process of breathing, but is very different from the process of respiration. *Ventilation involves the movement of air into and from the lungs by the process of bulk flow.* During inspiration and expiration the lung compartments are opened to the external environment and, therefore, to the pressure, temperature, and humidity of atmospheric air. The pressure differential that exists between atmosphere and alveolar air is crucial to the process of ventilation which can increase air flow through the lung from a mere 6 l/min at rest to over 150 l/min during maximal exercise, and in excess of 200 l/min during maximal voluntary breathing.[19,35]

A. ALVEOLAR VENTILATION

Due to the anatomical dead space, only 350 ml of "fresh" air reaches the respiratory zone. The volume of fresh air that reaches the respiratory zone of the lung is termed *alveolar ventilation* ($\dot{V}_A$). *The greater the depth of breathing, the less impact the anatomical dead space has on alveolar ventilation.*

B. MECHANICS OF VENTILATION

The process of ventilation exemplifies how biological function is often based on the application of physical principles. Ventilating air into the lungs, or *inspiration,* results from the expansion of the pleural cavity. This expansion lowers the pressure (relative to atmospheric pressure) within the pleural cavity and connected alveoli and airways of the lung, and air moves by bulk flow down the airways along the pressure gradient that has developed to the respiratory zone. During resting ventilation, inspiratory effort can reduce the pleural pressure from –5 to –7 cmH$_2$O (1 cmH$_2$O = 0.7352 mmHg), which returns to resting values at the end of expiration.

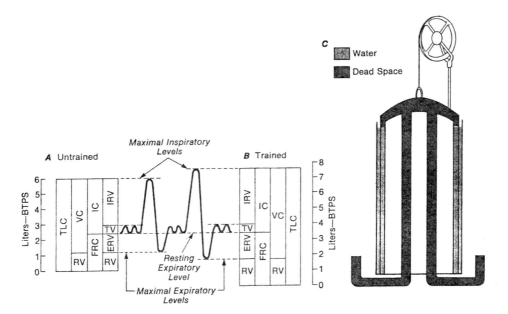

Figure 2 The volumes of the lung can be measured by spirometry. The total lung capacity includes a volume that cannot be exhalled from the lungs (residual volume, RV) and a volume that represents the maximal ability for lung inflation above RV (vital capacity, VC). During breathing, an average of 500 ml of air is inspired and expired from the lungs at rest and is termed tidal volume (TV). Lung volumes are known to increase with endurance training (A and B). C. The basic spirometer functions on the vertical displacement of an aluminum bell in water. (From Fox, Bowers, and Foss, *The Physiological Basis of Physical Education and Athletics*, 4th ed., 1988. With permission.)

During the expulsion of air from the lungs, or *expiration,* the reverse process occurs, whereby the constriction of the pleural cavity increases pressure within and surrounding the lungs, generating a pressure gradient from the lung to the atmosphere, thus forcing air from the lungs. These mechanical processes are driven by muscle contractions and, as will be explained in later sections, involve work resulting from the conversion of metabolic energy expenditure to mechanical energy (changes in pressure).

During resting ventilation, inspiration is driven by the contraction of the diaphragm which enlarges the lower regions of the lungs. Expiration begins with the relaxation of the diaphragm, and elastic recoil returns the diaphragm and lung to their original end-expiration positions and volumes. During more-forceful inspiration, such as is required during exercise, the diaphragm is assisted by the contraction of the external intercostal muscles, which function to raise and outwardly flair the rib cage, resulting in a further increase in lung volume and sustained decreases in pressure. *Added lung inflation can result from the contraction of the muscles of the neck* that have an origin on the sternum, on a clavicle, or on an upper rib and further raise and expand the rib cage, such as the scalene, superior serratus posterior, and sternocleidomastoid muscles. These added pressure changes within the lung increase the volume of air that enters the airways and lungs and further increase the work of inspiration. *The more rapid, large, and sustained the change in pressure, the greater the functional and metabolic demands on the inspiratory muscles.*

When the inspired volumes of air increase, enhanced expiration results form the elastic recoil of the rib cage. Added expiratory effort is obtained by the contraction of the internal intercostal, abdominal, transverse thoracic, and inferior serratus posterior muscles.

1. Pressure–Volume Relationships

Different changes in pressure and volume of the lungs exist for inspiration and expiration. During inspiration, the process of lung inflation is opposed by forces in the lung that resist inflation. These forces are best explained by modeling the alveolus as a sphere; the forces that resist inflation mainly comprise surface tension, as described by the law of Laplace.

$$P = 2T_s/r^4$$

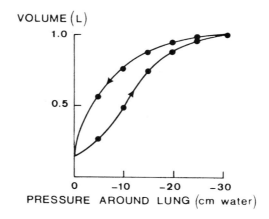

Figure 3 The relationship between the change in lung volume for given changes in intrathoracic pressure during inspiration and expiration can be graphed as a pressure–volume curve. The pressure–volume relationship differs for inspiration and expiration. The ability of a structure such as the lung to change volume for a given pressure differential is referred to as compliance. At low lung volumes, the lung is more compliant during expiration than inspiration, and vice versa. (From West, *Respiratory Physiology,* 3rd ed., 1990. With permission.)

The smaller the radius (r) of a sphere, the greater will be the surface tension (T_S) over the sphere and the greater will be the force that is required to overcome the pressure (P) within the sphere and cause inflation. Furthermore, this law indicates that as a sphere gets smaller, surface tension increases and would result in the expulsion of all air and the eventual collapse of the sphere. *These physical characteristics would prevent lung inflation from occurring and result in collapsed alveoli and airways.* Obviously, these conditions must be modified *in vivo* for the lungs to operate as they do!

The processes of inflation and deflation of the respiratory structures are aided by the presence of *surfactant.* Surfactant is produced by a subset of alveolar epithelial cells and is a mixture of phospholipids, proteins, and calcium ions.[31] Surfactant mixes with the fluid that bathes the alveolar membranes and results in the interruption of the water layer and a reduction in surface tension. For example, the surface tension of water = 70 dyn/cm², normal alveolar fluid (without surfactant) = 50 dyn/cm², and alveolar fluid with surfactant < 10 dyn/cm² (1 dyn/cm² = 0.1 N/m² = 0.750×10^{-3} mmHg).

The presence of surfactant makes it easier to inflate small alveoli. During inflation, the size of the alveoli surface area increases, and the concentration of surfactant decreases, so that *at higher lung volumes the resistance to inflation increases.* The latter event is not disastrous, as it promotes a more even inflation of neighboring alveoli and respiratory bronchioles and provides some elastic recoil force during the start of expiration.

As indicated in Figure 3, during inspiration the lung is able to inflate with minimal generation of negative intrapleural pressures and, therefore, has what is termed high *compliance.* Compliance is greatest during midinspiration and decreases at the start and end of inspiration, even for resting ventilation (tidal) volumes. During expiration compliance is reduced at higher lung volumes, yet remains stable at mid-to-low lung volumes.

The high compliance of the lung reduces the work of breathing. For example, a given volume of lung inflation requires one tenth of the work required to similarly inflate a balloon.[64] Data of the work of inspiration and expiration during rest and exercise conditions will be presented in the section on acute respiratory adaptations to exercise.

2. Regional Distribution of Ventilation

During the explanation of the mechanics of ventilation, it may have become obvious that the different muscles contributing to ventilation at different ventilation volumes may alter the regional inflation of the lung. For example, normal resting ventilation is accomplished by the contraction of the diaphragm, which is connected to the bottom of the pleural membranes and lungs. This ventilation pattern results in greater volume changes in the lower regions of the lung and, therefore, increases alveolar ventilation in these regions more than in the upper regions (Figure 4). Conversely, increased depth of breathing causes the added inflation of the lateral and upper regions of the lung because of the involvement of the flaring and elevation of the rib cage. A more even inflation of the lung results.

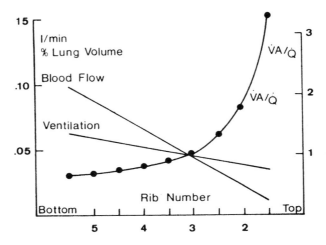

Figure 4   Due to the regional distribution of ventilation and blood flow, the ventilation–perfusion ratio ($\dot{V}_A/\dot{Q}$) for different levels of the lungs ranges from below to above 1. As explained in the text, exercise improves the $\dot{V}_A/\dot{Q}$ of the lung by making the ventilation and blood flow distribution throughout the lung more even. (From West, *Respiratory Physiology*, 3rd ed., 1990. With permission.)

3. Regional Distribution of Blood Flow

As the two lungs are located beside the heart, and extend vertically above the heart, a force exerted by the vertical column of blood, or *hydrostatic force,* exists to oppose blood flow to and perfusion of the upper regions of the lung. For the superior regions of the lung, this vertical distance can be as great as 30 cm, which amounts to a pressure differential of 23 mmHg,[32] which may equal or exceed pulmonary systolic blood pressure. Consequently, under resting conditions the greatest perfusion of the lung occurs near the lower regions, and practically zero flow occurs in the upper regions, as indicated in Figure 4.

C. RESPIRATION

The three main gases of air — nitrogen, oxygen, and carbon dioxide — all diffuse between the alveolar air and blood, but as gaseous nitrogen is not metabolized within the body, the latter two gases are of interest for normal physiological conditions. The process of gas exchange, or respiration, involves the movement of oxygen and carbon dioxide down pressure gradients that exist between pulmonary capillary blood and the air of the alveoli, and between capillary blood of the systemic circulation and the cells perfused by this blood. Consequently, the locations of respiration can either be in the lung, which is referred to as *external respiration,* or at the level of the systemic tissues, which is referred to as *internal respiration.*

1. External Respiration

The processes of external respiration result in the movement of gases between alveolar air and the pulmonary capillary blood. This exchange occurs via diffusion through a fluid medium that contains several membranes. The success of this diffusion depends on the characteristics of the gases for diffusion in an aqueous environment and on the nature of the diffusion medium within the lung.

a. Gas Partial Pressures in Atmospheric and Alveolar Air

Dry atmospheric air contains 20.93% oxygen 79.03% nitrogen, 0.03% carbon dioxide, and extremely small percentages of certain rare gases, such as argon, that make up the remaining 0.01%. When air contains moisture, or water vapor, the water vapor molecules force the gas molecules to disperse, resulting in an increases volume of air. For constant volumes of gas, the presence of water vapor occupies a pressure within the total gas pressure, and the pressures of the gases decrease.

Figure 5 presents the partial pressures of gases in air under standard conditions, in atmospheric air at a coastal location, and how these gas pressures change in the alveoli. When accounting for the relative humidity and temperature of the atmospheric gas sample, the actual pressure occupied by the true gases decreases from 747 to 729 mmHg. Within the alveoli, the pressure remains equal to atmospheric pressure, but as the air is warmed to 37°C and completely humidified (100% relative humidity), the partial pressure of water vapor increases to 47 mmHg. Consequently, the pressure remaining for the true gases is 700 mmHg.

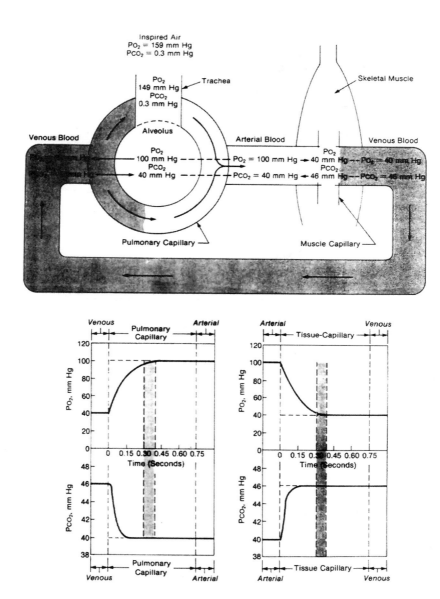

Figure 5 The partial pressures of oxygen and carbon dioxide in inspired air, air in the alveoli of the lung, and in pulmonary arterial and venous blood. As blood flows through the lung, gas partial pressures equilibrate. Due to the higher solubility of CO_2 compared with O_2, the time for equilibration is less for CO_2. This fact applies to both the lung and peripheral vasculature. (From Fox, Bowers, and Foss, *The Physiological Basis of Physical Education and Athletics*, 4th ed., 1988. With permission.)

Figure 6 illustrates the changes in oxygen and carbon dioxide partial pressures as air is exhaled from the lungs. Initially, there is no change in either gas partial pressure, as a large portion of the air in the anatomical dead space has not been intermixed with air from the respiratory zone. There is then a gradual increase in the partial pressure of carbon dioxide and a gradual decrease in the partial pressure of oxygen until the air near the end of expiration (*end-tidal*) reflects alveolar air. Interestingly, end-tidal air gas fractions are often used as an indirect measure of alveolar gas fractions. When the alveolar partial pressure of carbon dioxide (P_ACO_2) and respiratory exchange ratio (RER) are known, the alveolar partial pressure of oxygen (P_AO_2) can be calculated from the alveolar gas equation:

$$P_AO_2 = P_IO_2 - (P_ACO_2/RER) + [(P_ACO_2 \times F_IO_2 \times ((1 - RER)/RER)]$$

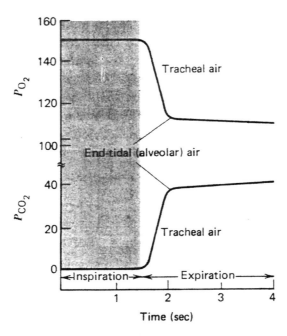

Figure 6   The changes in carbon dioxide and oxygen gas fractions in air during the progression from the start to the end of expiration. (From Brooks and Fahey, *Exercise Physiology: Human Bioenergetics and its Applications*, 1st ed., 1985. With permission.)

When no carbon dioxide is inspired, the right side of the equation can be removed.[64]

2. Diffusion of Gases

Once air is in the alveoli it is subject to gas diffusion from the alveoli to the blood, or vice versa. The factors that govern the direction and magnitude of diffusion are the diffusion capacity of each of the gases, their partial pressure gradient between the alveoli and blood, and the characteristics of the medium through which diffusion occurs.

a. Physical Properties of Oxygen and Carbon Dioxide

The exchange of gases within the lung and body involves movement along a pressure gradient that exists in both liquid and gas mediums and encompasses several membranes. The solubility and diffusability of gases through these membranes are therefore important for their ability for diffusion between the alveoli and blood (*blood–gas interface*) of the lung.

i. Lung Diffusion Capacity

Researchers and clinical pulmonologists have measured the diffusion capacities of certain gases for the blood–gas interface. Carbon dioxide and oxygen are not suited to the measurement of the lung diffusion capacity because the rate of diffusion is biased by their partial pressure gradients between the alveoli and blood. Conversely, carbon monoxide and nitrous oxide are suitable gases to use as they bind to hemoglobin within the lung with far greater affinity than oxygen, are not soluble, and therefore do not increase their respective blood partial pressures, and their exchange between the alveoli and blood is limited solely by diffusive properties.[30]

The diffusion capacity of the lung can therefore be measured by having a subject inhale a given volume of CO or N_2O, and the rate of disappearance of the gas in expired air is measured. As will be explained in later sections, the diffusion capacity of the lung increases from resting values during moderate exercise intensities, but may decrease during more-intense exercise.[51,52,58,59]

b. Gas Partial Pressure Gradients between Alveoli and Blood

Figure 5 illustrated the difference in gas partial pressures between alveolar air and the pulmonary capillary blood. A large gradient exists for the diffusion of oxygen from the alveoli to the blood, and a small gradient exists for the diffusion of carbon dioxide from the blood to the alveoli. When combined with

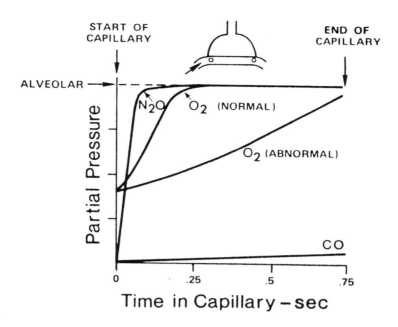

Figure 7 A comparison between nitrous oxide (N_2O), oxygen (O_2), and carbon monoxide (CO) for diffusion of gas across the blood–gas interface of the lung. For the normal lung, O_2 and N_2O are dependent on gas partial pressure gradients for diffusion; however, diffusion of CO is independent of partial pressure gradients. (From West, *Respiratory Physiology*, 3rd ed., 1990. With permission.)

the specific diffusive capacities for each gas, these partial pressure gradients result in similar diffusion profiles for oxygen and carbon dioxide (Figure 7). As blood flows through the pulmonary capillaries, the partial pressures of oxygen and carbon dioxide in the blood and alveoli reach an equilibrium after approximately 0.25 s under resting blood flow conditions (5 l/min). It is clear that the larger partial pressure for oxygen overcomes the low diffusability. The fact that alveolar and blood gas partial pressures reach equilibrium within the lung enables researchers to estimate arterial blood gas partial pressures from alveolar partial pressures.

3. Ventilation–Perfusion Relationships

For the lung to operate optimally in respiration, there would need to be a balance between ventilation and perfusion. Relative to blood flow, overinflation would cause the alveoli to be flushed with "fresh" air at a rate too high to maintain normal alveolar partial pressures. Conversely, underinflation would not provide adequate oxygen and remove adequate carbon dioxide. As previously explained, all regions of the lung are not ventilated or perfused equally, and, furthermore, when comparing ventilation and perfusion (Figure 4), it is clear that the changes in these capacities as one progresses from the bottom to the top of the lung are not identical. As imbalance in alveolar ventilation and perfusion would detrimentally affect gas exchange, *a measure of the effectiveness of lung respiration is the ventilation–perfusion ratio* (V_A/Q), which under optimal conditions would equal 1.0.

The V_A/Q equals the ratio between regional alveolar ventilation and blood flow and, due to measurement difficulty, is calculated as follows:

$$V_A/Q = 0.863 \times RER \times [(CaO_2 - CvO_2)/P_ACO_2]$$

This calculation needs to be made at several levels of the lung, and when the measurements required in this equation are completed in the vertical position, the results indicate that only a small region of the lung is at or close to V_A/Q unity. Apical gas exchange criteria reflect a relative overinflation and a resultant gas partial pressure profile that more resembles atmospheric air. Conversely, the basal regions of the lung reflect a relative underinflation and a resultant gas partial pressure profile that more resembles central mixed venous blood.

Table 1 Representative Concentrations of Hemoglobin and Oxygen-Carrying Capacity of the Blood in Males and Females, after Blood Doping, and When Anemic

Population/Condition	[Hb] (g/l)	ml O_2/l blood[a]
Males	140	183.8
Females	120	157.6
Blood doping	180	236.4
Anemia	<100	<131.3

[a] Assumes 98% Hb saturation and a blood pH = 7.4.

In damaged regions of the lungs, either ventilation or perfusion may be reduced, or completely absent. These regions would be extreme examples of alterations in V_A/Q and, when present, constitute regions of *physiological dead space.*

V. BLOOD GAS TRANSPORT

The equilibration of oxygen and carbon dioxide partial pressures between the alveoli and blood of the lung does not reflect gas volumes. To understand how gas partial pressures affect the volume of gases in blood, knowledge of how blood transports oxygen and carbon dioxide must be acquired.

A. OXYGEN TRANSPORT

Oxygen is transported in blood bound to a specialized protein, *hemoglobin,* which is located on the surface of red blood cells. Hemoglobin consists of four polypeptide chain domains (*globins*), that each have a *heme* prosthetic group which contain a central iron (Fe^{2+}) atom.[39] Each of these domains can bind one oxygen molecule, which amounts to the maximal binding of *1.34 ml of oxygen per gram of hemoglobin.* Table 1 presents representative hemoglobin concentrations for certain athletic populations and clinical conditions and the corresponding volume of oxygen transported at specific hemoglobin saturations. When the hemoglobin concentration equals 150 g/l, the following calculations result in the maximal volume of oxygen that can be transported in arterial blood.

$$\text{Blood Oxygen-Carrying Capacity} = 150 \text{ g/l} \times 1.34 \text{ ml/g}$$
$$= 201.0 \text{ ml/l}$$

Even if the hemoglobin concentration was accurate, there is never this much oxygen in arterial blood, as hemoglobin saturation is never 100%. The incomplete saturation is due to a combination of diffusion limitations resulting from an average inequality between the lung V_A/Q, a *pulmonary arterial to venous shunt* due to blood from the bronchioles that drain into the pulmonary veins without passing through the pulmonary capillaries of the respiratory zone, and a *cardiac shunt* involving the drainage of coronary venous blood into the left ventricle. The three deficiencies of pulmonary and cardiac circulation result in minor reductions in average sea-level arterial oxyhemoglobin saturation to 98% and a maximal blood oxygen-carrying capacity of 197.0 ml/l. For individuals who live above sea level, further decreases in hemoglobin saturation occur that are determined by the oxyhemoglobin dissociation curve.

Another small source of oxygen transport in blood is the volume of dissolved oxygen. Of course, due to the low solubility of oxygen this store is minimal and amounts to 0.03 ml O_2/l for every 1 mmHg of gas partial pressure, or 3 ml O_2/l at sea level.

1. Oxygen-Hemoglobin Saturation

At sea level, the P_AO_2 approximates 104 mmHg. For conditions that lower P_AO_2, such as altitude or air pollution, the partial pressure gradient between the alveoli and blood would decrease. Based on the low diffusion coefficient of oxygen and the data of Figure 9, this would be disastrous for the exchange of oxygen between alveolar gas and blood, preventing the ability to equilibrate P_AO_2 and PaO_2.[58]

Figure 8 illustrates the oxyhemoglobin dissociation curve, which essentially describes the change in hemoglobin saturation with a decrease in P_AO_2. For P_AO_2 values that range from 100 to 80 mmHg there

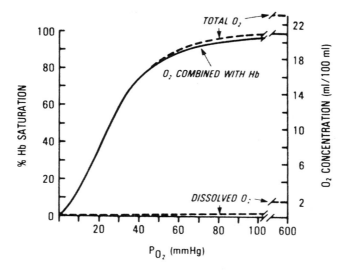

Figure 8   The relationship between the saturation of hemoglobin with oxygen and the partial pressure of arterial oxygen (PaO_2). The resulting curve is called the oxyhemoglobin dissociation curve. The curve is moved down and to the right during conditions that increase blood temperature, PCO_2, acidosis, and 2,3 DPG (see Figure 11). (From West, *Respiratory Physiology*, 3rd ed., 1990. With permission.)

is almost no reduction in the saturation of hemoglobin. As P_AO_2 decreases from 80 to 60 mmHg, hemoglobin saturation decreases from 94.9 to 89.3%, and for P_AO_2 values below 60 mmHg, dramatic decreases in hemoglobin saturation occur which can result in large decreases in arterial oxygen transport (Table 2).

a. Additional Factors that Alter Oxyhemoglobin Saturation

Apart from a decreased saturation when the PO_2 is reduced, dissociation of oxygen and hemoglobin occurs at given PO_2 values by increases in each of blood temperature, PCO_2, and 2,3 diphosphoglycerate (2,3 DPG) and by decreases in blood pH. These relationships are illustrated in Figure 8 and documented in Table 2.

Table 2   The Change in Oxyhemoglobin Saturation and Blood Oxygen-Carrying Capacity for Different Values of PO_2 and Blood pH

PO_2	O_2-Hb Saturation (%), at pH:			Concentration of Arterial Oxygen[a] (ml/l), at pH:		
	7.35	7.40	7.45	7.35	7.40	7.45
10	12.4	13.3	14.3	23.26	24.95	26.83
20	33.2	35.5	38.1	62.28	66.60	71.48
30	55.1	58.0	61.0	103.37	108.81	114.44
40	71.4	73.9	76.3	133.95	138.64	143.14
44	76.1	78.4	80.6	142.76	147.08	151.21
48	80.0	82.0	83.9	150.08	153.83	157.40
52	83.2	84.9	86.6	156.08	159.27	162.46
56	85.8	87.3	88.8	160.96	163.77	166.59
60	87.9	89.3	90.6	164.90	167.53	169.97
64	89.7	90.9	92.0	168.28	170.53	172.59
68	91.1	92.2	93.1	170.90	172.97	174.66
76	93.3	94.1	94.9	175.03	176.53	178.03
80	94.2	94.9	95.5	176.72	178.03	179.16
90	95.7	96.3	96.8	179.53	180.66	181.60
100	96.8	97.2	97.6	181.60	182.35	183.10

Adapted from Jones, N. L., *Blood Gases and Acid–Base Physiology*, 2nd ed., Thieme Medical Publishers, New York, 1987.

The molecule 2,3 DPG is a by-product of glycolysis in the red blood cell, and its production increases during conditions of low PO_2 (hypoxia).[39,41] The 2,3 DPG produced by the red blood cell binds to the deoxygenated form of hemoglobin and therefore assists the unloading of oxygen from hemoglobin.[39,41] Each of temperature, PCO_2, 2,3 DPG, and pH is a condition that changes at the level of the tissues, and the directions of these changes combine to decrease the affinity between oxygen and hemoglobin causing greater unloading of oxygen. The effect of temperature, pH, and PCO_2 on adjusting the oxyhemoglobin dissociation curve down and to the right is termed the *Bohr effect* in recognition of the scientist who first observed the phenomenon.[3,54]

B. CARBON DIOXIDE TRANSPORT

The volume of carbon dioxide stored in the body (blood and tissues) is approximately tenfold greater than oxygen stores,[36] and it is transported in the blood in several forms, some of which involve near equilibrium chemical reactions (Figure 9).

Although carbon dioxide has a greater solubility than oxygen, the majority of CO_2 is not dissolved in plasma or the red blood cell, but reacts with water and is converted to carbonic acid via the carbonic anhydrase–catalyzed reaction that occurs on the surface of red blood cells and inner walls of the vascular endothelium. Carbonic acid then dissociates to bicarbonate (HCO_3^-) and a free proton (H^+). The bicarbonate ions are transported in the plasma and under normal acid–base conditions the proton is bound to deoxygenated hemoglobin. The ability of hemoglobin to bind both carbon dioxide and protons is important for acid–base regulation of the blood.

The exchange in hemoglobin binding for carbon dioxide and oxygen is based on the change in the partial pressure of oxygen. When the partial pressure of oxygen increases, the affinity between hemoglobin and carbon dioxide decreases and carbon dioxide is forced from hemoglobin. This PO_2 effect on the ability of blood to store carbon dioxide is termed the *Haldane effect*.[37,54]

The changing content of blood CO_2 for a given PCO_2 can be graphed in a similar manner to the oxyhemoglobin dissociation curve. However, as the CO_2 content in blood is also dependent on the oxygen saturation of hemoglobin, as explained by the Haldane effect, a family of CO_2 dissociation curves exists (Figure 10). For normal function of the lung and normal acid–base conditions, the actual or "physiological" curve for CO_2 dissociation from hemoglobin spans the normal range of blood PCO_2 and connects the two lines that span the normal range of oxyhemoglobin saturation. The resulting CO_2 dissociation curve is therefore a small curve compared with the curve of oxyhemoglobin dissociation.

C. INTERNAL RESPIRATION

The exchange of gases at the cellular level is influenced by each of the Bohr and Haldane effects. In the tissues the partial pressure of oxygen is low (<5 mmHg during intense exercise) because of the reduction of oxygen in the electron transport chain, and the partial pressure of carbon dioxide is high because of metabolic production of CO_2. The additional characteristics of an increased temperature and low pH favor the dissociation of oxygen from hemoglobin, and, due to the Haldane effect, the affinity between hemoglobin and carbon dioxide increases.

The unloading of oxygen from hemoglobin is also aided by the molecule *myoglobin*. Myoglobin is found within skeletal muscle fibers and is a similar protein to hemoglobin in that it contains a *heme* prosthetic group which contains a central iron (Fe^{2+}) atom that binds oxygen.[39] At the cellular level of the circulation where oxygen is consumed and the partial pressure of oxygen in blood decreases, there is a sharp decrease in the affinity between oxygen and hemoglobin. For oxygen partial pressures less than 60 mmHg, myoglobin has a higher affinity for oxygen than does hemoglobin (Figure 11), which allows a unidirectional transfer of oxygen from hemoglobin to myoglobin within the muscle fibers.[3,62] *Myoglobin can therefore be viewed as a "go-between," transferring oxygen molecules between hemoglobin and the mitochondria within the muscle fiber.* The drastic decrease in oxygen and myoglobin affinity below an oxygen partial pressure of 10 mmHg is favorable because of the known decreases in intramuscular PO_2 below 5 mmHg during intense exercise. At these low PO_2 values, there is a much higher capacity for oxygen to be released from myoglobin for use in mitochondrial respiration. Having more myoglobin would increase the reservoir of oxygen stored within muscle fibers and also increase the ability of muscle to continue mitochondrial respiration during intermittent periods of *hypoxia* (low PaO_2) or *ischemia* (reduced blood flow).

The cellular removal of carbon dioxide is driven by the Haldane effect and the concentration gradient between the cells and capillary blood. As previously explained, the relatively high solubility and diffusability of carbon dioxide prevents diffusion limitation.

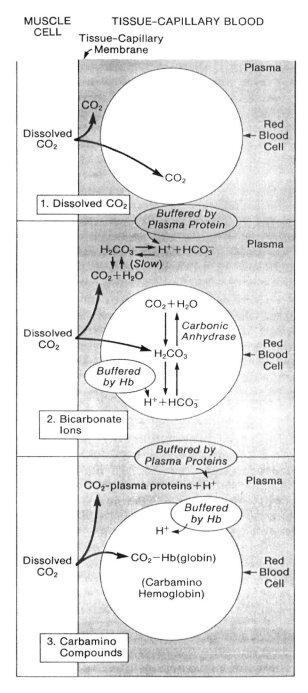

Figure 9 Carbon dioxide is transported in the blood dissolved in plasma and in the red blood cell, bound to hemoglobin and plasma proteins, and as bicarbonate (HCO_3^-). (From Fox, Bowers, and Foss, *The Physiological Basis of Education and Athletics*, 4th ed., 1988. With permission.)

VI. ACUTE ADAPTATIONS OF PULMONARY FUNCTION DURING EXERCISE

As previously explained, the start of exercise is accompanied by immediate increases in ventilation. The factors that regulate this increase are numerous and need to be explained. In addition, the changes in ventilation can be different for different types of exercise and are affected by the acidosis generated

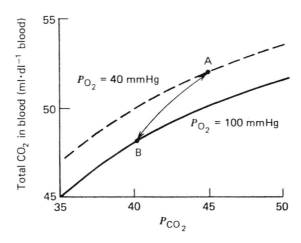

Figure 10 The relationships between the partial pressure of alveolar carbon dioxide (P_ACO_2) and the saturation of hemoglobin with CO_2 in blood. As the Haldane effect explains the role of PaO_2 on the affinity between hemoglobin and CO_2, there is a family of curves for the dissociation of CO_2 and hemoglobin based on the PaO_2. As the pressure gradient between P_ACO_2 and pulmonary PCO_2 is only 5 mmHg, the physiological range of CO_2 dissociation is small. (From Brooks and Fahey, *Exercise Physiology: Human Bioenergetics and its Applications*, 1st ed., 1985. With permission.)

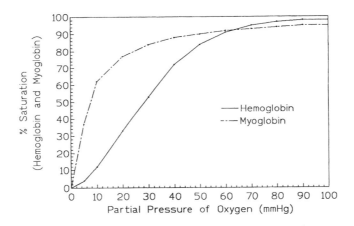

Figure 11 A comparison between oxyhemoglobin and oxymyoglobin dissociation curves.

during exercise at intensities above the lactate threshold. Low-to-moderate exercise intensities increase the effectiveness of external respiration, but for many individuals intense exercise can impair external respiration. Research has focused on how exercise affects the lung diffusion capacity and V_E/Q, and these results have provided valuable knowledge of lung function during exercise.

A. CONTROL OF VENTILATION DURING REST AND EXERCISE

The control of ventilation is an intricate and multifaceted regulatory characteristic of the human body. This is understandable given the importance of ventilation for maintaining optimal oxygen content of the blood, and for regulating blood acid–base balance. *Ventilation can be controlled by both voluntary and involuntary functions of the nervous system.* Neural controls exist in the central and peripheral nervous systems and exert their effects through input and alteration to central controls of inspiration and expiration. Pheripheral *chemoreceptors* also exist that convert chemical stimuli into action potentials that are relayed to the control locations within the central nervous system. Due to this anatomical diversity, an understanding of the anatomical distribution of the control sites involved in the regulation of ventilation is important. These multiple control systems combine to regulate ventilation, and their relative importance differs in the resting compared with the exercise state.

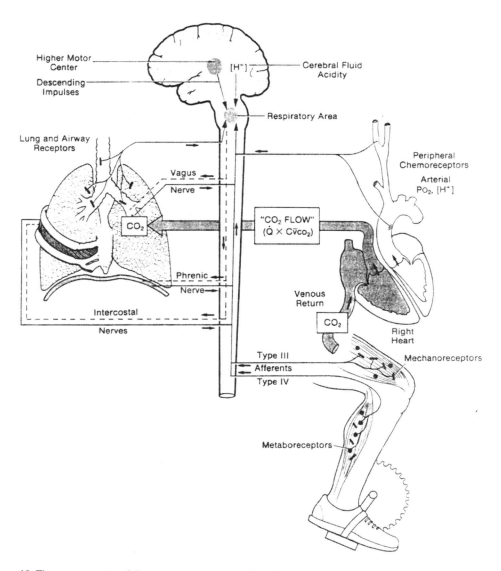

Figure 12 The components of the nervous system and cranial and systemic circulations that are involved in the regulation of ventilation. The respiratory center of the medulla (inset) comprises discrete neural regions responsible for inspiration, expiration, and their regulation. In the periphery, afferent nerves arise from the lungs, joints, muscles, and chemoreceptors, as explained in the text. (From Fox, Bowers, and Foss, *The Physiological Basis of Physical Education and Athletics*, 4th ed., 1988. With permission.)

1. Anatomical Organization of Ventilatory Control
a. Central Nervous System
The main components of the neural circuitry within the central nervous system that are involved in the control of ventilation are presented in Figure 12. A collection of nerves within the medulla of the lower brain functions as the *respiratory center*. Within the respiratory center are localized regions that specifically influence inspiration and expiration and, hence, are termed inspiratory and expiratory centers, respectively. As will be discussed, these two locations coordinate the sequence of inspiration and expiration during breathing.

Superior to the respiratory center are additional nerve regions, termed the *apneustic area* and the *pneumotaxic area,* that influence the function of the respiratory center. Basically, input from the apneustic area prolongs the duration of inspiration, while input from the pneumotaxic area shortens the duration of inspiration and thereby increases the frequency of breathing. In addition, nerves that originate in the cortex descend and innervate the respiratory center, as well as the apneustic and pneumotaxic areas, thus accounting for the voluntary control circuits of ventilation.

In close proximity to the respiratory center is a collection of nerve endings that are directly sensitive to hydrogen ions and indirectly sensitive to $PaCO_2$. The nerves from this location are termed *central chemoreceptors* and represent a method of ventilatory control based on a blood-borne, or *humoral,* factor. When the $PaCO_2$ increases, as it does only slightly during conditions of metabolic acidosis, the CO_2 penetrates the *blood–brain barrier,* forms carbonic acid in the cerebrospinal fluid, and then dissociates to HCO_3^- and H^+. As there is minimal bicarbonate in cerebrospinal fluid, even a small increase in $PaCO_2$ can decrease cerebrospinal fluid pH, which is detected by the central chemoreceptors.

b. Peripheral Nervous System

Nerves from the periphery return from various locations to influence the pattern of ventilation. Free nerve endings exist in joints and within skeletal muscle that return action potentials to the respiratory center during muscle contraction and even passive limb movement. In addition, animal research has revealed the presence of chemoreceptors in the lung that are sensitive to CO_2.[28] Increasing PCO_2 in the pulmonary capillary blood stimulates these receptors, and action potentials are returned to the respiratory center to stimulate an increase in ventilation. It is unclear whether or not similar receptors exist in the human lung.

Additional chemoreceptors are located in the periphery. Located on the superior wall of the aortic arch are chemoreceptors termed *aortic bodies,* and on the carotid arteries in the region of the carotid bifurcation are additional chemoreceptors termed *carotid bodies.* Both sets of peripheral arterial chemoreceptors are stimulated by increases in $PaCO_2$ and decreasing pH (increasing $[H^+]$), with the carotid bodies capable of additional stimulation by potassium and PaO_2.[9,45] However, decreases in PaO_2 only cause minor increases in ventilation until PaO_2 values are less than 65 mmHg, after which stimulation to ventilation increases abruptly.[31]

2. Controls of Ventilation at Rest

Normal resting breathing is characterized by infrequent shallow inspiratory and expiratory maneuvers. The transition between inspiration and expiration is controlled by a repetitive discharge of action potentials from the inspiratory center. Expiration involves the passive recoil of the diaphragm. During normal acid–base conditions, minimal additional regulation occurs from chemoreceptor stimulation.

3. Controls of Ventilation during Exercise

Exercise provides multiple stimuli for increases in ventilation. Depending upon exercise intensity, all the components of ventilatory control become influential in determining the ventilatory rate. Considerable research has been conducted to try and determine the most influential controls of ventilation during exercise, but the multiple regulation schemes have prevented the ability to rank each control system.

a. Neural Factors

The relative importance of central neural vs. peripheral neural controls of ventilation has been assessed by having humans exercise without intervention and exercise by artificial electrical stimulation.[7] Theoretically, the absence of voluntary control to muscle contraction would not have the conscious stimulation of the respiratory center and, therefore, should have a compromised ventilatory pattern. A similar model using individuals with complete spinal cord injury has been used for the same reasons.[8] Results have indicated that alveolar ventilation was optimal in either condition. As spinal cord injury prevents afferent nerve return to the central nervous system, additional factors were also concerned in regulating ventilation during exercise. Nevertheless, the role of neural factors in regulating ventilation has been extensively documented in animal research that is characterized by more-invasive procedures and better control of other ventilatory stimulants.[21,22,24]

b. Humoral Factors

A common model used with human subjects is to occlude blood flow from a limb, and then to exercise the muscles from the limb. Such a model prevents the removal of a metabolite stimulant to ventilation, such as carbon dioxide.[34] Such research has shown that ventilation still increases in a similar manner to exercise with intact circulation.

c. Neurohumoral Approach

A commonsense approach to the control of ventilation is to expect that multiple control systems function together. In 1954 a French physiologist named Dejours[15] postulated that at the start of exercise neural

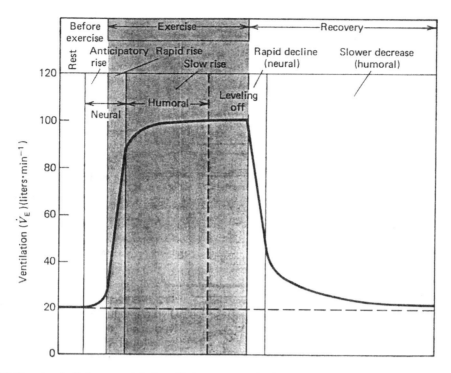

Figure 13 The classic Dejours model of ventilation expressed relative to the change in ventilation from rest to submaximal steady exercise. The initial increase in ventilation and the rapid decrease in ventilation when exercise is stopped are rapid and are explained by the neural components of regulation. The fine-tuning of ventilation during exercise is believed to be due to humoral components of ventilation regulation. (From Brooks and Fahey, *Exercise Physiology: Human Bioenergetics and its Applications*, 1st ed., 1985. With permission.)

mechanisms were of most importance, and then humoral factors fine-tuned the neural controls to provide a steady state ventilatory profile (Figure 13). Consequently, as steady state exercise implies being at an intensity below the lactate and ventilatory thresholds, the humoral factors were not determined by increasing $PaCO_2$, decreasing pH, or exercise-induced hypoxemia.[24] Recent evidence of lung CO_2 receptors that respond to increasing VCO_2 and alveolar CO_2 exchange may provide the functional explanation of a humoral effect of ventilatory control without hypercapnia and acidosis.[28]

When exercise intensity increases above the lactate or ventilatory thresholds, acidosis develops and is accompanied by small increases in $PaCO_2$. These stimuli exert action on the peripheral and central chemoreceptors, resulting in increased neural input to the respiratory center and increased ventilation. A general depiction of the changes in postulated humoral mediators of ventilation during incremental exercise is presented in Figure 14. The increase in ventilation occurs with increasing acidosis and is effective in reducing $PaCO_2$ and higher ventilatory rates. This response is paradoxical, given the belief that increasing $PaCO_2$ is a potent stimulator of ventilation. However, due to the multiple ventilatory stimulants that increase ventilation during exercise, the hyperventilation results in the removal of CO_2 from the blood and reduces $PaCO_2$ as a means to combat the increasing acidosis.

B. VENTILATION DURING TRANSITIONS FROM REST TO STEADY STATE EXERCISE

As with oxygen consumption, the increase in ventilation during exercise is abrupt, exponential, and proportional to exercise intensity. Steady state ventilation is attained earlier than is steady state VO_2 for a given bout of exercise (Figure 14), which is understandable given the effectiveness of both the neural and humoral controls of ventilation. The increase in ventilation is due to increases in each of tidal volume and breathing frequency.

The transition period following the increase in intensity is associated with slight increases in $PaCO_2$ and decreases in PaO_2,[63] which indicate that, although rapid, the increase in ventilation is still insufficient

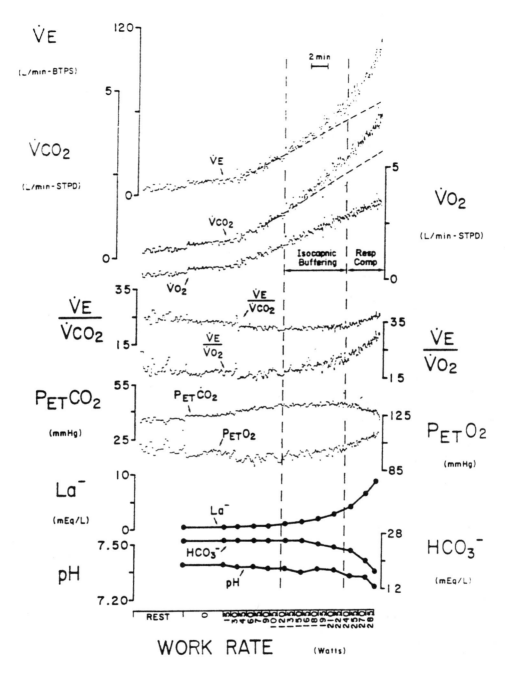

Figure 14 The changes in the humoral stimulants of ventilation during incremental exercise to fatigue. The intensity corresponding to a nonlinear deviation in the increase in ventilation and the point where V_E/VO_2 increases is termed the ventilation threshold. (From Wasserman and Casaburi, in *Lung Biology and Health Disease*, V52, Whipp and Wasserman, Eds., 1991, 409. With permission.)

to overcome the instantaneous demands of the onset of exercise. Once again, as with oxygen consumption, ventilation continues to increase during intensities that are above the intensity at the lactate threshold.

Recent research has shown that increased ventilation rates are associated with the enlargement of the trachea during expiration,[35] which would decrease resistance to air flow. When this is combined with the dilation of the bronchi and bronchioles resulting from neural and circulatory catecholamine stimulation, the conducting zone of the lung is actually a very responsive component of the pulmonary system and therefore should not be viewed as a rigid structure.

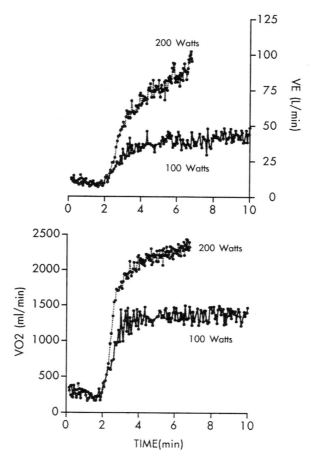

Figure 15 The increase in ventilation and oxygen consumption during different rest to steady state exercise intensities. (From Wasserman and Casaburi in Lung Biology in Health and Disease, V52, Whipp and Wasserman, Eds., 1991. With permission.)

Numerous studies have shown that both ventilation and perfusion of the lungs increase during exercise and become more evenly distributed throughout the lung.[11,13,18,19] Based on the previous discussion of V_A/Q, these responses improve the V_A/Q of the lung and, therefore, improve the process of external respiration.

Ventilation during submaximal exercise at given loads is also known to differ for different types of exercise.[29,44] Arm or upper-body exercise causes a relatively larger ventilation compared with cycling, and static exercise also causes ventilation to be larger than dynamic exercise. Data from Paek and McCool[44] also indicate that tidal volumes, inspiratory times, and end-expiratory lung volumes may also differ between different types of exercise; however, their data were normalized to ventilation and not metabolic load (VO_{2max}). Finally, posture during exercise is also known to affect ventilation, which has been of interest when studying different positions of the upper body during cycling.

C. VENTILATION DURING INCREMENTAL EXERCISE

The increase in ventilation and oxygen consumption during an incremental cycle ergometry exercise test are presented in Figure 15. The variables V_E/VO_2 and V_E/VCO_2 are the ventilatory equivalents for oxygen and carbon dioxide, respectively, and are obtained by dividing the VO_2 or VCO_2 into V_E. During the initial intensities, ventilation increases linearly with intensity and VO_2, and PaO_2 remains stable.

After an individually specific intensity, the increase in V_E deviates from linearity, and this point in time coincides with an abrupt increase in V_E/VO_2. Approximately 2 min later, V_E/VCO_2 begins to increase, and this time delay has been explained by the large storage capacity of the body for CO_2 and the initial similarity between increased ventilation and VCO_2.[10]

1. Ventilatory Threshold

The exercise intensity at which there is a simultaneous deviation from linearity in ventilation and an increase in V_E/VO_2 is termed the *ventilatory threshold* (VT).[4,10,23,27,38,43,55,61,65,67] Other measures can also be used to detect this point, such as an exponential increase in VCO_2 or RER, and an abrupt increase in blood acidosis. However, Caiozzeo et al.[10] have demonstrated that *the joint V_E and V_E/VO_2 criteria are most sensitive in detecting the VT.*

The traditional explanation of the VT is that as exercise intensity increases, the abrupt increase in lactate acidosis that occurs after the lactate threshold causes an increase in blood acidosis and $PaCO_2$. Both the acidosis and the increased $PaCO_2$ stimulate the chemoreceptors to induce increased ventilation. This mechanism has been interpreted by many physiologists as evidence for the lactate and ventilatory thresholds to occur at a similar exercise intensity.

a. Is the Ventilation Threshold Identical to the Lactate Threshold?

Numerous studies have been conducted to compare the lactate threshold and the VT.[23,27,43,61] Researchers have concluded that the two measures are identical;[10,14,60,61,65] however, others have concluded that the two measures can differ under certain conditions and that the two criteria should not be used interchangeably.[1,27,32,43] Factors that can cause the two measures to deviate are altered carbohydrate nutrition, certain exercise test protocols, enzyme deficiency diseases, methodological error, exercise training, and altered states of sympathetic stimulation.[1,26,27,43,67] Gladden et al.[27] have estimated that the variation in relative exercise intensity between the two measures may be larger than 8% of VO_{2max} which would be significant when using the measures to prescribe a training exercise intensity.

2. Mechanics and Metabolic Costs of Ventilation during Exercise

As alveolar ventilation increases, there are increased metabolic demands placed on the muscles of inspiration and expiration. Both the frequency of ventilation and the tidal volume increase during increases in exercise intensity and ventilation, and that increased ventilation during high ventilation rates is due to continued increases in the frequency of breathing and a plateau in tidal volume.

Various mechanical changes also occur as ventilation and exercise intensity increase. As intensity increases, so too does each of the volume of air remaining in the lung after expiration, peak inspiratory pleural pressure, and the work of breathing. Interestingly, dynamic compliance decreases as exercise intensity increases, and this can be explained by the improved compliance of the lung at higher end-expiratory volumes.

The exponential nature of the increased work of breathing during exercise is predominantly due to the cost of expiration at higher ventilation rates, as the flow rate during expiration is then limited by the constriction of the smaller airways.[35]

a. Do the Muscles of Ventilation Fatigue during Exercise?

The large increase in the work of breathing could cause respiratory muscle fatigue during maximal exercise. However, results indicate that for endurance-trained individuals the ability to generate inspiratory negative pleural pressures during maximal exercise is similar to the pleural pressures generated during maximal voluntary inspiratory maneuvers.[35] However, whether or not untrained individuals have near-optimal respiratory muscle and ventilatory function during fatiguing exercise remains to be researched.

Final comment needs to be given to the specific type of exercise performed. Some exercises, such as swimming and deep water exercise, have the upper body submerged in water, which provides an increased external pressure (compression) to the thoracic cavity. This would theoretically decrease the work of expiration, but cause ventilation to occur at a lower end-expiratory volume and reduced compliance, and therefore potentially increase the work of inspiration. Whether or not these changes would cause respiratory muscle fatigue and affect the effectiveness of ventilation is unclear.

3. Exercise-Induced Hypoxemia

The partial pressure (PaO_2) and concentration of oxygen (CaO_2) in arterial blood remain stable in most individuals during all intensities of exercise. High altitude can reduce PaO_2 and CaO_2 due to the lowered partial pressure of oxygen, or *hypoxia,* resulting in a reduced CaO_2, or *hypoxemia.* Interestingly, numerous reports have documented hypoxemia during exhausting exercise at sea level in individuals with healthy lungs.

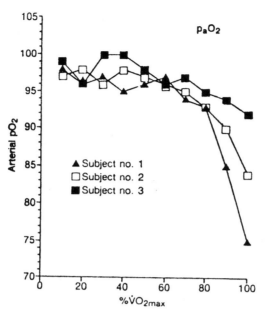

Figure 16 The decrease in oxyhemoglobin saturation (hypoxemia) and blood oxygen content during incremental exercise in individuals with different $\dot{V}O_{2max}$ capacities. For individuals with increasing $\dot{V}O_{2max}$, there are larger reductions in oxyhemoglobin saturation, and indicate inadequacies in lung function. (From Powers, Martin, and Dodd, *Sports Med.,* 16(1):14–22, 1993. With permission.)

In 1984 it was observed that highly trained endurance athletes experience significant reductions in CaO_2, and this condition was termed *exercise-induced hypoxemia.*[16] Figure 16 reveals the change in arterial oxyhemoglobin saturation in individuals of different cardiorespiratory endurance fitness during an incremental exercise test to volitional fatigue. The more endurance trained the athlete, the larger is the reduction in CaO_2, which indicates that for these individuals the lungs are not functioning optimally during intense exercise. Powers et al.[46,47,51] have shown that exercise-induced hypoxemia occurs in approximately 50% of well-trained endurance athletes during intense intensities above 80% VO_{2max}.

As the healthy lung was always thought to function optimally during exercise, the initial explanation for this phenomenon was an imbalance between cardiac output and maximal pulmonary blood flow. It was assumed that endurance athletes were trained to the point where their central blood volume and maximal cardiac output had exceeded the ability of their lungs to maintain pulmonary blood flow at a velocity required to equilibrate P_AO_2 and PaO_2. The velocity of blood flow in the pulmonary capillaries is important, as a high velocity would decrease the time of a given red blood cell within the blood–gas interface, termed the *pulmonary transit time,* and risk inequilibration. The time required for equilibration between P_AO_2 and PaO_2 in the healthy lung is believed to be 350 to 400 ms.[59]

Warren et al.[59] measured pulmonary transit time in individuals known to exhibit exercise-induced hypoxemia. Although pulmonary transit time decreased during increases in exercise intensity, it did not reach critical levels in these subjects, indicating that the traditional explanation of exercise-induced hypoxemia was inaccurate. The remaining explanations of inadequate hyperventilation, increasing venoarterial shunt, a decrease in lung diffusion capacity, or ventilation–perfusion inequality required investigation. Inadequate ventilation would prevent the oxygenation of arterial blood and also limit the removal CO_2 from the blood. As there is no increase in $PaCO_2$ in individuals who experience hypoxemia, inadequate hyperventilation does not appear to be the cause.[35,48,50,51] In facet, Johnson et al.[35] have shown that highly trained endurance athletes ($VO_{2max} > 70$ ml/kg/min) reach the maximal mechanical limits of alveolar ventilation during maximal exercise yet have an increasing P_AO_2 and a decreasing $PaCO_2$ during the development of arterial hypoxemia.[35] At rest, the venoarterial shunt of the lung and heart account for 50% of the difference between P_AO_2 and $PaCO_2$, and researchers have estimated that the same could be true for exercise.[51] However, if a shunt explanation was valid, then inspiring hyperoxic gas during exercise should not dramatically improve the hypoxemia. Dempsey et al.[16] and Powers et al.[46,48,50] have shown that breathing hyperoxic gas does relieve the hypoxemia. The combined evidence presented above suggests that processes involved in the exchange of oxygen in the lung, such as diffusion limitations or ventilation–perfusion inequality, must be the cause(s).

VII. CHRONIC ADAPTATIONS

The lungs and pulmonary circulation do not express the degree of long-term adaptation to exercise as was evident for the neuromuscular function and skeletal muscle energy metabolism. Efforts have been made to verify whether or not respiratory muscles can adapt to exercise training and improve lung function during exercise.[49] However, although respiratory muscles can adapt to exercise, it appears that their function remains near optimal, and there are no signs to support superior lung function in the trained compared with the untrained state.

Numerous studies have shown that the VT improves with endurance training.[14,26,61] As the causes for this improvement are more determined by muscular and cardiovascular function, no comment will be given for this response in this chapter.

REFERENCES

1. Anderson G. S. and E. C. Rhodes. The relationship between blood lactate and excess CO_2 in elite cyclists. *J. Sports Sci.* 9:173–181, 1991.
2. Bastacky J. B. and J. Goerke. Pores of Kohn are filled in normal lungs: low-temperature scanning electron microscopy. *J. Appl. Physiol.* 73(1):88–95, 1992.
3. Baumann R., H. Bartels and C. Bauer. Blood oxygen transport. In Farhi L. E. and S. M. Tenney, Eds. *Handbook of Physiology,* Section 3: *The Respiratory System,* Volume 1: *Gas Exchange,* 147–172, American Physiological Society, Bethesda, 1987.
4. Beaver W., K. Wasserman and B. Whipp. A new method for detecting anaerobic threshold by gas exchange. *J. Appl. Physiol.* 60(6):2020–2027, 1986.
5. Bennett F. A role for neural pathways in exercise hyperpnea. *J. Appl. Physiol.* 56(6):1559–1564, 1984.
6. Boutellier U. and P. Piwko. The respiratory system as an exercise limiting factor in normal sedentary subjects. *Eur. J. Appl. Physiol.* 64:145–152, 1992.
7. Brice A. G., H. V. Foster, L. G. Pan, A. Funahashi, T. F. Lowry, C. L. Murphy and M. D. Hoffman. Ventilatory and $PaCO_2$ responses to voluntary and electrically induced leg exercise. *J. Appl. Physiol.* 64(1):218–225, 1988.
8. Brice A. G., H. V. Foster, L. G. Pan, A. Funahashi, M. D. Hoffman, C. L. Murphy and T. F. Lowry. Is the hyperpnea of muscular contractions critically dependent upon spinal cord afferents. *J. Appl. Physiol.* 64(1):226–233, 1988.
9. Busse M., N. Maassen and H. Konrad. Relation between plasma K^+ and ventilation during incremental exercise after glycogen depletion and repletion in man. *J. Physiol.* 443:469–476, 1991.
10. Caiozzeo V. J., J. A. Davis, J. F. Ellis, J. L. Azus, R. Vandagriff, C. A. Prietto and W. C. MccMaster. A comparison of gas exchange indices used to detect the anaerobic threshold. *J. Appl. Physiol.* 53(5):1184–1189, 1982.
11. Capen R. L., W. L. Hanson, L. P. Latham, C. A. Dawson and W. W. Wagner, Jr. Distribution of pulmonary transmit times in recruited networks. *J. Appl. Physiol.* 69(2):473–478, 1990.
12. Cerretelli P. and P. E. Di Prampero. Gas exchange in exercise. In Farhi L. E. and S. M. Tenney, Eds. *Handbook of Physiology,* Section 3: *The Respiratory System,* Volume 1: *Gas Exchange,* 297–339, American Physiological Society, Bethesda, 1987.
13. Cotton D. J., F. Taher, J. T. Mink and B. L. Graham. Effect of volume history on changes in DL_{CO}^{SB}-3EQ with lung volume in normal subjects. *J. Appl. Physiol.* 73(2):434–439, 1992.
14. Davis J. A., P. Vodak, J. Wilmore, J. Vodak and P. Kurtz. Anaerobic threshold and maximal aerobic power for three modes of exercise. *J. Appl. Physiol.* 41(4):544–550, 1976.
15. Dejours P. Control of respiration in muscular exercise. In Fenn W. O. and H. Rahn (Eds.), *Handbook of Physiology,* Section 3: *Respiration,* Volume 1, 631–648, American Physiological Society, Washington, 1964.
16. Dempsey J. A., P. G. Hanson and K. S. Henderson. Exercise-induced arterial hypoxemia in healthy persons at sea level. *J. Physiol.* 355:161–175, 1984.
17. Dempsey J. A., G. Mitchell and C. Smith. Exercise and chemoreception. *Am. Rev. Respir. Dis.* 129:31–34, 1984.
18. Dempsey J. A., E. Virdruk and G. Mitchell. Pulmonary control systems in exercise: update. *Fed. Proc.* 44:2260–2270, 1985.
19. Dempsey J. A. Is the lung built for exercise. *Med. Sci. Sports Exercise* 18(2):143–155, 1986.

20. Derion T., H. J. B. Guy, K. Tsukimoto, W. Schaffartzik, R. Prediletto, D. C. Poole, D. R. Knight and P. D. Wagner. Ventilation-perfusion relationships in the lung during head-out water immersion. *J. Appl. Physiol.* 72(1):64–72, 1992.
21. Eldridge F., D. E. Millhorn and T. G. Waldrop. Exercise hyperpnea and locomotion: parallel activation from the hypothalamus. *Science.* 211:844–846, 1981.
22. Eldridge F., D. E. Millhorn, J. P. Kiley and T. G. Waldrop. Stimulation by central command of locomotion, respiration, and circulation during exercise. *Respir. Physiol.* 59:313–317, 1985.
23. Farrel S. W. and J. L. Ivy. Lactate acidosis and the increase in V_E/VO_2 during incremental exercise. *J. Appl. Physiol.* 62(4):1551–1555, 1987.
24. Favier R., D. Desplanches, J. Frutoso, M. Grandmontagne and R. Flandrois. Ventilatory and circulatory transients during exercise: new arguments for a neurohumoral theory. *J. Appl. Physiol.* 54(3):647–653, 1980.
25. Fencl V. and D. E. Leith. Stewart's quantitative acid–base chemistry: applications in biology and medicine. *Respir. Physiol.* 91:1–16, 1993.
26. Gaesser G. A. and D. C. Poole. Lactate and ventilatory thresholds: disparity in time course of adaptations to training. *J. Appl. Physiol.* 61(3):999–1004, 1986.
27. Gladden L. B., J. W. Yates, R. W. Stremel and B. A. Stamford. Gas exchange and lactate anaerobic thresholds: inter- and intraevaluator agreement. *J. Appl. Physiol.* 58(6):2082–2089, 1985.
28. Green J. and N. Schmidt. Mechanism of hyperpnea induced by changes in pulmonary blood flow. *J. Appl. Physiol.* 56:1418–1422, 1984.
29. Grucza R., Y. Miyamoto and Y. Nakazonto. Kinetics of cardiorespiratory response to rhythmic-static exercise in men. *Eur. J. Appl. Physiol.* 61:230–236, 1990.
30. Guenard H., N. Varene and P. Vaida. Determination of lung capillary blood volume and membrane diffusing capacity in man by the measurements of NO and CO transfer. *Respir. Physiol.* 70:113–120, 1987.
31. Guyton A. C. *Textbook of Medical Physiology.* (8th Ed.), W.B. Saunders Co., Philadelphia, 1991.
32. Hagberg J. M., E. F. Coyle, J. E. Carroll, J. M. Miller, W. M. Martin and M. H. Brooke. Exercise hyperventilation in patients with McArdles disease. *J. Appl. Physiol.* 52(4):991–994, 1982.
33. Hlastala M. P. Diffusing capacity heterogeneity. In Farhi L. E. and S. M. Tenney (Eds.), *Handbook of Phyiology, Section 3: The Respiratory System,* Volume 1: *Gas Exchange,* 217–232, American Physiological Society, Bethesda, 1987.
34. Innes J. A., I. Solarte, A. Huszczuk, E. Yeh, B. J. Whipp and K. Wasserman. Respiration during recovery from exercise: effects of trapping and release of femoral artery blood flow. *J. Appl. Physiol.* 67(6):2608–2613, 1989.
35. Johnson B. D., K. W. Saupe and J. A. Dempsey. Mechanical constraints on exercise hyperpnea in endurance athletes. *J. Appl. Physiol.* 73(3):874–886, 1992.
36. Jones N. L. Blood gases and acid–base physiology. 2nd Ed., Thieme Medical Publishers, Inc., New York, 1987.
37. Klocke R. A. Carbon dioxide transport. In Farhi L. E. and S. M. Tenney, (Eds.) *Handbook of Physiology,* Section 3: *The Respiratory System,* Volume 1: *Gas Exchange,* 173–198, American Physiological Society, Bethesda, 1987.
38. Koike A., D. Weiler-Ravell, D. K. McKenzie, S. Zanconato and K. Wasserman. Evidence that the metabolic acidosis threshold is the anaerobic threshold. *J. Appl. Physiol.* 68(6):2521–2526, 1990.
39. Loat C. E. R. and E. C. Rhodes. Relationship between the lactate and ventilatory thresholds during prolonged exercise. *Sports Med.* 15(2):104–115, 1993.
40. Lehninger A. L. *Principles of Biochemistry.* Worth Publishers, Inc., New York, 1982.
41. Mairbaurl H., W. Schobersberger, W. Hasibeder, G. Schwaberger, G. Gaesser and K. R. Tanaka. Regulation of 2,3-DPG and Hb-O_2-affinity during acute exercise. *Eur. J. Appl. Physiol.* 55:174–180, 1986.
42. McCool F. D., M. B. Hershenson, G. E. Tzelepis, Y. Kikuchi and D. E. Leith. Effect of fatigue on maximal inspiratory pressure-flow capacity. *J. Appl. Physiol.* 73(1):36–43, 1992.
43. Neary P. J., J. D. MacDougall, R. Bachus and H. A. Wenger. The relationship between lactate and ventilatory thresholds: coincidental or cause and effect? *Eur. J. Appl. Physiol.* 54:104–108, 1985.
44. Paek D. and D. McCool. Breathing patterns during varied activities. *J. Appl. Physiol.* 73(3):887–893, 1992.
45. Paterson D. Potassium and ventilation during exercise. *J. Appl. Physiol.* 72(3):81–82, 1992.
46. Powers S. K., S. Dodd, J. Lawler, G. Landry, M. Kirtley, T. McKnight and S. Grinton. Incidence of exercise-induced hypoxemia in the elite endurance athlete at sea level. *Eur. J. Appl. Physiol.* 58:298–302, 1988.
47. Powers S. K. and J. Williams. Exercise-induced hypoxemia in highly trained athletes. *Sports Med.* 4:46–53, 1987.
48. Powers S. K., J. Lawlor, J. A. Dempsey, S. Dodd and G. Landry. Effects of incomplete pulmonary gas exchange on VO_{2max}. *J. Appl. Physiol.* 66(6):2491–2495, 1989.
49. Powers S. K., J. Lawlor, D. Criswell, S. Dodd, S. Grinton, G. Bagby and H. Silverman. Endurance-training-induced cellular adaptations in respiratory muscles. *J. Appl. Physiol.* 68(5):2114–2118, 1990.
50. Powers S. K., D. Martin, M. Cicale, N. Collop, D. Huang and D. Criswell. Exercise-induced hypoxemia in athletes: role of inadequate hyperventilation. *Eur. J. Appl. Physiol.* 65:37–42, 1992.
51. Powers S. K., D. Martin and S. Dodd. Exercise-induced hypoxemia in elite endurance athletes: incidence, causes and impact on VO_{2max}. *Sports Med.* 16(1):14–22, 1993.
52. Reuschlein P. S., W. G. Reddan, J. Burpee, J. B. L. Gee and J. Rankin. Effect of physical training on the pulmonary diffusing capacity during submaximal work. *J. Appl. Physiol.* 24(2):152–158, 1968.
53. Roselli R. J., R. E. Parker and T. R. Harris. A model of unsteady-state transvascular fluid and protein transport in the lung. *J. Appl. Physiol.* 56(5):1389–1402, 1984.

54. Seeley R. R., T. D. Stephens and P. Tate. *Anatomy and Physiology.* Times Mirror/Mosby College Publishing, St. Louis, 1989.

55. Skinner J. S. and T. H. McLellan. The transition from aerobic to anaerobic metabolism. *Res. Q. Exercise Sport.* 51(1):234–248, 1980.

56. Stewart P. A. Modern quantitative acid–base chemistry. *Can. J. Physiol. Pharmacol.* 61:1444–1461, 1983.

57. Terrados N., E. Jansson, C. Sylven and L. Kaijser. Is hypoxia a stimulus for synthesis of oxidative enzymes and myoglobin? *J. Appl. Physiol.* 68(6):2369–2372, 1990.

58. Torre-Bueono J. R., P. D. Wagner, H. A. Saltzman, G. E. Gale and R. E. Moon. Diffusion limitation in normal humans during exercise at sea level and simulated altitude. *J. Appl. Physiol.* 58(3):989–995, 1985.

59. Warren G., K. J. Cureton, W. F. Middendorf, C. A. Ray and J. A. Warren. Red blood cell pulmonary transit time during exercise in athletes. *Med. Sci. Sports Exercise* 23(12):1353–1361, 1991.

60. Wasserman K. and M. B. McIlroy. Detecting the threshold of anaerobic metabolism in cardiac patients during exercise. *Am. J. Cardiol.* 14:844–852, 1964.

61. Wasserman K., B. J. Whipp, S. N. Koyal and W. L. Beaver. Anaerobic threshold and respiratory gas exchange during exercise. *J. Appl. Physiol.* 35(2):236–243, 1973.

62. Wasserman K., B. J. Whipp and R. Casaburi. Respiratory control during exercise. In Cherniak N. S. and J. G. Widdicombe. (Eds.) *Handbook of Physiology,* Sections 3: *The Respiratory System,* Volume II: *Control of Breathing,* 595–620, American Physiological Society, Bethesda, 1986.

63. Weissman M. L., P. W. Jones, A. Oren, N. Lamarra, B. J. Whipp and K. Wasserman. Cardiac output increase and gas exchange at the start of exercise. *J. Appl. Physiol.* 52(1):236–244, 1982.

64. West J. B. *Respiratory Physiology — the Essentials.* 4th Ed., Williams and Wilkins, Baltimore, 1990.

65. Whipp B. and S. Ward. Physiological determinants of pulmonary gas exchange kinetics during exercise. *Med. Sci. Sports Exercise* 22:62–71, 1990.

66. Williams J. H., S. K. Powers and M. Kelly Stewart. Hemoglobin desaturation in highly trained athletes during heavy exercise. *Med. Sci. Sports Exercise* 18(2):168–173, 1986.

67. Yeh M. P., R. M. Gardner, T. D. Adams, F. G. Yanowitz and R. O. Crappo. "Anaerobic threshold": problems of determination and validation. *J. Appl. Physiol.* 55(4):1178–1186, 1983.

Chapter 4

Neuromuscular Function and Adaptation to Exercise

George Salem and Jack E. Turman, Jr.

CONTENTS

0-8493-4593-6/97/$0.00+$.50

I. EXERCISE AND THE NEUROMUSCULAR SYSTEM

This chapter will provide an overview of the structure and function of the nervous and muscular systems. Considering the scope of these two topics, we will pay special attention to components of the neuromuscular system related to movement and exercise and to the adaptations observed in this system after exercise training.

II. STRUCTURE AND FUNCTION OF THE NERVOUS SYSTEM

A. ORGANIZATION OF THE NERVOUS SYSTEM

The vertebrate nervous system is divided into two major divisions, the central nervous system (CNS) and the peripheral nervous systems (PNS). The CNS contains neuronal networks for integration and decision making, and the peripheral nervous system acts as a conduit to transmit information from the periphery (muscles, skin, and viscera) to the CNS or from the CNS to the periphery, to affect muscle contraction.

The human CNS is divided into four areas, the cerebrum, brain stem, cerebellum, and spinal cord. The CNS is well protected by bone; the cerebrum, cerebellum, and brain stem are protected by the skull, while the spinal cord is protected by the canal of the vertebral column. Additionally, the CNS is protected by three connective tissue membranes called meninges — the dura, arachnoid, and pia mater. In addition to the skeletal and connective tissue covering, the CNS is cushioned by cerebrospinal fluid (CSF).

Several components of the CNS play important roles in exercise and movement. Areas of the cerebrum include the cerebral cortex and the basal ganglia. In addition, at the base of the cerebrum, there are diencephalic nuclei which consist of the thalamus, hypothalamus, and subthalamic nuclei. The brain stem is divided (rostral to caudal) into the midbrain, pons, and medulla oblongata. The medulla has a critical role in the integration of neuronal signals related to exercise and contains neurons which directly affect the cardiorespiratory response to exercise. The medulla also contains motor neurons which innervate pharyngeal and laryngeal muscles which are important in the mechanics of breathing. The cerebellum can be divided into three functional areas — the vestibulocerebellum, which has a role in balance and postural responses, the spinocerebellum, which acts in the error detection and correction of ongoing movements, and the cerebrocerebellum, which is involved in the initiation of movement and the storage of motor commands. The spinal cord contains the motor neurons which innervate skeletal muscle. Of special interest here are those neurons which assist in the mechanics of respiration. Phrenic motor neurons originate in the midcervical region of the spinal cord and innervate the diaphragm. The internal and external intercostal muscles receive their innervation from thoracic motor neurons, and abdominal muscles receive innervation from thoracic and lumbar motor neurons.

The PNS consists of a series of spinal and cranial nerves that transmit motor (efferent) signals to muscle and sensory (afferent) signals to the CNS from receptors located in muscle and skin, as well as those in the eye, ear, and nose. The PNS has two divisions, the somatic peripheral system and the autonomic peripheral system. The somatic system transmits sensory input from skin, muscle, and joint receptors to the CNS, as well as motor signals to skeletal muscle. The autonomic system transmits sensory input from receptors located within the viscera and blood vessels, as well as motor signals to smooth and cardiac muscle. The autonomic PNS is further divided anatomically into two divisions, the sympathetic (associated with the thoracic and lumbar regions of the spinal cord) and the parasympathetic (associated with the brain stem and the sacral region of the spinal cord) divisions.

B. NEURONS AND SYNAPSES

Neurons are the individual signaling components of the nervous system and come in a variety of shapes and sizes. Although neurons contain many similarities to other cell types, including intracellular organelles and morphology, the neuron has processes that are uniquely adapted to serve its primary role as a signaling unit. Signaling occurs intracellularly from one region of the neuron to another and intercellularly, from one neuron to another. The components of the neuron which provide for this signaling make them unique in comparison with other cell types.

The axon of a neuron is a thin, cylindrical process that originates from the cell body. Axons can branch profusely and travel a distance of micrometers to meters before ending as terminal boutons forming synaptic contacts. The structure of the axon is formed by its cytoskeleton which consists of microfilaments, microtubules, and neurofilaments. These filaments are polymeric structures made up of repeating units of the protein tubulin. The filaments play an important role in the life of a neuron by transporting proteins intracellularly. Proteins can travel from soma to terminal (anterograde direction) to be used as neurotransmitters or from terminal to cell body (retrograde direction) to be resynthesized for metabolic or neurotransmitter purposes.

Signaling that occurs between neurons arises with the production of action potentials. Action potentials are initiated at the proximal region of the axon, the axon hillock, provided sufficient membrane depolarization occurs in this area. Action potentials are then propagated along either myelinated or unmyelinated axons toward the terminal boutons. In nonmyelinated axons the conduction of the action potential is continuous because of the uniform distribution of voltage-gated sodium channels, voltage-gated potassium channels, and nongated sodium and nongated potassium channels over the plasma membrane. In contrast, saltatory conduction of action potentials is observed in myelinated axons because of the intermittent concentrations of voltage-gated sodium channels existing between myelinated regions.

Dendrites are usually shorter, thicker neuronal processes arising from the soma. Classically, dendrites are considered to be an input site for the neuron; however, it is now accepted that dendrodendritic synapses occur throughout the CNS. Some dendrites have short projections, called dendritic spines, that arise from the shaft of the dendrite; there are also enlarged areas of the dendritic shaft called dendritic swellings. Dendritic spines and swellings serve as sites of synaptic integration.

The synapse is the site of contact between two neurons or between a neuron and muscle. In the CNS, synapses can be chemically or electrically mediated. Chemically mediated synapses have a presynaptic and postsynaptic component and a synaptic cleft separating them. Information transfer in a chemically mediated synapse is unidirectional, flowing from the presynaptic component across the synaptic cleft to the postsynaptic component. The presynaptic components (terminal boutons) contain a high density of mitochondria and presynaptic vesicles. These vesicles contain a neurotransmitter that is released upon depolarization of the plasma membrane of the terminal. Following its release, the neurotransmitter binds to appropriate receptors on the subsynaptic membrane of the postsynaptic component. The subsynaptic membrane is an electron-dense structure situated adjacent to the vesicle-filled presynaptic component. The subsynaptic membrane contains receptors for the neurotransmitters released and proteins that are involved in the transduction of the chemical signal into the electrical signal. The response elicited in the postsynaptic cell is related to the receptors that are utilized in the neurotransmission. The activation of membrane receptors can either facilitate the postsynaptic cell by creating an excitatory postsynaptic potential (EPSP) or inhibit the cell via the production of an inhibitory postsynaptic potential (IPSP). In chemically mediated synapses, there is a variability in the temporal component of the IPSP or EPSP which lasts from milliseconds to hours.

Electrical synapses between neurons occur via low-resistance connections termed gap junctions. Gap junctions are essentially cell-to-cell pores that allow the flow of ions to pass freely from cytoplasm to cytoplasm. Signal transfer in electrical synapses occurs with little attenuation, because there is minimal leakage of current into the extracellular space. Electrical synapses differ from chemical synapses in that they are bidirectional and transfer information with little to no synaptic delay. This type of synaptic connection also provides for the synchronization of a population of neurons which may be important in rhythmical behaviors such as respiration.

C. SOMATIC RECEPTORS AND REFLEXES

Nervous system processing of sensory information begins with the facilitation of a sensory receptor. Sensory receptors are specialized tissues located throughout the body that respond to mechanical (thermal, noxious), chemical, visual, or auditory stimuli. Each sensory receptor has a distinct receptive field and functions by transforming the stimulus energy into electrical energy which is used by all neurons in the nervous system. The sensory receptor is a component of the primary sensory neuron — the first neuron utilized in the transmission of sensory information. Primary sensory neurons converge on secondary sensory neurons located in the CNS. Secondary sensory neurons then relay their information on to higher-order neurons located in subcortical relay nuclei. Neurons in these nuclei have a large receptive field in comparison with primary sensory neurons because they receive indirect information from a variety of sensory receptors. An essential relay nuclei utilized in sensory transmission is the thalamus, a bilateral structure that exists rostral to the midbrain. All sensory pathways (except olfaction) make synaptic connections with thalamic neurons. Thalamic neurons, in turn, make synaptic connections in primary sensory regions of the cerebral cortex. Neurons in the primary sensory regions and association areas of the cerebral cortex are critical for the perception of sensory information.

The intensity and duration of a stimulus are represented by the number of action potentials, or neuronal code, observed in the primary sensory neuron following the introduction of the stimulus. In regard to intensity, there is a direct relationship among the strength of the stimulus, the number of activated receptors, and the number of resultant action potentials. Coding of stimulus duration is more variable between receptors. Sensory receptors display an ability to adapt to constant stimulation; however, the response can be either slow or rapid. Pacian corpuscles, located in subcutaneous tissue, are rapidly adapting mechanoreceptors that will respond at the onset and termination of the stimulus. In contrast, a Merkel receptor, located in the skin, is an example of a slowly adapting mechanoreceptor that will continue to discharge throughout the duration of the stimulation. The adaptation displayed by sensory receptors is dependent upon the non-neural tissue properties of the receptor and on the membrane excitability of the sensory neuron.

There is a wide array of sensory receptors which are compartmentalized into exteroceptors, interoceptors, and somatic receptors. Exteroceptors relay information to the CNS about external events, including vision, audition, smell (olfaction), touch, and taste; these will not be discussed in this review. Interoceptors provide input about the internal state of the viscera and blood vessels, and these will be discussed in the section on the autonomic nervous system (ANS). Somatic receptors convey information about pain, proprioception, touch, and thermal sense. Information about pain, touch and thermal sense will not be discussed in this review; however, proprioceptive receptors are discussed below.

All primary sensory neurons relaying proprioceptive information from the body have their cell bodies in the dorsal root ganglion which is a part of the dorsal root carrying afferent information into the spinal cord. There are two primary mechanoreceptors that are sensitive to limb movement, joint capsule afferents and muscle spindles. Joint capsule afferents are sensitive to extremes of joint angles and play a role primarily during limb movement and have little role when the limb is at rest. The critical sensory receptor for proprioception is the muscle spindle. The muscle spindle is located in parallel with muscle fibers. The spindle is capable of displaying a static and dynamic response and is sensitive to minute changes in muscle length. The muscle spindle is capable of encoding for both static and dynamic responses because of its unique morphology (Figures 1A and B). The spindle is made up of *intrafusal* fibers called the nuclear bag, which are further broken down into static and dynamic bag fibers, and nuclear chain fibers. The nuclear chain fibers have a high viscosity and code for static conditions, and the bag fibers are less viscous and thereby are more sensitive to small changes in length. The decreased viscosity of the dynamic bag fibers allows them to code for the velocity of length change as well. The muscle spindle receives afferent innervation by group Ia and II fibers. Group Ia afferents wrap around the central portion of all intrafusal fibers while the group II fibers wrap around the central portion of nuclear chain and static bag fibers. The stretch of a muscle spindle is the appropriate stimulus for activation of a muscle spindle; the stretch activates stretch-sensitive channels that depolarize the receptor membrane and result in action potential production. When the stretch is released, afferent firing decreases.

The spindle is provided efferent innervation by gamma motor neurons. The endings of gamma motor neurons are located at polar ends of the spindle where contractile proteins exist. Activation of gamma motor neurons results in a stretch of the central portion of the spindle, thereby activating spindle afferents. This efferent innervation is also responsible for biasing the muscle spindle during shortening contractions so muscle length can be perceived by the CNS. The recruitment of alpha motor neurons during active contractions is accompanied by the recruitment of gamma motor neurons located in the motor neuronal pool. This coactivation of alpha and gamma motor neurons allows the spindle to respond to length and velocity changes and thereby provide sensory feedback to the CNS about such changes. This coactivation and sensory feedback system allows for postural control of both limb and axial musculature and for fluid, controlled movements.

Another important kinesthetic receptor is the Golgi tendon organ (GTO). This receptor is sensitive to the force production of muscle. The GTO is located in the musculotendinous junction, is in series with its muscle fibers, and receives afferent innervation by group Ib fibers. There is a direct relationship between the code of a Ib fiber and the force production of a muscle.

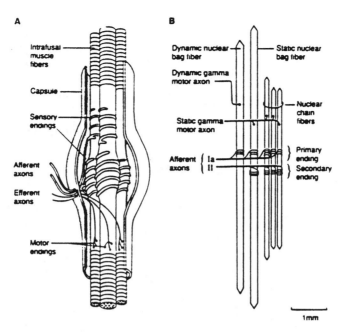

Figure 1 A, Basic morphology of a muscle spindle indicating regions of afferent and efferent innervation and region of intrafusal muscle fibers. B, Schematic illustrating the nuclear bag and chain fibers and the afferent and efferent innervation pattern of muscle spindle components. (From Kandel, E. R., Schwartz, J. H., Jessell, T. M., *Principles of Neural Science*, 3rd ed., Elsevier, New York, 1991. With permission.)

Both the muscle spindle and the GTO play roles in spinal reflexes. Reflexes are rapid, involuntary movements or responses of the nervous system that are under little to no voluntary control. They involve the introduction of a sensory stimulus and a motor response; the size of the response is directly related to the size of the sensory stimulus. Spinal reflexes are those that have the motor circuitry necessary to elicit the response located in the spinal cord. The simplest of spinal reflexes is the stretch reflex. This is a monosynaptic reflex that is elicited with the stretch of a muscle. The stretch activates the muscle spindle which triggers an action potential in the Ia fiber. The Ia fiber monosynaptically excites homonymous alpha motor neurons in the spinal cord and also makes synaptic contact with Ia inhibitory interneurons — which inhibit the antagonistic motor neuronal pool.

The function of the GTO-mediated reflex is to prevent excessive development of muscle tension. The function is met by a negative feedback circuit. The Ib afferents make synaptic contact with Ib inhibitory interneurons in the spinal cord. These interneurons inhibit alpha motor neurons innervating the homonymous muscle. Muscle force regulation helps prevent microruptures at the musculotendinous junction. The Ib inhibition is arranged so that it is most powerful on large motor neurons that innervate fast glycolytic fibers (large tension-producing fibers).

D. AUTONOMIC NERVOUS SYSTEM

Whereas the somatic PNS provides motor and sensory innervation to skeletal muscle, the ANS provides motor and sensory innervation to smooth and cardiac muscle. The ANS has two divisions, sympathetic and parasympathetic. Both divisions innervate the same organs, usually with competing results (Figure 2, Table 1). One of the distinctions between the somatic PNS and the ANS is the efferent innervation provided by both. Motor innervation of skeletal muscle requires a group of motor neurons; these cells are located in the ventral horn of the spinal cord, and their terminals end on groups of muscle fibers. For the ANS, however, motor innervation of smooth or cardiac muscle requires two neurons, pre- and postganglionic neurons (Figure 3). Preganglionic neurons have large diameter, myelinated axons and use acetylcholine (ACh) as a neurotransmitter. The second neuron is called the postganglionic neuron, whose axons are generally unmyelinated and have small diameters. Postganglionic neurons in the sympathetic division use norepinephrine as a neurotransmitter, and postganglionic neurons in the parasympathetic division use ACh as a neurotransmitter.

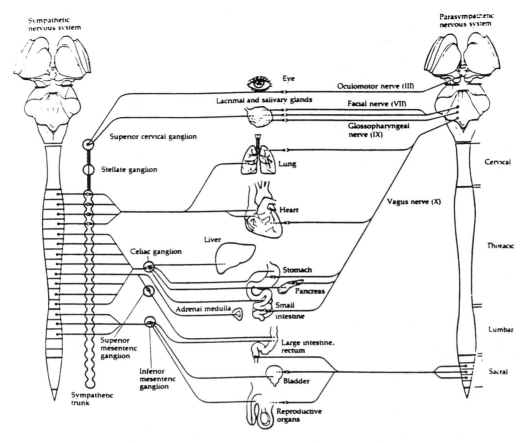

Figure 2 Schematic illustrating the innervation of visceral organs by the sympathetic and parasympathetic divisions of the ANS. The sympathetic system is illustrated on the left and the parasympathetic system is illustrated on the right half of the diagram. (From, Martin, J. H., *Neuroanatomy, Text and Atlas*, Elsevier, New York, 1989. With permission.)

1. Sympathetic Division

We will first provide a detailed review of the sympathetic system, focusing primarily on sympathetic ganglia associated with the thoracic vertebrae, since they are involved in responses to exercise. Sympathetic preganglionic neurons are located in the intermediolateral nuclei of the spinal cord gray matter extending from T1 to L2. Postganglionic cells are located in either the sympathetic ganglion, located adjacent to the lateral aspect of the vertebral column, or are found in the prevertebral ganglion. Sympathetic ganglia are connected by vertically connecting rami which form a single line called the sympathetic chain. A sympathetic chain exists on both sides of the vertebral column. There are two sympathetic ganglia associated with each vertebral body except in the cervical region. The sympathetic ganglia for the eight cervical segments are "fused" together to form three cervical ganglia, called the superior, middle, and inferior (or stellate) cervical ganglia. Sympathetic ganglia are also connected to each spinal nerve by two rami — the white ramus and gray ramus. These rami play a role in the innervation of smooth or cardiac muscle.

The sympathetic PNS also includes prevertebral ganglia. These ganglia are located anterior to the vertebral bodies and adjacent to the abdominal aorta. Three pairs of prevertebral ganglia pertinent to this review are named after the branches of the abdominal aorta in a rostral-to-caudal fashion: celiac, superior mesenteric, inferior mesenteric. The celiac ganglia are located anterior to the L1 vertebral body and surround the celiac artery. The greater, lesser, and lumbar splanchnic nerves connect regions of the sympathetic chain with the celiac, superior mesenteric, and inferior mesenteric ganglia, respectively. The basic function of these prevertebral ganglia is to provide sympathetic motor innervation for the organs of the abdominal cavity. The postganglionic axons from the celiac ganglia are targeted for the

Table 1 The Resultant Effects of Either Sympathetic or Parasympathetic Stimulation on Organ Function

Responses of Selected Effector Organs to Autonomic Innervation		
Effector Organ	**Sympathetic Stimulation**	**Parasympathetic Stimulation**
Heart	Increased heart rate (β_1)[a]	Decreased heart rate
	More contractile force (β_1)	Reduced contractile force
	More output volume (β_1)	Reduced output volume
Coronary Arteries		
Direct effect (innervation)	Superfacial constriction (α)	Slight dilation
	Deep vessel dilation (β_2)	
Indirect effect (metabolic)	Generalized vasodilation	Generalized constriction
Systemic Blood Vessels		
Skeletal muscle	Mostly vasodilation (β_2)	No detectable response
Integument	Vasoconstriction (α)	Dilation (face blushing)
Visceral organs	Vasoconstriction (α)	Vasodilation
Nasal mucosa	Vasoconstriction (α)	Vasodilation
Eye		
Iris	Dilation (mydriasis) (α_1)	Constriction (miosis)
Ciliary muscle	Relaxation (far vision) (β)	Contraction (near vision)
Tarsal muscles	Contraction (α)	—
Lacrimal gland	Vasoconstriction (α)	Secretion of tears and vasodilation
Integument		
Erector pili mm.	Contraction (α)	—
Apocrine glands	Secretion (α)	—
Sweat glands	Palms of hands (α), rest of body (Mr-AChR)[b]	—
Respiratory System		
Bronchioles	Dilation (β_2)	Constriction
Bronchial glands	Decreased secretion (β_1)	Increased secretion
	Increased secretion (β_2)	
Salivary Glands	Mucus secretion (α)	Serous secretion
	Vasoconstriction (α)	Vasodilation
Gastrointestinal Tract		
Peristalsis	Inhibition (α_1)	Stimulation
Sphincters	Contraction (α)	Relaxation
Blood flow	Vasoconstriction (α)	Vasodilation
Intrinsic glands	—	Increased secretion
Liver	Glycogenolysis and gluconeogenesis	Glycogenesis
Pancreas		
Acinar cells	Decreased secretion (α)	Increased secretion
Islet (β) cells	Decreased secretion (α_2)	—
	Increased secretion (β_2)	—
Urinary Bladder		
Detrusor muscle	—	Contraction
Sphinctor muscle	Contraction (α)	Relaxation
Reproductive Organs		
Male	Smooth muscle component of ejaculation (α)	Erection of penis
		Accessory gland secretion
Female	Smooth muscle component of orgasm; cervical dilation	Engorgement of clitoris and bulbs of vestibule
		Glandular secretion

[a] Adrenergic receptor type is indicated in parentheses.
[b] Most sweat gland innervation is cholinergic with muscarinic receptors (see text).

Source: From Burt, A. B., *Textbook of Neuroanatomy,* W.B. Saunders, Philadelphia, 1993. With permission.

liver, stomach, small intestine, and kidney. Postganglionic fibers from the superior mesenteric ganglia are targeted primarily for the large intestine, while postganglionic fibers from the inferior mesenteric ganglia are targeted for the colon, bladder, and uterus.

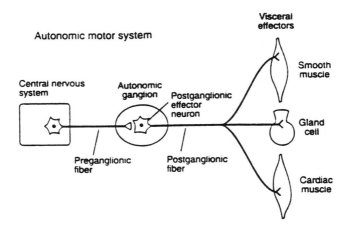

Figure 3 This illustrates the two-neuron circuit that is utilized by the ANS to control smooth muscle, cardiac, or gland function. (From Kandel, E. R., Schwartz, J. H., Jessell, T. M., *Principles of Neural Science*, 3rd ed., Elsevier, New York, 1991. With permission.)

The efferent innervation of smooth or cardiac muscle begins with the myelinated axon of the preganglionic neuron traveling through the ventral root into the spinal nerve and then exiting the spinal nerve to join the white ramus. From the white ramus, the preganglionic axon enters the sympathetic ganglion. Once in the sympathetic ganglion, the preganglionic axon follows one of three routes to provide motor innervation of smooth or cardiac muscle; the axon (1) synapses with a postganglionic neuron in the ganglion (the postganglionic unmyelinated axon then travels via the gray ramus to join the spinal nerve toward the target organ), (2) travels through the ganglion into a vertical ramus to synapse with a postganglionic neuron in a more rostral or caudal sympathetic ganglion (this postganglionic axon will join the spinal nerve at that respective segment), or (3) travels through the ganglion, enters a peripheral nerve, and then synapses with a postganglionic neuron in one of the prevertebral ganglion (from here the postganglionic axon will join a peripheral nerve to innervate the target organ).

The sympathetic PNS also provides sensory innervation of the internal organs. Receptors of the autonomic system are called interoceptors. Interoceptors are located within blood vessels, the heart, and abdominal organs. These receptors are responsible for sensing changes in blood pressure, distension of the bladder, distension of the stomach, and other important sensations from internal organs. The receptor is innervated by an axon of a visceral afferent, and the cell body of this afferent is located in the dorsal root ganglion. The axon of the visceral afferent enters the sympathetic ganglion (via a peripheral nerve); the axon travels through the ganglion (there is no synapse) and exits via the white ramus. Once in the white ramus, the axon enters the spinal nerve and then enters the dorsal root. The axon of the visceral afferent terminates and synapses with an interneuron in the dorsal horn of the spinal cord.

Activation of the sympathetic motor circuit prepares the body for flight or fight. Stimulation of the sympathetic system results in a higher heart rate, a dilation of bronchioles to increase air flow, an increased rate of respiration, an inhibition of smooth muscle contraction to slow or stop digestion, an inhibition of urination, a simultaneous vasodilation to increase the blood flow to heart and skeletal muscle, and vasoconstriction to reduce blood flow to the gut and skin.

2. Parasympathetic Nervous System

The parasympathetic division of the ANS has its preganglionic components located in the brain stem and sacral regions of the spinal cord. This review will concentrate on the brain stem components of the parasympathetic system because of its relation to cardiorespiratory control. Parasympathetic postganglionic cells are located in peripheral ganglia or the target organ. Stimulation of parasympathetic activity stabilizes or regulates autonomic activity by lowering heart rate, decreasing air flow, lowering the rate of respiration, facilitating smooth muscle contraction for digestion, facilitating urination, simultaneously vasoconstricting heart and skeletal muscle vessels, and vasodilating visceral and skin vessels.

Four cranial nerves provide parasympathetic innervation, they are the oculomotor (CN III), facial (CN VII), glossopharyngeal (CN IX), and vagus (CN X) nerves. This review will concentrate on vagus nerve activity because it is responsible for approximately 75% of all parasympathetic activity. Its parasympathetic components innervate the smooth muscles and glands of the pharynx, larynx, and thoracic and abdominal viscera. The parasympathetic component that innervates the heart arises from the nucleus ambiguus in the medulla, and innervation of the bronchial tree and abdominal viscera arises from the dorsal nucleus of the vagus nerve in the medulla. The postganglionic neurons are found in the target organs and not in a peripheral ganglion. The vagus nerve also carries visceral sensory information. Vagal sensory neurons innervate interoceptors, including pressure receptors (to monitor blood pressure), chemoceptors of the aortic artery (to monitory blood gases), and stretch receptors of the lungs (to monitor lung inflation). Signals from these interoceptors help regulate blood pressure, heart rate, and respiration.

3. Autonomic Nervous System and the Hypothalamus

The primary function of the hypothalamus is to regulate homeostasis by influencing both the autonomic and endocrine systems. Its complex role in regulating the output of the pituitary gland is beyond the scope of this review, but its role in regulating the ANS is critical in the study of exercise. The hypothalamus serves as the "master controller" of the ANS by coordinating signals to the parasympathetic and sympathetic systems. For example, stimulation of the anterior hypothalamus excites the parasympathetic system, causing a decrease in heart rate and blood pressure, while stimulation of the posterior hypothalamus excites the sympathetic system, causing an increase in heart rate and blood pressure. Regulation of body temperature is another example of this dual control. Special hypothalamic cells act as "thermostat sensors" monitoring the temperature of the blood flowing through the capillaries. When temperature increases, thermosensitive cells in the anterior hypothalamus respond — facilitating heat-loss mechanisms such as sweating and cutaneous vasodilation. When blood temperature decreases, thermosensitive cells in the posterior hypothalamus respond — facilitating heat-gain mechanisms such as cutaneous vasoconstriction and shivering.

Hypothalamic control of autonomic responses utilizes descending fiber tracts originating in hypothalalmic nuclei. Control of heart rate depends upon neurons that originate in the hypothalamus and terminate on brain stem neurons involved in regulating the cardiorespiratory system. These brain stem neurons can form either inhibitory or excitatory synaptic connections with neurons in the nucleus ambiguus which give rise to the vagus nerve, while other brain stem neurons in this region form inhibitory or excitatory connections with preganglionic neurons of the sympathetic system. Thus, the hypothalamus regulates heart rate by controlling the output of preganglionic neurons via brain stem neurons. The location and nature of these cells will be discussed later.

E. MOTOR SYSTEMS AND MOTOR CONTROL

There are three hierarchical levels of motor control: the spinal cord, motor pathways originating from the brain stem, and motor areas of the cerebral cortex. These three areas interact in both hierarchical and parallel fashions (Figure 4). The cerebral cortex has input over brain stem nuclei giving rise to motor pathways. Both the cortex and brain stem influence interneuronal and motoneuronal networks of the spinal cord, which are responsible for reflexes utilized in voluntary movements. The parallel nature of these systems results in an overlap of motor information in the CNS — which becomes critical following a lesion to one of these areas.

The spinal cord has been discussed in the context of reflexes and the ANS; however, it is important to emphasize that the spinal cord contains motor neurons which have direct synaptic contact with skeletal muscle. Further, the spinal cord houses important interneuronal networks involved in the execution of reflexes. These interneuronal networks are also utilized in the production of rhythmical movements such as walking and respiration. They receive input from primary sensory neurons and from descending systems originating in the cerebral cortex or brain stem. Neurons comprising these networks make synaptic contact with alpha motor neurons to formulate alternating, rhythmical movements. This is executed by the facilitation of one pool of motor neurons with the simultaneous inhibition of its antagonists.

There are four major groups of motor tracts that originate in the brain stem and terminate on interneurons or motor neurons of the spinal cord: the vestibulospinal tracts (medial and lateral), the reticulospinal tracts (medial and lateral), the tectospinal tract, and the rubrospinal tract. The vestibulospinal tracts originate from vestibular nuclei located at the pontomedullary junction. Neurons which give rise to this tract receive input from the vestibular apparatus located in the inner ear and the vestibulocerebellar system. Functionally, this tract helps in the reflex control of balance and posture. The reticulospinal tracts originate from the reticular formation making up the central core of the brain stem. Neurons comprising these tracts form excitatory and inhibitory connections with spinal motor

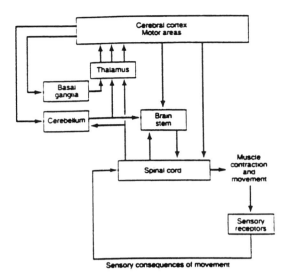

Figure 4 The three levels of motor control (cerebral cortex, brain stem and spinal cord) are illustrated in relation to the basal ganglia, cerebellum, and sensory systems which act to influence the motor control and planning. (From Kandel, E. R., Schwartz, J. H., Jessell, T. M., *Principles of Neural Science*, 3rd ed., Elsevier, New York, 1991. With permission.)

neurons and interneurons. The tracts function in the control of posture and in the suppression of spinal reflexes during voluntary movement. The tectospinal tract originates in the superior colliculus of the midbrain and connects with motor neurons and interneurons in the cervical region of the spinal cord. This tract helps coordinate head and eye movements. The rubrospinal tract originates from the red nucleus in the midbrain and assists in the control of distal musculature operating in fine movements.

Motor regions of the cerebral cortex are responsible for the planning and execution of complex movements and fine motor control. The primary motor cortex, located in the precentral gyrus of the frontal lobe, gives rise to the corticospinal (cortex–spinal cord connections) and corticobulbar (cortex–brain stem connections) tracts. The corticospinal tract exerts control over the spinal motor neurons, and the corticobulbar tracts exert control over the cranial nerve motor and sensory nuclei (i.e., facial nucleus, trigeminal nuclei, and hypoglossal nucleus). The corticospinal tract is the largest descending fiber tract and exerts contralateral control. Neurons in the premotor cortex and in the somatosensory cortex also contribute to the corticospinal tract. Other important regions of the cortex that process motor information include the premotor cortex, the supplementary motor area, and the prefrontal association cortex. These regions do not play a role in the execution of the motor command but are critical in the planning and storage of complex motor plans.

These three levels of motor control receive a variety of important inputs that modify their neuronal output. Sensory input is important at each level, providing a means of feedback about what is occurring and important clues about the environment. Sensory feedback is not only utilized in reflexes but is also used to modify the output of interneuronal networks responsible for rhythmical movements. Sensory feedback is also used in the planning of complex motor acts. In addition to sensory feedback, the cerebellum and the basal ganglia have important roles influencing the output of motor systems.

The cerebellum is involved in three arenas of motor control. It acts as a comparator to assist in the error detection/correction of ongoing movements. It does this by receiving sensory feedback from the spinal cord via the spinocerebellar tracts and by receiving a copy of the original motor plan from the motor cortex. The cerebellum sends output to the red nucleus of the midbrain to affect the ongoing movement via the rubrospinal tract. The cerebellum also affects control of posture and balance by receiving input from the vestibular apparatus in the inner ear and from the vestibular nuclei located at the pontomedullary junction. The cerebellum then processes this information and relays its output to the vestibular nuclei (primarily the lateral vestibular nuclei) which give rise to the lateral vestibulospinal tract. Finally, the cerebellum helps initiate movement by influencing the premotor and motor areas of the cerebral cortex.

The basal ganglia are a subcortical collection of five nuclei consisting of the caudate, putamen, globus pallidus, substantia nigra, and subthalamic nucleus. Unlike the cerebellum, the basal ganglia do not have direct or indirect connections with the spinal cord and have few connections with brain stem nuclei involved in motor control. Instead, output from the basal ganglia is directed to the ventral anterior or ventral lateral regions of the thalamus. Here, thalamocortical tracts directed to the prefrontal, premotor, or motor cortices relay the motor information. Basal ganglia input comes from regions throughout the entire cerebral cortex and from the intralaminar nuclei of the thalamus. The input from the cortex is topographically organized to effectively execute specific behavioral functions, with the putamen receiving most of the motor information. Efferent and afferent connections of the basal ganglia support the contention that the basal ganglia assist in the planning of complex motor strategies and are tied to the cognitive aspects of motor control. This is in contrast to the cerebellum which plays a role in the execution of movement as suggested by its direct or indirect input to brain stem nuclei and spinal cord centers related to movement.

F. RESPONSES TO EXERCISE

Exercise results in stressing the many systems which act in concert to maintain homeostasis. The CNS has the role of regulating and coordinating the response of these systems to provide optimal performance during exercise. The nervous system receives feedback, both in the form of neural codes and blood-borne information regarding the status of the organism. After integrating this sensory information, the CNS provides regulatory output via the sympathetic and parasympathetic systems and by controlling the alpha and gamma motor neuron excitability. Examining the scope of mechanisms utilized by the nervous system to regulate all systems challenged by an exercise bout is beyond the scope of this chapter; therefore, we will briefly focus on nervous system regulation of the cardiorespiratory system during exercise.

The response of the cardiorespiratory system is so rapid that it is thought to be the result of purely neural control mechanisms.[1] The first phase of the cardiorespiratory system response to exercise occurs within 15 s after the initiation of an exercise bout. During the second and third phase of the response, both neural and humoral systems act in concert to exert control on the cardiorespiratory system. The control networks utilized by the nervous system in phase 1 will be the focus of this section. The two critical networks operating in phase 1 are mechanical feedback reflexes that originate in the active muscle and a feedforward motor plan that is generated by the CNS.[1] During phases 2 and 3, feedback mechanisms arising from neuronal afferents in the lungs, heart, carotid bodies, muscle chemoreceptors, arterial baroreceptors, and thermoreceptors act directly on the CNS — influencing its output.

The organization of sensory afferent neurons arising in the muscle provides rapid feedback to the CNS regarding changes in the muscle environment. In addition to the proprioceptive fibers discussed above, there exists a group of thin, free nerve endings that are responsive to changes in muscle activity during an exercise bout. These fibers are called group III and IV fibers. They are small in diameter and have slower conduction velocities than group I and II fibers. Group III fibers are associated with collagen structures in the muscle, and group IV fibers are associated with blood and lymphatic vessels.[2] Specific stimuli for group III and IV fibers include muscle contraction, stretch, and/or changes in potassium, bradykinins, and arachidonic acid concentrations.[3] Following stimulation of these fibers, investigators have observed increases in blood pressure, heart rate, and contractility, and a redistribution of blood flow toward the working muscle and selected areas of the brain.[4-7]

Anatomically, group III and IV fibers are well connected with areas of the nervous system that are related to exercise control. These fibers have synaptic connections with neurons in the spinal cord[8] which in turn form synaptic connections with neurons in the cardiorespiratory control centers of the brain stem, including the lateral reticular nucleus[9] and cells of the lateral tegmental field.[10] Group III and IV fibers also form connections with neurons in the nucleus tractus solitarius[8] of the medulla. This connection with the nucleus tractus solitarius is critical as neurons located there form synapses with neurons in other regions of the CNS responsible for regulating cardiovascular responses.

Much of the evidence for the CNS control over an exercise response in humans is circumstantial.[1] However, two regions of the CNS were implicated as locations of central command. The subthalamic nucleus appears to play a role in increasing blood pressure, heart rate, and ventilation.[11] Likewise, stimulation of a neuronal population adjacent to the subthalamic nucleus, called the fields of Florel, can result in the increase of blood pressure, heart rate, phrenic nerve activity, and bronchodilator response.[12-14] The presence of these two centers implies that a redundancy is built into the CNS for the control of cardiorespiratory responses, in case of injury to one of these neuronal centers. Inputs to these regions include the motor regions of the cerebral cortex[11] utilized in voluntary movements, and from regions including and surrounding the hypothalamus.[15]

In summary, it appears that there is a central control mechanism originating in the subthalamic region of the brain and a peripheral feedback mechanism originating in group III and IV muscle afferents that together operate to cause the rapid response of the nervous system to exercise. However, Waldrop et al.[16] and Rybicki et al.[14] demonstrated that if both of these systems were stimulated the result was not the algebraic sum of the two, but that some neuronal integration had taken place. The ventrolateral region of the medulla is considered to be the region where the integration takes place. Neurons in this region of the brain stem have synaptic connections with sympathetic preganglionic neurons in the spinal cord[17] and inhibitory synaptic connections with nucleus ambiguus neurons that result in the withdrawal of vagal tone of the heart.[18-19] This area of the medulla also contains the respiratory centers that have connections with phrenic motor neurons and spinal interneuronal networks that help regulate the mechanics of respiration.[20] Because of its afferent and efferent connections, this region of the medulla is also a critical region responsible for executing a central command over the cardiorespiratory system during exercise, and its concerted effort with neurons in the subthalamic region and fields of Florel initiate appropriate systemic responses.

III. STRUCTURE AND FUNCTION OF THE MUSCULAR SYSTEM

Perhaps the most intriguing tissue in the human body, skeletal muscle has the ability to actively develop tension and physically shorten. Muscles are composed of numerous cells containing intricately arranged contractile proteins, which when stimulated are able to produce tension by repetitively altering their configuration in the presence of ATP and Ca^{++}. Activated muscles are able to affect human movement by attaching to the skeleton of the body and controlling skeletal-arthrodial action.

A. GROSS STRUCTURE OF SKELETAL MUSCLE

The functional unit of skeletal muscle is the multinucleated myofiber or muscle cell. Muscle cells are cylindrical structures which vary in thickness from 10 to 100 µm and in length from a few centimeters to more than 30 cm.[21] Each muscle fiber is surrounded by a plasma membrane — the sarcolemma. In addition to separating the cytoplasm (sarcoplasm) of the cell from the surrounding external fluids, the sarcolemma is capable of carrying an electrical charge that is required for muscular contraction. Each muscle cell is surrounded by a fine sheath of areolar connective tissue — the endomysium. Groups of muscle fibers are bundled into fascicles and bound by another connective tissue sheath — the perimysium. Fascicles are further bound by a dense connective tissue called the epimysium, which surrounds the entire muscle (Figure 5A, B, and C).

B. NEUROMUSCULAR JUNCTION

The neuromuscular junction is the bridge between the nervous and musculoskeletal systems. Here, axonal endings of the motor neuron terminate at approximately the middle of each muscle fiber. Each muscle fiber has only one neuromuscular junction and, hence, can be affected by only one motor neuron. The axonal ending and muscle fiber sarcolemma are separated by a small fluid-filled space, the synaptic cleft. When a nerve impulse reaches the axonal terminal ending, synaptic vesicles, containing the neurotransmitter ACh, fuse with the axonal membrane. ACh is released into the synaptic cleft and binds to ACh receptors located in the highly invaginated motor end plate on the sarcolemma — potentially depolarizing the sarcolemma.

C. ULTRASTRUCTURE OF SKELETAL MUSCLE

The ultrastructure of skeletal muscle has been exhaustively studied by light and electron microscopy, and by biochemical and histochemical analyses.[22-24] Each muscle fiber contains a large number of rodlike structures called myofibrils, which are arranged in parallel and span the entire length of the muscle cell (Figure 5D). When viewed under a light microscope, a repeating pattern of light and dark bands is visible along the length of each myofibril. These striations are due to the optical characteristics of the myofibril contractile proteins — actin and myosin. These small protein strands are arranged in a regular overlapping pattern, permitting the attachment of actin and myosin during the process of contraction.

The dark bands along the myofibril are formed by the thick myosin filaments and the thin actin filaments. They are called A bands because they are anisotropic (i.e., the bands are not of uniform

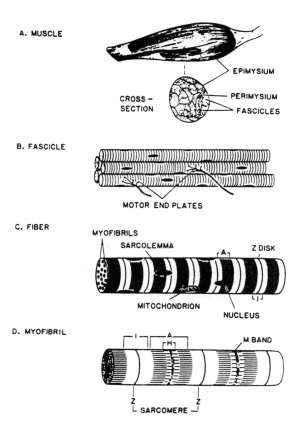

A. MUSCLE

EPIMYSIUM

CROSS-SECTION

PERIMYSIUM

FASCICLES

B. FASCICLE

MOTOR END PLATES

C. FIBER

MYOFIBRILS

SARCOLEMMA

Z DISK

A

MITOCHONDRION

NUCLEUS

D. MYOFIBRIL

I

A

H

M BAND

Z   Z

SARCOMERE

Figure 5   Gross and fine structure of skeletal muscle. (From Jensen, D., *The Principles of Physiology*, 2nd ed., Appleton-Century-Crofts, New York, 1980. With permission.)

darkness). Within the A band is the lighter H zone, where only myosin filaments can be identified. Contrastingly, the isotropic or I band is composed entirely of actin filaments and is the lightest band of the myofibril (Figure 6).

Myosin and actin filaments are anchored by dense proteins which appear as lines along the myofibril. The actin filaments are anchored to the Z line which divides the myofibril into functional units called sarcomeres. Myosin filaments are anchored to M lines which can be found at the center of each sarcomere (Figure 6).

When viewed in cross section, each muscle fiber reveals a three-dimensional pattern of thin and thick filaments. Six actin filaments form a hexagonal array about each myosin filament, allowing each actin filament to be bridged by three separate myosin filaments (Figure 7). Note in Figure 7 that cross sections along the length of a sarcomere reveal different thick and thin filament patterns. For example, a cross-sectional cut through the I band shows only the actin filaments, while a cross-sectional cut through the dark region of the A zone shows both actin and myosin filaments.

When treated with trypsin, myosin molecules of the thick filament yield both a heavy subunit, heavy meromyosin (HMM), and a light subunit, light meromyosin (LMM) (Figure 8). The LMM subunit is thought to be structural in function — anchoring to the M line. The HMM subunit consists of both a globular subfragment (S_1) and a linear subfragment (S_2). The S_2 fragment appears to bind S_1 to LMM, whereas the S_1 fragment appears to be the site of cross-bridge attachment and ATPase activity.[24]

D. MUSCULAR CONTRACTION AND THE SLIDING FILAMENT THEORY

During muscular contraction, actin filaments are "pulled" past the myosin filaments altering the length of the sarcomere and its regions. The Z lines are pulled closer together, and the I band and H zone shorten (Figure 6). This is the basis of the sliding filament theory of contraction which was first proposed by H. E. Huxley and is the most accepted theory of muscular contraction.[25,26]

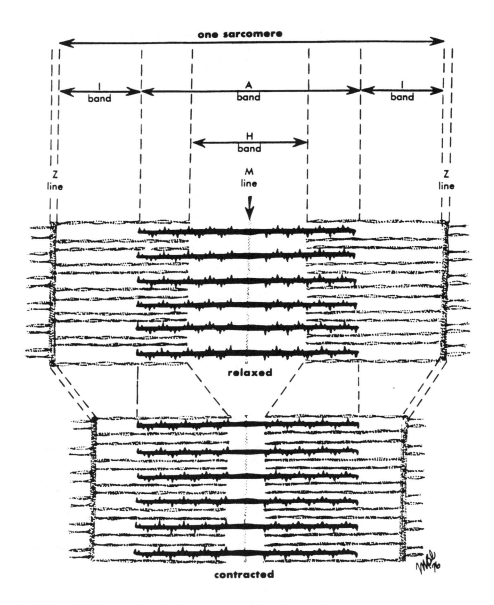

Figure 6 Schematic diagram of a single sarcomere while relaxed and contracted. As the thin actin filaments slide past the thick myosin filaments, the I and H bands shorten, whereas the A band remains a constant length. (From Crouch, J. E., *Functional Human Anatomy,* 4th ed., Lea & Febiger, Philadelphia, 1985. With permission.)

1. Initiation of Muscular Contraction

Muscular contraction is initiated by the release of ACh from the motor neuron at the neuromuscular junction. The binding of ACh with the motor end plate of the muscle causes the depolarization of the sarcolemma and the conduction of an action potential along the membrane. This electrical charge is transmitted to the sarcoplasmic reticulum of the muscle fiber via a system of transverse tubules (T tubules) which run perpendicularly from the surface of the cell into the central areas of the muscle fiber (Figure 9). Propagation of the action potential down the T tubules triggers the release of Ca^{++} from the sarcoplasmic reticulum — a modified endoplasmic reticulum consisting of a network of interconnected tubules surrounding each myofibril.

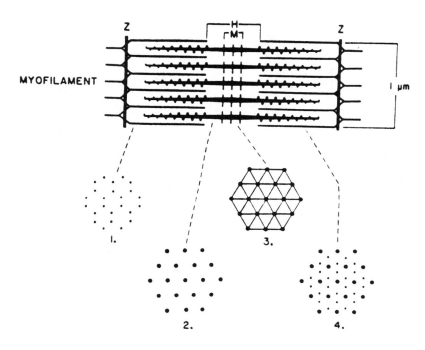

Figure 7 Ultrastructure of skeletal muscle. Transverse cross sections through the different sarcomere zones will reveal different patterns of contractile proteins. Note in 4 that each myosin filament is surrounded by six actin filaments. (From Jensen, D., *The Principles of Physiology,* 2nd ed., Appleton-Century-Crofts, New York, 1980. With permission.)

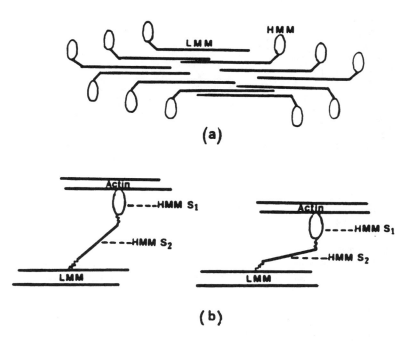

Figure 8 Proposed ultrastructure of myosin. (a) Aggregation of LMM and HMM. (b) HMM subfragments including the globular fragment S_1 and the linear fragment S_2. (From Gowitske, B. and Milner, M., *Scientific Basis of Movement,* 3rd ed., Williams and Wilkens, 1988. With permission.)

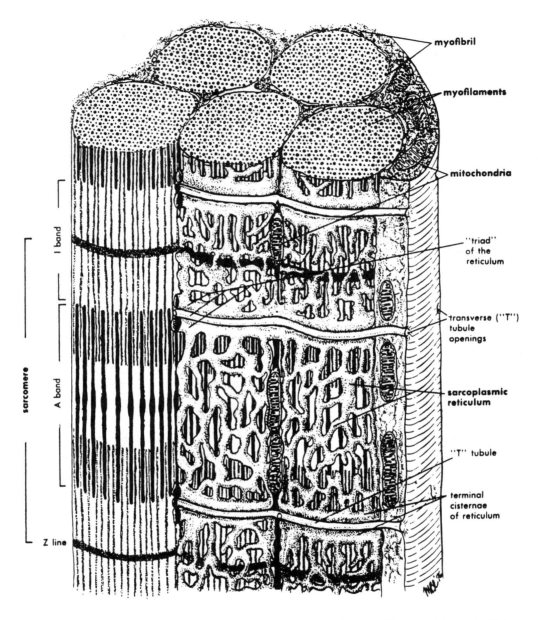

Figure 9 Transverse tubule and sarcoplasmic reticulum systems of mammalian skeletal muscle. Note the relationship of the T tubules to the myofilaments. (From Crouch, J. E., *Functional Human Anatomy,* 4th ed., Lea & Febiger, Philadelphia, 1985. With permission.)

2. Contraction Mechanism

In the absence of Ca++, myosin-binding sites on actin are physically blocked by tropomyosin molecules, and the muscle is relaxed. The release of Ca++ from the sarcoplasmic reticulum, however, starts a cascade of events beginning with the physical movement of the tropomyosin molecule and ending in the development of muscular force.

Released calcium ions bind to the molecule troponin, causing the calcium–troponin complex to change its orientation and physically move tropomyosin away from the myosin-binding site on the actin protein. When the tropomyosin barrier is removed, S_1 components of the thick myosin filaments (myosin heads) bind with actin — a process called cross-bridge attachment. Once attached, the myosin head pivots from

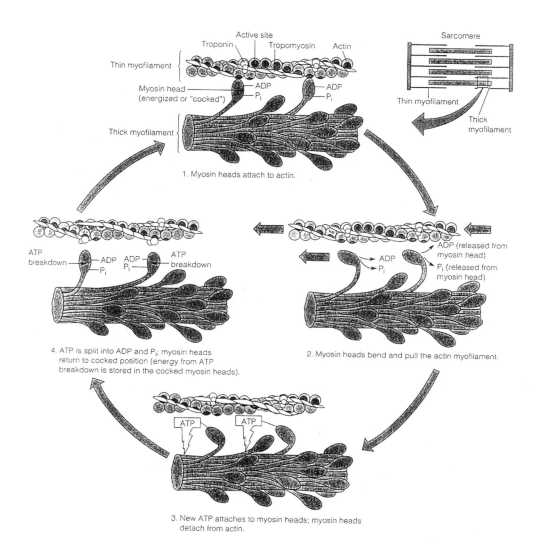

Figure 10 Sequence of events, beginning with cross-bridge attachment, during muscular contraction. Adjacent actin and myosin filaments are used to illustrate the interactions of the myofilaments. (From Stalheim-Smith and Fitch, *Understanding Human Anatomy and Physiology*, West Publishing, Minneapolis/St. Paul, 1993. With permission.)

its high-energy configuration to a low-energy configuration and pulls the actin filament toward the center of the sarcomere. During its reconfiguration, the myosin head releases ADP (low energy, adenosine diphosphate) and inorganic phosphate (Pi). Cross-bridge detachment occurs as a new ATP molecule binds with the myosin head. Finally, the myosin head returns to its "cocked" or high-energy position as ATP is hydrolyzed to ADP and Pi by the enzyme ATPase (Figure 10). The hydrolytic activity of myosin is thought to be influenced by low-molecular-weight polypeptide chains called "light chains." These light chains, which differ between fiber types, may be responsible for the contraction characteristics of fast- and slow-twitch muscle fibers.

This cycle repeats itself until the calcium ions are actively transported back into the sarcoplasmic reticulum — halting the muscular contraction. This series of events, from propagation of the action potential along the sarcolemma to the actual sliding of the thin filaments past the thick filaments, is called excitation-contraction coupling.

E. ORGANIZATION OF MUSCLE
1. Motor Units
Each motor neuron innervates several muscle fibers, and each stimulatory impulse will stimulate all of the muscle fibers the neuron innervates. The motor neuron and all of the muscle fibers it innervates is called a motor unit. Each motor unit has several important characteristics related to the number of muscle fibers within the motor unit, the muscle fiber contraction velocities, and the muscle fiber metabolic properties.

The degree of motor unit control is inversely related to the number of muscle fibers within the motor unit. For example, motor units in muscles involved in fine, discrete motor tasks (e.g., movements of the eye) have a small number of muscle fibers per motor unit. Conversely, muscles involved in gross movements (e.g., movements of the limbs) may contain over 1000 muscle fibers per motor unit. Further, all muscle fibers within a given motor unit have the same contraction and metabolic properties, and although there is a continuum of muscle fiber contraction speeds and metabolic properties, three traditional categories of muscle fiber (motor unit) types have been identified.[27-29]

2. Muscle Fiber Types
Type I slow-oxidative (SO) fibers have relatively slow contraction speeds because of their slow ATPase activity. These fibers are innervated by smaller slower motor neurons which are easily stimulated. They have a high mitochondrial content and a high capacity for aerobic metabolism. These fibers are well vascularized and contain a high content of myoglobin — which increases the rate of oxygen diffusion into the cells. Type I SO fibers are fatigue resistant and therefore are the predominant muscle fiber type found in postural muscles which support the body against the force of gravity. These fibers are also the predominant muscle fibers found in endurance athletes.

Type IIa fast-oxidative-glycolytic (FOG) fibers have relatively fast contraction speeds because of their fast ATPase activity. These fibers are innervated by larger faster motor neurons which are more difficult to stimulate. They have a high mitochondrial content and a high capacity for both aerobic and anaerobic metabolism. These fibers are well vascularized and contain a high content of myoglobin. Type IIa FOG fibers are fatigue resistant (although less so than type I fibers) and are the predominant fibers in middle distance athletes, where both speed and endurance are important attributes.

Type IIb fast-glycolytic (FG) fibers have the fastest contraction speeds because of their fast ATPase activity. These fibers are innervated by the largest motor neurons, which do not depolarize easily. They have a low mitochondrial content, a low capacity for aerobic metabolism, but a high capacity for anaerobic metabolism. Type IIb fibers produce the greatest amount of force, fatigue easily, and are the predominant fibers in the leg muscles of sprint athletes.

F. MUSCLE CONTRACTION CHARACTERISTICS
1. Muscle Twitch
When skeletal muscle fibers are stimulated with a single, brief stimulus, they will quickly contract and then relax. This phenomenon, usually measured *in vitro*, is called a muscle twitch and can be separated into three distinct phases. The first phase is called the latent period. During the latent period, which lasts just a few milliseconds, no force response can be measured. It is during this period that the events of excitation–contraction coupling occur. The next phase is the period of contraction (10 to 100 ms).[30] During this phase, the muscle actively develops tension; however, as we will see, the muscle may shorten, lengthen, or remain the same length. The final phase is termed the period of relaxation. During this phase, tension which was developed in the previous phase gradually returns to zero.

2. Graded Muscle Responses
Fortunately, animals and humans have the ability to "grade" their muscular responses to meet the needs of their tasks. For example, we do not need to use the same amount of force to pick up an egg as we do to pick up a heavy garbage can. Although the same muscles may be used in both tasks (i.e., wrist and finger flexors), the force produced during each task is regulated and monitored by joint and muscle receptors of the nervous system. The nervous system in turn recruits the correct number of motor units, at just the right firing frequency, to achieve our goal (i.e., not break the egg). In general, there are two mechanisms by which muscular force can be graded: (1) by increasing the firing rate of the motor neuron to achieve wave summation and tetanus and (2) by increasing the number of motor units during a contraction — a process called motor unit summation.

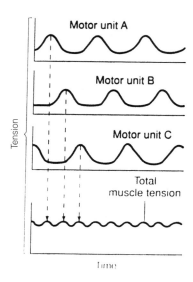

Figure 11 Asynchronous motor unit summation results in a nearly constant tension produced by muscle. (From Spence, A. P. and Mason, E. B. *Human Anatomy and Physiology,* 4th ed., West Publishing, Los Angeles, 1992. With permission.)

3. Wave Summation and Tetanus

In vivo, motor neurons rarely transmit a single stimulatory impulse. Rather, motor neurons transmit volleys of impulses with each impulse followed closely by another. These volleys typically occur before the muscle fiber has had time to relax, resulting in a summation of individual twitches — a process called wave summation. If the volleys occur fast enough, the muscle will be in a state of sustained contraction or tetanus. Wave summation is possible because subsequent contractions occur before the sarcoplasmic reticulum has actively removed Ca^{++} ions from the sarcoplasm. The additional Ca^{++} ions increase the number of cross-bridge attachment sites available for myosin head binding. The result is an increase in the magnitude and duration of the motor unit force.

4. Motor Unit Summation

Muscular force may also increase by increasing the number of motor units recruited during a muscular contraction. As with wave summation, motor units may be summed to increase the force produced by the muscle. Typically, the smallest motor units are recruited first because their neurons are most excitable. When additional force is required, larger motor units become activated and muscle tension increases.

Motor unit recruitment must be staggered or asynchronous in order to achieve a smooth, sustained contraction (Figure 11). As some motor units are activated, others are relaxed. Activated motor units then relax, while the relaxed motor units become active. This asynchronous behavior results in a smooth, sustained contraction of the entire muscle — even during weak contractions involving a limited number of motor units.

5. Types of Contraction

During excitation–contraction coupling, contractile elements (actin and myosin) develop an "internal" muscle tension independent of the external length changes of the muscle. The relationship, however, between this internal tension and the external loading of the muscle will determine whether the muscle shortens, lengthens, or remains the same length. If the external load on the muscle is less than the internal force generated by the contractile elements, the muscle will shorten. This type of contraction is called a concentric contraction. Conversely, if the internal force is less than the external load, the muscle will lengthen. This type of contraction is called an eccentric contraction. Finally, if the internal and external forces are equivalent, the muscle will remain the same length. This is called an isometric contraction. During most activities a combination of concentric, eccentric, and isometric contractions occur. For example, during the squat exercise (or other closed-chain exercises), an eccentric contraction occurs as the weight is lowered toward the ground, the hip and knee flex, and the ankle dorsiflexes. During this downward phase, the hip and knee extensors and ankle plantar flexors are actively lengthening to slow the movement and prevent the body and resistance from crashing to the floor. During the ascension phase of the exercise, a concentric contraction is utilized. The same muscles must now actively shorten to "lift" the resistance from the lower position. Additionally, postural muscles of the vertebral column (abdominals and erector spinea) are recruited isometrically to stabilize the spine and prevent unwanted vertebral flexion and hyperextension. Similar combinations of contractions occur during walking, running, jumping, and even during open-chain isolation exercises.

6. Series Elastic Contributions

During muscular contractions, energy is stored in series elastic components of the musculoskeletal complex. Series elastic components are those connective tissues located between the muscle and the external load (i.e., tendon). When muscle contractile elements are activated, the series elastic components are stretched, much like a spring, and store potential energy. The amount of stretch and potential energy is greatest during eccentric contractions. For example, when an eccentric contraction is followed by a concentric contraction, energy stored in the series elastic components is released, contributing to the force of the concentric contraction. During locomotion, series elastic energy contributions reduce the overall metabolic costs of movement.[31]

7. Length/Tension Relationship

The amount of tension developed by skeletal muscle is related to the length of the muscle immediately preceding the contraction. Each skeletal muscle produces its maximum active tension at a specific "optimal" length. At lengths less than or greater than optimum, muscular contractions result in a decreased active force output. The relationship between active tension and muscle length is related to myofilament overlap, because force production is proportional to the number of cross bridges between actin and myosin proteins (Figure 12). When muscle contractions are initiated at greater than optimum lengths, the amount of overlap between myosin and actin is reduced and active force production decreases. When muscle contractions occur at less than optimum lengths, interference between actin filaments and compression of the myosin filaments against the Z lines of the sarcomere also limits the amount of force produced. Fortunately, sarcomere lengths in relaxed muscle (2.0 μm) are at or close to optimal lengths.[32]

8. Force/Velocity Relationship

During concentric contractions, increased loading decreases the velocity of muscle shortening. For example, the speed with which you can move a barbell during an concentric overhead press will be faster when the load is light, and slower when the load is heavy. If the loading equals the maximum force production of the muscle, the velocity of shortening will be zero, and the contraction will be isometric. If the loading exceeds the maximum force produced by the muscle, the muscle will lengthen. Here, the velocity will be negative and will decrease with increasing load.

G. SKELETAL MUSCLE ADAPTATIONS TO TRAINING

While exercise, in general, can increase muscular size, strength, and endurance, specific activities and exercises effect specific changes in muscle morphology and energy metabolism. Endurance and "aerobic" activities tend to increase the oxidative capacity and resistance to fatigue of muscle fibers, with type IIa fibers being most responsive. Conversely, high-intensity exercise (e.g., resistance training) produces muscular hypertrophy and strength gains, with type IIb fibers being most responsive. The following sections detail the specific muscle property changes that occur with endurance and resistance training.

1. Endurance Training

Mitochondria are the sites of oxidative metabolism in the muscle fiber, and endurance training has been shown to significantly increase mitochondrial content and oxidative enzymes. For example, electron microscopy studies have shown that both the number and size of the mitochondria increase with endurance training.[33-35] Furthermore, muscle homogenate and isolated mitochondrial studies document that endurance training increases the ability of a muscle to oxidize fatty acids, ketones, and pyruvate with a potential twofold increase in the level of aerobic system enzymes.[29,36,37] These adaptations significantly increase the oxidative capacity of the muscle fiber.

The myoglobin content of muscle can increase by as much as 80% as a result of endurance training.[38] Combined with the training-related increases in capillary density,[39] these changes significantly increase

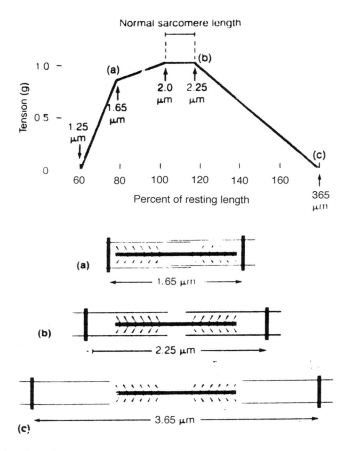

Figure 12 Length/tension relationship in skeletal muscle. Maximum muscular force is produced at sarcomere lengths between 2.0 and 2.25 μm (b). At lengths less than 2.0 μm (a), interference between actin filaments and compression of the myosin filaments against the Z lines of the sarcomere limit force production. At lengths greater than 2.25 μm (c), the amount of overlap between myosin and actin is reduced and active force production decreases. (From Marieb, E. N., *Human Anatomy and Physiology*, 2nd ed., Benjamin/Cummings, Menlo Park, CA, 1992. With permission.)

muscle fiber oxygen content and facilitate mitochondrial diffusion. Eased diffusion is consistent with the increased oxidative capabilities of the muscle cell.

2. Resistance Training

The adaptations that occur in muscle, as a result of resistance training, are variable and influenced by genetic, nutritional, environmental, neurological, and exercise-specific factors. For example, muscle fiber density and composition of resistance-athlete specialists are related to the types of events in which these athletes compete. World-class bodybuilders, who utilize high-volume, moderate-to-high-intensity resistance programs, have a relatively greater number of type I fibers than Olympic and power lifters.[40] It remains to be determined, however, if these differences are training related or genetically predetermined.

Muscle growth in response to resistance training occurs primarily through hypertrophy of individual muscle fibers.[41] Recent animal studies, however, suggest that the number of muscle fibers may also increase (hyperplasia) with resistance training.[42] While these findings have not been repeated in humans, cross-sectional studies indicate that bodybuilders may have an increased number of muscle fibers when compared with Olympic and power lifters.[43]

Resistance training may also affect the metabolic properties of the muscle. For example, resistance training has been shown to increase resting muscle cell ATP, CP (high energy, creatine phosphate), and glycogen stores.[44] Resistance training has also been shown to decrease the mitochondrial volume density in muscle; however, these changes typically reflect increased myofibril volume — not decreases in mitochondrial volume.[45]

Finally, resistance training does not appear to affect muscle contraction velocities, and contraction times in humans remain unchanged even after 4 months of dynamic resistance training, three times per week.[46]

3. Muscle Fiber Type

Fiber type proportions are genetically determined, and certain muscles, due to genetic factors, have either more type I (slow-twitch) fibers, type II (fast-twitch) fibers, or an equal proportion of type I and type II fibers. Vastus lateralis (VL) is an often studied "mixed fiber" muscle, typically containing 50% type I fibers and 50% type II fibers. Sprinters, however, tend to have a higher percentage of type II VL fibers, while endurance athletes tend to have a higher percentage of type I VL fibers. These differences are likely genetically determined — predisposing an athlete to one or the other sporting conditions.

Conversion of type II fibers to type I fibers as a result of exercise training has not been shown to occur,[47] but conversion of IIb (fast-twitch white, glycolytic) to IIa (fast-twitch red, oxidative) can happen with endurance training.[39] Some forms of endurance training can produce complete conversion of type IIb fibers to type IIa fibers, and the adaptive increases in oxidative capacity appear greater in the type II fibers than in the type I fibers.[48]

REFERENCES

1. Turner, D. L., Cardiovascular and respiratory control mechanisms during exercise: an integrated view, *J. Exp. Biol.*, 160, 309, 1991.
2. von During, M., Andres, K. H., and Schmidt, R. F., Ultrastructure of fine afferent fibre terminators in muscle and tendon of the cat, in *Sensory Receptor Mechanisms*, Hamann, W. and Iggo, A., Eds., World Scientific Publications Company, Singapore, 1984, 15.
3. Kaufman, M. P., Rotto, D. M., and Rybicki, K. L., Pressor reflex responses to static muscular contraction: its afferent arm and possible neurotransmitters, *Am. J. Cardiol.*, 62, 58E, 1988.
4. McCloskey, D. I. and Mitchell, J. H., Reflex cardiovascular and respiratory responses originating in exercising muscle, *J. Physiol.* (London), 224, 173, 1972.
5. Mitchell, J. H., Reardon, W. C., and McCloskey, D. I., Reflex effects on circulation and respiration from contracting skeletal muscle, *Am. J. Physiol.*, 233, H374, 1977.
6. Crayton, S. C., Aung-Din. R., Fixler, D. E., and Mitchell, J. H., Distribution of cardiac output during induced isometric exercises in dogs, *Am. J. Physiol.*, 236, H218, 1979.
7. Waldrop, T. G. and Mitchell, J. H., Effects of barodenervation on cardiovascular responses to static muscular contraction, *Am. J. Physiol.*, 249, H710, 1985.
8. Kalia, M., Mei, S. S., and Kao, F. F., Central projections from ergoreceptors (C fibres) in muscle involved in cardiopulmonary responses to static exercise, *Circ. Res.* (Suppl. 1), 48, 48, 1981.
9. Iwamoto, G. A., Parnavelas, J. G., Kaufman, M. P., Botterman, B. R., and Mitchell, J. H., Activation of caudal brainstem cell groups during the exercise pressor reflex in the cat as elucidated by 2-[14C] deoxyglucose, *Brain Res.*, 304, 178, 1984.
10. Iwamoto, G. A., Waldrop, T. G., Bauer, R. M., and Mitchell, J. H., Pressor response to muscular contraction in the cat: contributions by caudal and rostral ventrolateral medulla, in *Progress in Brain Research,* Vol. 81, Ciriello, J., Caverson, M. M., and Polosa, C., Eds., Elsevier Biomedical, New York, 1989, 253.
11. Hobbs, S. L., Central command during exercise: parallel activation of the cardiovascular and motor systems by descending command signals, in *Circulation, Neurobiology and Behavior*, Smith, O. A., Galosy, R. A. and Weiss, S. M., Eds., Elsevier Biomedical, New York, 1982, 216.
12. Eldridge, F. L., Millhorn, D. E., Kiley, J. P., and Waldrop, T. G., Stimulation by central command of locomotion, respiration and circulation during exercise, *Respir. Physiol.*, 59, 313, 1985.
13. McCallister, L. W., McCoy, K. W., Connelly, J. C., and Kaufman, M. P., Stimulation of H fields of Florel decreases total lung resistance in dogs, *J. Appl. Physiol.*, 65, 2156, 1988.
14. Rybicki, K. J., Stremel, R. W., Iwamoto, G. A., Mitchell, J. H., and Kaufman, M. P., Occlusion of pressor responses to posterior diencephalic stimulation and muscular contraction, *Brain Res. Bull.*, 22, 305, 1989.
15. Spyer, K. M., The central nervous system organization of reflex circulatory control, in *Central Regulation of Autonomic Functions*, Loewy, A. D., Spyer, K. M., Eds., Oxford University Press, New York, 1990, 168.
16. Waldrop, T. G., Henderson, M. C., Iwamoto, G. A., and Mitchell, J. H., Regional blood flow responses to static muscular contraction, *Am. J. Physiol.*, 249, H710, 1985.
17. Caverson, M. M. and Ciriello, J., Ventrolateral medullospinal neurons involved in the control of the circulation, in *Organization of the Autonomic Nervous System: Central and Peripheral Mechanisms*, Ciriello, J., Calaresu, F. R., Renaud, L. P., and Polosa, C., Eds., Alan R. Liss, New York, 1987, 227.
18. Machado, B. H. and Brody, M. J., Role of nucleus ambiguus in the regulation of heart rate and arterial pressure, *Hypertension*, 11, 602, 1988.

19. Machado, B. H. and Brody, M. J., Mechanisms of pressor response produced by stimulation of nucleus ambiguus, *Am. J. Physiol.*, 259, R955, 1990.

20. Feldman, J. L., Neurophysiology of respiration in mammals, in *Handbook of Physiology. The Nervous System,* vol. 4, Bloom, F. E., Ed., American Physiological Society, Bethesda, MD, 1986, 463.

21. Fisher, A. G. and Jensen, C. R., *Scientific Basis of Athletic Conditioning,* 3rd ed., Lea & Febiger, Philadelphia, 1990, 4.

22. Åstrand, P. O. and Rodahl, K., *Textbook of Work Physiology: Physiological Bases of Exercise,* 2nd ed., McGraw Hill, New York, 1977, 37.

23. Henriksson, J. and Reitman, J. S., Quantitative measures of enzyme activities in type I and type II muscle fibers of man after training, *Acta Physiol. Scand.,* 97, 392, 1976.

24. Huxley, H. E., The mechanism of muscular contraction, *Science*, 164, 1356, 1969.

25. Huxley, H. E., The mechanism of muscular contraction, *Sci. Am,* 1213, 18, 1965.

26. Huxley, A. F., Muscular contraction, *J. Physiol.,* 23, 1, 1974.

27. Burke, R. E. and Edgerton, V. R., Motor unit properties and selective involvement in movement, *Exercise Sports Sci. Rev.,* 3, 31, 1975.

28. Spence, A. P. and Mason, E. B., *Human Anatomy and Physiology,* 4th ed., West Publishing, Los Angeles, 1992, 266.

29. McArdle, W. D., Katch, F. I., and Katch, V. L., *Exercise Physiology: Energy, Nutrition, and Human Performance,* 3rd ed., Lea & Febiger, Philadelphia, 1991, 359.

30. Marieb, E. N., *Human Anatomy and Physiology,* 2nd ed., Benjamin/Cummings, Menlo Park, CA, 1992, 263.

31. Hill, A. V., The series elastic component of muscle. *Proc. R. Soc. Biol.,* 137, 273, 1950.

32. Jensen, D., *The Principles of Physiology,* 2nd ed., Appleton-Century-Crofts, New York, 1980, 92.

33. Morgan, T. E., Cobb, L. A., Short, F. A., Ross, R., and Gunn, D. R. Effect of long-term exercise on human muscle mitochondria., *Muscle Metabolism during Exercise,* Perrow, B. and Saltin, B., Eds., Plenum Press, New York, 1971.

34. Hoppler, H., Lüthi, P., Claasen, H., Weibel, E. R., and Howald, H., The ultrastructure of normal human skeletal muscle: a morphometric analysis on untrained men, women, and well-trained orienters, *Pfluegers Arch.,* 344, 217, 1973.

35. Baldwin, K. M., Klinkerfuss, G. H., Terjung, R. L., Molé, P. A., and Holloszy, J. O., Respiratory capacity of white, red, and intermediate muscle: adaptive response to exercise, *Am. J. Physiol.,* 222, 373, 1972.

36. Winder, W. W., Baldwin, K. M., and Holloszy, J. O., Enzymes involved in ketone utilization in different types of muscle: adaptation to exercise, *Eur. J. Biochem.,* 47, 461, 1974.

37. Gollnick, P. D. and King, D. W., Effect of exercise and training on mitochondria of rat skeletal muscle., *Am. J. Physiol.,* 216, 1502, 1969.

38. Pattingale, P. K. and Holloszy, J. O., Augmentation of skeletal muscle myoglobin by programs of treadmill running., *Am. J. Physiol.,* 213, 738, 1967.

39. Zernicke, R. F., Salem, G. J., and Alejo, R., Endurance training, in *Sports Medicine the School-Age Athlete*, Reider, B., Ed., W.B. Saunders, Philadelphia, 1991, chap. 1.

40. Tesch, P. A., Thorsson, A., and Kaiser, P., Muscle capillary supply and fiber type characteristics in weight and power lifters, *J. Appl. Physiol.,* 56, 35, 1984.

41. McDonagh, M. J. and Davies, C. T. M., Adaptive responses of mammalian skeletal muscle to exercise with high load., *Eur. J. Appl. Physiol.,* 52, 139, 1984.

42. Gonyea, W. J., Role of exercise in inducing increases in skeletal muscle fiber number, *J. Appl. Physiol.,* 48, 421, 1980.

43. Tesch, P. A. and Larsson, L., Muscle hypertrophy in body builders, *Eur. J. Appl. Physiol.,* 49, 310, 1982.

44. MacDougall, J. D., Ward, G. R., Sale, D. G., and Sutton, J. R., Biochemical adaptation of human skeletal muscle to heavy resistance training and immobilization, *J. Appl. Physiol.,* 43, 700, 1977.

45. Haupt, H., Strength training, in *Sports Medicine the School-Age Athlete,* Reider, B., Ed., W.B. Saunders, Philadelphia, 1991, chap. 2.

46. DeLorme, T. L., Ferris, B. G., and Gallagher, J. R., Effect of progressive exercise on muscular contraction time, *Arch. Phys. Med.*, 33, 86, 1952.

47. Holloszy, J. O. and Booth, J. W., Biochemical adaptations to endurance exercise in muscle, *Ann. Rev. Physiol.*, 38, 273, 1976.

48. Chi, M. M.-Y., Hintz, C. S., Coyle, E. F., Martin III, W. H., Ivy, J. L. Nemeth, P. M., Holloszy, J. O., and Lowry, O. H., Effects of detraining on enzymes of energy metabolism in individual human muscle fibers, *Am. J. Physiol.,* 244, C276, 1983.

Chapter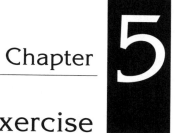

Gender, Aging, and Exercise

Roy J. Shephard

CONTENTS

0-8493-4593-6/97/$0.00+$.50

I. INTRODUCTION

Much of our current knowledge of exercise physiology has been obtained from observations on young adult males. It is important to recognize that both acute and chronic responses to exercise differ between women and men, and also between young and older adults. The present chapter will examine the nature of these differences, pointing out their practical implications for both exercise testing and the prescription of physical activity.

II. GENDER

A. DIFFERENCES BETWEEN MALES AND FEMALES

The extent of inherent physiological differences between males and females is an extremely controversial issue, with important practical implications for performance on the sports field and in traditional male occupations. Some feminists would argue that much if not all of the commonly described gender differences in body form, physiological characteristics, and athletic performance are the result of parallel differences in both opportunities and encouragement to practice physical activity and sport.[1-4] Attention is drawn to the shrinking gap between male and female records in many types of competition;[5] it is further suggested that the currently available range of events favors male dominance, but nevertheless the time may not be too distant when women will outperform men in a number of categories of athletic competition. Realists point to the added burden of fat carried by the female. This offers a significant disadvantage in most events except long-distance swimming. Reserves of body fat seem more resistant to the metabolic demands of exercise in women than in men.[6,7] However, a fair part even of the usually anticipated fat differential disappears in response to prolonged involvement in endurance running.[8]

Women are frequently excluded from both heavy employment and vigorous athletic competition on the grounds of average gender differences in physical characteristics. However, such an approach ignores the large within-sex differences in these same characteristics. Thus, the weakest males at any given age are not as strong as the strongest of the female contenders, and top female athletes often resemble sedentary or even athletic males more closely than they do their female peers. If indeed it is important to exclude individuals with inadequate physical or physiological characteristics from a certain type of sport or employment on grounds of safety or poor job performance, equity demands that such exclusions be based upon an objective testing of the individual rather than physiological norms derived from group averages. Some progress has been made in the development of performance-related tests for various occupations over the past decade, but unfortunately most of the current options still lack the precision to allow a valid classification of physical ability in an individual worker.[9]

A further problem in discussing gender differences of exercise physiology is a lack of agreement on appropriate methods for the standardization of laboratory data. Men are generally some 10 cm taller and 15 to 20 kg heavier than women. However, there is little agreement as to whether data such as peak muscle forces and maximal oxygen intake should be expressed per unit of $(height)^2$, per $(height)^3$, per kilogram of body mass, or per kilogram of lean mass.[10] If total body mass is adopted as the criterion, this immediately places most women at a disadvantage, since a higher proportion of the body mass is fat in female subjects. Again, many measurements of muscular performance examine torque (the product of muscle force and the length of the lever arm) rather than force per se, so that limb length becomes an issue as well as muscle bulk.

Matching of the sexes for fitness is a difficult practical issue when designing many exercise experiments. For example, it is well known that a person's level of fitness influences the rate of sweat production at any given core temperature. Thus, if we wish to examine whether or not exercising women sweat more than their male peers, the two subject groups should be matched for fitness. Some authors have chosen to equate subjects on the basis of maximal oxygen intake per kilogram of body mass. However, both in well-trained international athletes and in sedentary adults, the average aerobic power is less in women than in men. Thus, the adoption of this tactic compares fit women with unfit men. If we were to examine the best athletes of each sex, the comparison would again be somewhat biased, since the female competitors are generally drawn from a smaller pool of interested individuals. At the other extreme, if we were to compare sedentary individuals of both sexes, it again remains arguable that the women are at a disadvantage because sociocultural factors have restricted their physical activity in work and leisure from an early age. Currently, the best approach is probably to match subjects per kilogram of lean mass,[10] but plainly we will not have a definitive answer to many of the questions regarding gender differences until opportunities for physical activity have been equalized for the general population of both sexes.

Table 1 Typical Physical Characteristics
of Young Women and Men

Variable	Female	Male
Height (cm)	162	175
Body mass (kg)	57	74
Lean mass (kg)	41.9	58.8
Body fat (%)	26.4	20.6
Fat mass (kg)	15.1	15.2
Essential fat (kg)	6.8	2.1
Bone mass	6.8	10.5

Based in part on data of Canada Fitness Survey of
1981[14] and data of Katch and Katch.[15]

B. MORPHOLOGICAL DIFFERENCES AND SIMILARITIES

With the specific exception of the sex organs, there are only minor differences of anthropometric characteristics between girls and boys through to the age of puberty. At puberty, females show a substantial increase in body fat, whereas in males the dominant change is an increase of muscle. At maturity, males have a substantially larger muscle mass, and greater cardiac dimensions, than females, but there are no consistent sex differences in the relative proportions of slow- and fast-twitch muscle fibers.[11,12]

The mature female has a smaller thorax, a larger abdomen, a broader and shallower pelvis, shorter legs, and a lower relative center of gravity than the male. The bones are smaller and lighter in structure,[13] reducing the average density of the lean body compartment (a key figure in hydrostatic determinations of body fat). Some of the accumulation of fat in the female is culturally imposed, but nevertheless the minimum quantity of essential fat associated with good health (Table 1) seems to be substantially larger than in the male (probably 10 to 12% rather than 3% of body mass).[16] Because there has been an excessive emphasis upon the physical appearance of females, it may be useful to estimate their minimal desirable body mass. Katch and Katch[15] have suggested that this can be calculated as Mass (kg) = 1.11 (Height, m) $\times$ (D/33.5)^2, where D is the sum (in cm) of 12 diameters (biacromial, chest, bi-iliac, bitrochanteric, R + L knees, R + L ankles, R + L elbows, and R + L wrists).

The morphometric differences seen between the average male and the average female carry some biomechanical consequences. The broader hips and a marginally lower center of gravity tend to give greater stability to the female, facilitating gymnastic performance, but reducing performance in high jumping. Women's shoulders tend to be narrower and with a greater slope, and the upper arms hang less vertically; however, the concept of an increased carrying angle at the elbows, and resulting problems in throwing, has been challenged as a poorly documented fallacy.[17] Any gender differences in throwing performance are attributable rather to a shorter lever arm and lesser arm strength in the female. A greater angulation of the lower limbs, with an inward slope of the thighs toward the knees affects gait patterns and the mechanical efficiency of movement, possibly increasing the woman's likelihood of problems of patella tracking during running.[18] The shorter limb length also limits stride frequency and thus peak running speeds.[19]

C. PHYSIOLOGICAL DIFFERENCES AND SIMILARITIES

The commonly encountered gender differences in physiological responses to exercise are mainly quantitative rather than qualitative in nature. They stem partly from underlying morphological differences and partly from the culturally imposed differences in exercise participation that have already been discussed.

1. Aerobic Power

Prior to puberty, gender-related differences of maximal oxygen intake[20] seem due almost entirely to sociocultural factors. The gender discrepancy widens at puberty. Given that the absolute value for peak oxygen transport is a power function of body size,[21,22] the greater height of males could account for at least 30% of their ultimate advantage. A second important factor is a gender difference in blood hemoglobin concentration (typically 13.8 g/dl in a woman, but 15.6 g/dl in a man). The lower values of the typical female apparently arise from a combination of a menstruation-related iron deficiency,[23] lower blood levels of androgenic steroids, and in some cases deliberate dietary restriction. For every

Table 2 Maximal Oxygen Intake of Top-Level Female and Male Competitors in Various Endurance Sports (expressed in ml/[kg·min])

Sport	Women	Men	Female Disadvantage
Cross-country skiing	63	82	23%
Distance cycling	63	78	19
Orienteering	60	77	22
Pentathlon	50	74	32
Distance running	62	82	24
Speed-skating	53	79	33
Swimming	58	70	17

See Shephard[26] for detailed supporting references.

liter of blood that is pumped by the heart, a typical man can carry to the working tissues a 13% greater quantity of oxygen than a female subject. Finally, because the skeletal muscles of a woman are smaller than those of a man, they tend to contract at a larger fraction of their maximal voluntary force; thus, at any given absolute work rate the vascular impedance-limiting cardiac ejection is greater in the female than in the male.[24] The absolute aerobic power as measured on a treadmill or cycle ergometer is at least 30 to 40% smaller in a woman than in a man of similar age. Gender differences in the peak oxygen transport during aerobic arm exercise are of a similar order.[25]

The substantial physiological disadvantages of the woman are offset by a lighter body mass; she thus performs a smaller total amount of work in any task that involves a displacement of body mass. If maximal oxygen intake values are expressed per kilogram of body mass, the gender discrepancy narrows to less than 20% in young adults. Claims that there is no gender difference in the aerobic power of highly trained young endurance athletes seem unwarranted (Table 2), but by the normal age of retirement there is little difference of relative aerobic power between typical representatives of the two sexes.[26]

Oxygen transport is closely related to muscle mass, and gender differences of aerobic power are smallest if data are expressed per kilogram of lean tissue mass.[10,27] Such a calculation eliminates the penalty associated with the larger fraction of essential body fat in a woman. However, the practical significance of oxygen transport per kilogram of lean mass is unclear. Weight-supported tasks demand a certain level of absolute aerobic power, and weight-dependent tasks require a specific oxygen transport per kilogram of total body mass. Thus, depending on the activity to be performed, the aerobic power of male and female subjects should be compared either in absolute units or per kilogram of body mass.

2. Anaerobic Power and Capacity
The anaerobic power of a subject reflects mainly local stores of phosphagen energy in the active muscles. Because women are less muscular than men, a substantial disadvantage of anaerobic power might be envisaged. Estimates based on tests of absolute muscle power, such as all-out cycle ergometry (Wingate test) and peak lactate readings, suggest that women on average attain only 68 to 73% of male values.[28] However, much if not all of this disadvantage disappears if the anaerobic task is performed against body mass (for example, the Margaria staircase sprint).[5,29]

The ventilatory threshold is apparently reached at a similar fraction of maximal oxygen intake in women as in men.[30] Peak blood lactate concentrations are some 20% lower in average women,[28] but in well-trained athletes the differences are small.[30] The oxygen deficit repayment is smaller in women than in men,[31] although this difference also disappears if values are expressed per kilogram of body mass.

3. Muscle Strength
There are substantial (20 to 30%) differences of absolute muscular strength between women and men,[5,13,32] but values for leg extension and quadriceps force become almost identical when expressed per kilogram of body mass.[13] Values come closest to the male level in the case of the hip flexors and extensors, and the discrepancies are larger for the muscles of the chest, shoulders, arms, and forearms.[32] Moreover, although women are able to increase muscle strength by training, they show little of the increase in muscle bulk seen when male subjects engage in a similar regimen.[33,34]

Perhaps the most striking gender difference is in the time required to reach peak force. Although the muscles of a woman apparently contain more fast-twitch fibers than those of a man, it still takes almost twice as long for the woman to reach 70% of peak force.[13] On the other hand, women seem better able to store elastic energy in the stretched muscles.

4. Coordination and Motor Performance

It seems generally accepted that women have greater flexibility[14] and better fine motor skills than men, although it has been suggested that this advantage may result from differences in play patterns imposed from an early age, rather than from an inherent physiological difference.[35] Other factors contributing to the better coordination of the female are the lower center of gravity and the shorter average limb length. Reaction times of the female are similar to those of male peers, but because of shorter limb lengths and less-powerful muscles, movement times are substantially slower in women than in men.[36,37]

5. Tolerance of Thermal Stress

Because of a greater thickness of subcutaneous fat, women have some advantage over men in activities involving severe cold exposure, particularly distance swimming.[38,39] However, the advantage is less than might at first appear, since the women have a larger surface area/body mass ratio,[40] and a lower peak rate of heat production;[41] the core-to-surface temperature gradient depends on the heat flux per unit area of skin surface. Moreover, some of the insulation in a cold environment is derived from poorly perfused muscle rather than superficial fat, and in this respect the male has an advantage over the female.[42] Women apparently begin to shiver at a higher core temperature than men[43] and seem less able to generate heat through nonshivering thermogenic mechanisms;[44] possibly, this helps to conserve depot fat for the needs of reproduction and lactation.

Many of the gender-related differences noted in the cold operate in the opposite sense during exposure to hot and humid conditions. The greater surface area/body mass ratio gives the woman an advantage over a man in a hot environment, but the rise of core temperature may still be greater in a woman than in a man during performance of a given absolute quantity of work, since the increase of rectal temperature depends on the relative intensity of exercise (expressed as a percentage of maximal aerobic power). There are difficulties in matching men and women for aerobic fitness, and until this is achieved with confidence, it seems premature to discuss gender differences in the rate of sweat production or other indices of heat tolerance. Some recent studies suggest that at any given fraction of an individual's aerobic power, the severity of heat stress is rather similar for men and for women.[45,46]

In desert conditions, where the environment is hotter than skin temperature, the woman suffers a disadvantage; she gains more heat than a man for a given exposure because she has a larger relative body surface area. If male subjects exercise at a higher absolute rate than females under hot and dry conditions, they tend to produce more sweat than the women.[47]

D. PHYSICAL PERFORMANCE AND MENSTRUATION

The luteal phase of the menstrual cycle is associated with a substantial increase in resting body temperature (about 0.5°C), but this seems to have remarkably little impact upon physiological responses to submaximal exercise, even when the activity is performed in the heat.[48] The high blood levels of progesterone that develop during the luteal phase increase the ventilatory response to a given intensity of exercise, but this does not appear to influence the overall maximal oxygen intake.[49] Possibly, a larger fraction of the oxygen intake is consumed by the chest muscles, leaving less oxygen for the muscles that are performing external work.

Water retention may lead to a small increase of body mass during the premenstrual phase of the cycle, and in theory this could lead to a small increase in the oxygen cost of activities involving a displacement of body mass. Intraocular pressure may also rise in the premenstrual phase, and this could impair activities requiring a high level of visual acuity.[50] Potential treatments include fluid restriction and the administration of diuretics or small doses of progesterone during the latter part of the menstrual cycle. Simple reaction times are unaffected by premenstrual changes, but one report has noted a small decrease in hand steadiness,[51] and various anecdotes suggest an association between premenstrual tension and an increased proneness to accidents.

A number of athletes manipulate the timing of menstruation to avoid its coincidence with major competition, but many others maintain a full schedule of training and competition through all phases of the menstrual cycle. A heavy menstrual flow may sometimes impose practical problems of personal hygiene for a day or so, but there is now a strong consensus that physical performance shows remarkably little change over the course of a normal menstrual cycle. The performance of events requiring strength may show a small improvement during the premenstrual phase, and at this stage there may be a minor deterioration in the performance of activities requiring intense concentration or cooperation with other players. However, it is plainly impossible to conduct double-blind observations on physical performance over the menstrual cycle, and it is thus unclear how far any reported changes are a psychological response to socially conditioned expectations rather than a consequence of underlying physiological and biochemical phenomena.

E. EFFECTS OF EXERCISE ON MENSTRUAL FUNCTION

A number of reports have suggested that moderate exercise is helpful in relieving dysmenorrhea, possibly by altering the balance of prostaglandins[52] or improving overall mood state.

Participation in top-level gymnastics, figure skating, and prolonged endurance events is frequently associated with delayed menarche. The affected athlete is often dissatisfied with her current body image; the individual concerned thus has an inadequate intake of food energy and a very low percentage of body fat.[53,54] However, in sports that favor the petite competitor,[55] the deliberate selection of late maturers by coaches is a further factor contributing to late menarche. In a few unfortunate instances there may even have been a deliberate delaying of normal maturation by "doping" procedures.

The onset of irregular menstruation or the development of a temporary amenorrhea are common concomitants of heavy training, particularly when such training is associated with a negative energy or nitrogen balance and the stress of intense competition. Prior[56] has argued that parallel events, including a suppression of sperm production, can be seen in male endurance competitors, and that the entire phenomenon is a normal reproductive response to a relative shortage of food supply. Normal menstruation is resumed when training is moderated or the food intake is increased. A weakening of bone structure is one possible negative factor associated with menstrual disturbances. Women who have never had regular menstrual cycles show, on average, an acute 17% deficit of bone density; it has yet to be decided how readily a normal bone density is restored once the women halt intense competition.[57] Injuries are certainly more common in athletes with disturbed menstruation, although it is hard to separate out the mechanical effects of exposure to intense and prolonged training from the consequences of a lesser secretion of estrogens in the affected individuals.

If an athlete's menstruation becomes irregular, the sports physician should first rule out causes other than exercise (including pregnancy!). If an exercise-induced energy deficit is responsible, a normal cycle can usually be restored by a combination of counseling, a 10% reduction of training volume, and an increase of food intake sufficient to induce a modest (2 kg) increase of body mass. If anovulation or amenorrhea persists for longer than 3 to 6 months, medroxyprogesterone can be administered 14 days monthly, and calcium intake should also be increased to the level recommended for menopausal women (1500 mg/day).

F. EXERCISE DURING PREGNANCY

Most authorities now agree that it is beneficial to continue moderate physical activity throughout pregnancy, although it is plainly advisable to avoid contact sports and activities where there is a risk of falling.

Moderate physical activity has no adverse effect upon the fetus.[58] It may speed the course of labor,[59] and the long-term condition of the mother is improved.[60] The increase of blood volume may even improve athletic performance during the first few months of pregnancy, although this advantage is later offset by a significant increase of body mass. The energy supply of the fetus is in general well protected against the added metabolic demands of maternal exercise, but repeated bouts of very vigorous physical activity can lead to some reduction of birth weight.[61] During the first trimester of pregnancy, there is some increase in the risk of teratogenic effects if exercise is pushed to a level inducing significant hyperthermia (>38.9°C). The hazard of abnormal fetal development has been shown directly in exercising animals, and a parallel risk has been inferred in humans on the basis of adverse responses to the fevers induced by infectious diseases.[62]

In the late stages of pregnancy, the increase of body size and mass, plus a restriction of abdominal breathing make vigorous exercise quite difficult. If physical activity is performed while lying supine, the fetus may shift to a position where maternal venous return is compromised. The mother's ligaments also show greater laxity of ligaments, and this may increase the risk of musculoskeletal injuries.[63] About half of pregnant women elect to reduce their training schedules beyond the 28th week of gestation. At this stage, it is often helpful to introduce weight-supported activities such as swimming, aquabics, and running in water.[64]

Late in pregnancy, overvigorous exercise may reduce placental perfusion, causing fetal bradycardia; this is presumably a sign of temporary hypoxia, although its impact upon fetal development has yet to be decided.[65] Exercise-induced hemoconcentration compensates at least partially for any decrease of placental blood flow during heavy physical activity.[66] The fetus is dependent on glucose as its energy source, and it is thus important to ensure that a heavy and sustained bout of maternal exercise does not induce hypoglycemia. There is some evidence that (perhaps as a means of protecting the fetus from hypoglycemia) pregnancy reduces the ability of the mother to metabolize carbohydrate;[67] if so, this could possibly limit the ability of the mother to perform anaerobic activities during pregnancy.

Following delivery, the energy demands of regular exercise do not appear to impair lactation. Indeed, cross-sectional comparisons suggest that relative to their sedentary peers, women who choose to exercise regularly secrete larger volumes of milk with a higher energy content;[68] this may be due to enhanced levels of serum prolactin, or a relief of postpartum depression in the exercisers.[69] The competitive performance of international athletes is sometimes enhanced following recovery from pregnancy. Klaus and Noack[70] suggested that the heavy circulatory demands of gestation offered the equivalent of 9 months of rigorous conditioning!

III. AGING

A. THEORIES OF AGING

Aging and ultimate death are characteristic of all organisms. The course of human aging can be described in empirical terms. In some organs such as the brain, cells die and are not replaced. In other tissues, the cell constituents change — for example, cross-linkages develop between adjacent collagen fibrils, decreasing elasticity and facilitating mechanical injury of the affected tissue. The blood vessels become progressively affected by atherosclerosis and arteriosclerosis, decreasing the potential oxygen supply to all of the body organs. Partly as a consequence of this hypoxia, and partly because of local cellular changes, the function of most organs shows a progressive, age-related deterioration.[71] In some individuals, death is the result of a sudden disturbance of local blood flow (a "heart attack" or a massive cerebral hemorrhage). In others, there is a cancerous change of cells (reflecting in part a deterioration of the body's immune system). But commonly, death occurs from an infection or an environmental stress that a younger person with larger functional reserves would withstand successfully.

Mechanisms underlying the aging process are less clear, and indeed some biometricians have merely regarded aging as "an increased probability of death."[72] Other authors have sought metaphors to provide a useful description of events.[73] Possible hypotheses[74,75] include an accumulation of "wear and tear" which exceeds the reparative capacity of the body, a progressive development of autoimmunity, and errors in cell division, associated with exposure to endogenous or exogenous mitogens. Some have even argued that the aging process is "biologically programmed," to avoid the hazard of overpopulation.

1. Chronological Age

Adult life can be divided into young, middle, and old age. On average, young adulthood covers the period from 20 to 35 years. Biological function and physical performance are then at the subject's peak. The typical individual is busy establishing a career, marrying, and raising young children.

During young middle age (35 to 45 years), life-style generally becomes more static, and physical activity often begins to wane, with some accumulation of body fat. Active pursuits may continue to be shared with the developing family, but there is less urgency to impress either an employer or persons of the opposite sex with physical appearance and performance capabilities. During later middle age (45 to 65 years), women reach the menopause, and there is also a substantial but less definitive decrease in the male production of sex hormones. Career opportunities have commonly peaked, responsibility for any children rapidly diminishes, and a larger disposable income often allows an older married couple to depute the energy-demanding tasks of daily living such as garden maintenance or snow clearance to service contractors. The decline in physical condition thus continues and may accelerate.

Old age is commonly divided into three phases.[75] In early old age (65 to 75 years), some subjects show a modest increase of physical activity, in an attempt to fill the free time resulting from retirement. By middle old age (75 to 85 years), many people have developed some physical disability from a combination of a progressive deterioration in general condition and an accumulation of specific chronic ailments such as rheumatoid arthritis or a minor stroke. In the final stage of very old age (over 85 years), there is a progressive development of total dependency, as the individual loses the ability to undertake the basic activities of daily living unaided. A typical expectation for the senior citizen is thus of a final

8 to 10 years of partial disability, and as much as a year of total dependency.[76] Women live longer than men, but unfortunately they also experience a longer terminal period of disability.

2. Biological Age

Although the chronological categories noted above provide a good overall indication of the course of aging, there are wide interindividual differences in functional status at any given chronological age. Indeed, in terms of the usually measured fitness variables (maximal oxygen intake, muscle strength, and flexibility), the best-preserved 65-year-old individual may outperform a very sedentary 25-year-old person. The implication is that whether an investigator is assessing fitness for continuing employment or is recommending an exercise prescription, it is important to base decisions upon biological rather than chronological age. It further emphasizes the truth that dependency is not an inevitable concomitant of aging. Regular physical activity cannot alter the intrinsic rate of aging to any great extent, but because it maximizes the individual's potential at any given calendar age, it can reduce a person's biological age by as much as 10 to 20 years.[77]

Unfortunately, there is no very satisfactory method of determining biological age. Given the association between aging and the likelihood of death, one approach[78] has been to examine a person's lifestyle; from this information, the investigator can calculate an appraised age, corresponding to the chances of dying within 10 years from the 12 main causes of death for that particular age and sex category. Studies of this type have suggested that involvement of individuals in a vigorous endurance training program may improve their personal life-style, and thus reduce their appraised age.[79] Others have attempted to combine various anthropometric, physiological, and psychological measurements, such as graying of the hair, loss of skin elasticity, a decrease of vital capacity, and a decrease of reaction time, into a global index of biological age.[80] Difficulties arise because the different biological systems do not necessarily age at the same rates, and there is no simple method of combining such disparate sets of data; often, attempts to determine biological age from functional measurements provide no more than a complicated and inaccurate method of assessing chronological age.

B. AGING AND BASAL METABOLIC RATE

Many reports have suggested that aging is associated with a decrease of basal metabolic rate, when this is expressed in its traditional units (kJ per m^2 of body surface). On average, there is a 10% decrease from early adulthood to the age of retirement, and a further 10% decrease during the retirement years.[81] Some early authors inferred that this was due mainly to a decrease of cellular enzyme activity and/or a failure of cellular repair mechanisms.[82] However, a more important factor is an age-related alteration in body composition. The body surface used in the traditional calculation is not measured, but rather is estimated from a nomogram based upon height and body mass. Aging is usually associated with a small (2 to 4 cm) decrease of height (from a combination of kyphosis and vertebral collapse) and a larger (5 to 10 kg) increase of body mass (as muscle and other lean tissue is replaced by a storage of metabolically inert depot fat). After allowing for the age-related increase in adipose tissue, the decrease in metabolism is only 10%, even into the seventh and eighth decades of life.[83]

However, the reduction in basal metabolism for the body as a whole reaches the larger, 20% figure, and food intake must be correspondingly reduced if obesity is not to occur. This in turn leads to a reduced intake of protein and other key nutrients, particularly calcium. Many very old people lead extremely sedentary lives, and the combination of a low basal metabolism and a very limited amount of deliberate energy expenditure can give rise to dietary deficiencies — particularly an inadequate intake of calcium.[84] An important by-product of a physical activity program for the older senior is an increased intake of key nutrients without recourse to the provision of synthetic dietary supplements.

C. AGING AND OXYGEN TRANSPORT

In general, the maximal oxygen intake declines steadily by about 5 ml/[kg·min] per decade from age 25 to age 65 years, with some possible acceleration of the rate of loss subsequent to retirement (Figure 1).[75] It is difficult to be certain how far the loss of aerobic power is an inevitable consequence of aging, and how far it is secondary to a decrease of habitual physical activity, since ordinary people become progressively more sedentary as they become older, and even athletes tend to reduce the rigor of their training. There have indeed been occasional claims that an active person can sustain an unchanged maximal oxygen intake for many years.[85] However, critical evaluation of the supporting data suggests that once subjects who are enrolled in an exercise program have realized any immediate training response, they resume a normal age-related loss of aerobic power. Even in athletes who maintain their daily training

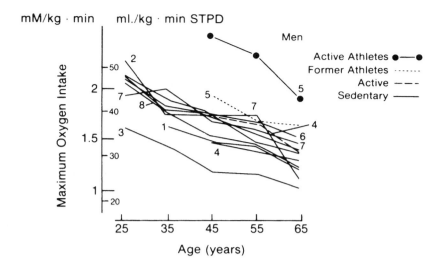

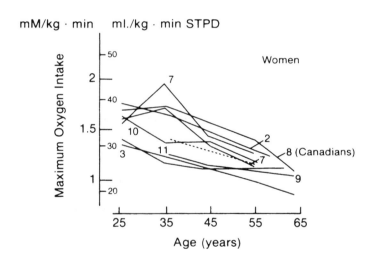

Figure 1 Cross-sectional data on the aging of aerobic power in men and women. STPD = standard temperature and pressure, dry gas. (Based largely upon data accumulated by K.H. Sidney, reproduced from Shephard, R.J., *Physiology and Biochemistry of Exercise,* Praeger Publications, New York, 1982. With permission. See original for details of references.)

volume, the rate of decrease of maximal oxygen intake is only a little slower than in the general population.[86] Potential causes of the aging of aerobic power could include a decrease of maximal heart rate, stroke volume and/or arteriovenous oxygen difference.

1. Maximal Heart Rate

There is a progressive decrease of maximal heart rate with aging (Figure 2), probably reflecting mainly a decreased chronotropic response to catecholamines. Early reports suggested that the peak heart rate for large muscle exercise was approximated by the equation (220 – age in years); this would imply a peak value of about 155 beats/min at age 65 years.[87] More recent research has suggested that the well-motivated sedentary 65-year-old can attain peak heart rates of 170 beats/min or more during uphill treadmill running, although weakness of the leg muscles may lead to somewhat lower maxima (around 160 beats/min) during cycle ergometry.[88,89] Peak values are further reduced if exercise is terminated by breathlessness (in chronic chest disease) or ischemia affecting the pacemaker (in the sick sinus syndrome).

DECLINE OF MAXIMUM HEART RATE WITH AGE IN HEALTHY MEN*

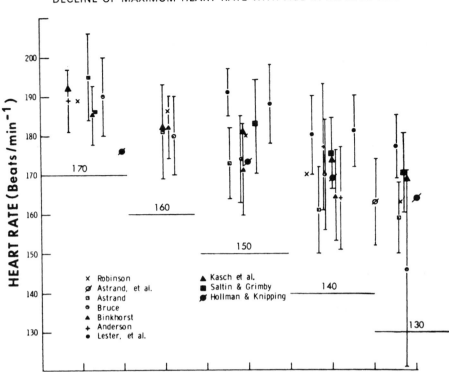

Figure 2   Decrease of maximal heart rate with age. (Based upon data accumulated by S.M. Fox, J.S. Carol. *Med. Assoc.* 65(12), Suppl. 1, p. 77, 1969. With permission. See original for details of references.)

2. Maximal Stroke Volume

Weisfeldt and associates[90] argued that if care was taken to exclude subjects with silent myocardial ischemia (by a combination of exercise electrocardiography and rigorous radionuclide screening), then a typical 65-year-old subject was able to compensate fully for the decrease of maximal heart rate by an increase of end-diastolic volume and thus cardiac stroke volume. However, their view was not confirmed by other laboratories.[91] During submaximal exercise, the stroke volume may be greater than in a younger adult, but the current consensus is that the older person has difficulty in sustaining stroke volume as maximal effort is approached.

There are many constraints upon the function of the older heart during vigorous exercise. Venous filling is impaired, due to a poor peripheral venous tone, varicosities, and a slower diastolic relaxation of the ventricular wall. The sensitivity of the myocardium to catecholamines is reduced, so that there is a lesser inotropic increase of contractility during vigorous effort. The after-loading of the ventricle also rises in older adults, in part because of hypertension and a loss of arterial elasticity and in part because of attempts to sustain perfusion through weak muscles that are contracting at a large fraction of their peak voluntary force. Finally, in some instances ventricular contractility is impaired by silent myocardial ischemia.

3. Maximal Arteriovenous Oxygen Difference

The maximal arteriovenous oxygen difference also tends to decrease with age, from perhaps 140 to 150 ml/dl in a young adult to 120 to 130 ml/dl in a senior citizen. This change reflects not so much a decreased peripheral extraction of oxygen in the working muscles as the direction of a larger fraction of the total cardiac output to regions of the body (the skin and the viscera) where oxygen extraction is

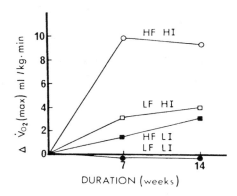

Figure 3 Response of 65-year-old subjects to self-selected aerobic training regimen. HI = high-intensity exercise (heart rate 130–140 beats/min), LI = low-intensity exercise (heart rate 110–120 beats/min). HF = high frequency (more than 2 sessions per week), LF = low frequency (less than 2 sessions per week). (From Sidney, K. H. and Shephard, R. J. *Med. Sci. Sports* 10, 125–131, 1978. With permission.)

quite limited.[75] Nevertheless, the end result is that the oxygen consumption per liter of cardiac output diminishes in an older individual.

4. Functional Consequences

Various authors[92-94] have shown that (depending on the nature of the task and the working environment) the average person becomes fatigued if they must sustain exercise for a long period at more than 33 to 50% of maximal oxygen intake. Thus, the aging of oxygen transport progressively restricts the ability of the individual to undertake the normal activities of daily living.[77]

The minimal aerobic power compatible with full independence is probably in the range 12 to 14 ml/[kg·min]. The functional capacity of many seniors drops below this threshold around 80 years of age. Often, the final critical factor precipitating dependence is a period of bed rest for some intercurrent illness.

5. Training Response

It is quite possible for seniors to augment their maximal oxygen intake by as much as 10 ml/[kg·min] by an appropriately graded aerobic training program (Figure 3).[95] In effect, training reduces the biological age of the oxygen transporting system by the equivalent of 20 years. Thus, a lack of aerobic power should not limit the independence of an active, well-trained individual unless she or he survives to an age of 100, rather than 80 years. Such survival is not particularly likely. Aerobic training eliminates premature disability, but it has little influence on the prospects for survival beyond the age of 80 years.[96] Rather, there is what Fries[97] has termed a "squaring" of the morbidity and mortality curves, and the majority of well-trained individuals live in good health until shortly before a normal age of death. Thus, activity patterns in late middle age are quite strong predictors of the likelihood of institutionalization as a senior (Table 3).[98]

Because the initial fitness of an old person is quite low, aerobic condition can be improved by a relatively low intensity of training. Gains are greatest if a 65-year-old subject can sustain a heart rate of 130 to 140 beats/min, but useful if slower progress is seen with heart rates of 110 to 120 beats/min, provided that the training is undertaken regularly.[95] In the frail elderly, heart rates rarely exceed 85 beats/min, and some response may then be anticipated even with activities inducing a heart rate of only 100 beats/min.

D. AGING AND THE MUSCULOSKELETAL SYSTEM

Aging leads to a progressive decrease of muscle strength and a loss of flexibility in the joints.

1. Muscle Function

Most muscle groups show a peaking of strength around the age of 25 years, a plateau through 35 or 40 years of age, and then an accelerating decline of function, so that some 25% of peak force is lost by the age of 65 years (Figure 4).[75] There is an associated decline in muscle mass, apparently with a selective

Table 3   To Illustrate the Relationship between Reported Physical Activity at Age 50 Years and Dependency during Retirement

Current Status	Reported Activity at Age 50 yr[a]
No disability (n =286)	9.3 ± 0.6
Minor disability (n = 126)	8.1 ± 0.7
Major disability (n = 173)	7.7 ± 0.7
Institutionalized (n = 25)	4.1 ± 1.3

[a] Arbitrary units, mean ± SE

Table developed from the findings of Shephard and Montelpare.[98]

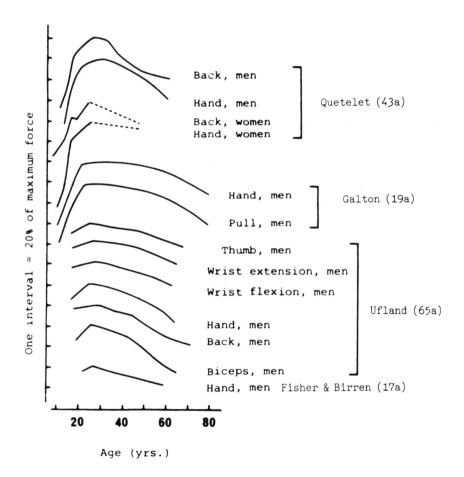

Figure 4   Influence of aging upon the isometric force of selected muscle groups. (Based on data accumulated by M.B. Fisher and J.E. Birren, *J. Appl. Psychol.* 31, 490-497, 1949. With permission. See original for details of references.)

decrease in the cross section if not the numbers of type II fibers.[99] However, because muscle biopsy specimens are not always representative of an entire muscle, it is still somewhat unclear whether there is a general hypotrophy of skeletal muscle or a selective hypoplasia and degeneration of type II fibers, associated with a loss of nerve terminal sprouting.[100]

Other possible causes of functional loss include a deterioration of end-plate structures, with impaired excitation–contraction coupling, and decreased fiber recruitment. Both contraction time and half-relaxation time become longer in older individuals, and there is a decrease of maximal contraction velocity. The functional changes are more obvious in the legs than in the arms, but it is unclear whether this is due to some inherent biological mechanism or whether there is merely a greater decrease in use of the legs with aging. Muscular endurance (measured at a fixed fraction of the individual's maximal voluntary force) tends to increase with age, in part because of the larger proportion of type I fibers and in part because weaker muscle contractions restrict perfusion less than in a younger individual.

As retirement continues, the progressive loss of strength begins to impede everyday living. It becomes difficult to carry a 5-kg bag of groceries, to open a jar of conserves or a vial of medicine, and even to lift the body mass from a chair or a toilet seat.[75] The male/female strength ratio is unchanged in the elderly, so that women are likely to be limited by a loss of muscle strength at an earlier age than men.

At one time, it was thought dangerous to commend programs of resisted exercise to the elderly, as it was feared that the resulting rise of blood pressure during contractions might provoke a heart attack. However, recent studies have emphasized that provided the subject avoids performing a Valsalva maneuver and individual contractions are held for no more than a few seconds at 60% of peak voluntary force, the rise of blood pressure is no greater than would be observed during a typical bout of cycle ergometer exercise.[101] Moreover, as little as 8 weeks of resisted training can yield dramatic increases in the strength of 90-year-old subjects.[102] Protein synthesis proceeds much more slowly than in a younger adult, and it is uncertain how much muscle hypertrophy is possible in seniors. However, cross-sectional comparisons between active and inactive individuals suggest that much of the wasting of lean tissue can be avoided by practicing a regular program of resisted exercise into old age.[102] The strengthening of muscles further enhances function in the frail elderly by stabilizing osteoarthritic joints, reducing the risk of falls, and lessening the extent of dyspnea.

2. Flexibility

The flexibility of the major joints deteriorates progressively as age-related changes develop in the structure of the connective tissues. In particular, the elasticity of tendons, ligaments, and joint capsule is decreased by cross-linkages between adjacent fibrils of collagen.[103]

The functional consequences have been documented most fully for the simple "sit and reach test," which measures the flexibility of the hips and lower back (Figure 5). Over the normal span of working life, Canadian subjects show a decrease of some 8 to 10 cm in the ability to reach toward their toes.[104]

The restriction in the range of joint movement becomes yet more pronounced during the retirement years, and eventually independence is threatened by the inability of the subject to climb into a car or a normal bath, to ascend a small step in a house, or to undertake the movements required for dressing and combing the hair.[75]

It is generally believed that flexibility can be conserved and/or improved by gently taking the main joints through their full range of motion each day, although there is little documentation of the extent of functional gains that may be expected from such therapy. If muscle weakness and arthritis are already advanced, such activities are best attempted in warm water. Buoyancy then supports body weight, and the warmth increases the flexibility of the joints.

3. Osteoporosis

There is a progressive decrease in the calcium content and a deterioration in the organic matrix of the bones as a person becomes older. However, as with many facets of the aging process, the dividing line between normality and a pathological change is unclear, and it is also uncertain how far a decline of habitual physical activity contributes to the usually observed age-related calcium loss. Changes are usually more marked in women than in men. This seems due in part to sex differences in the hormone profile and in part to a lower total energy intake and thus a smaller intake of calcium and good-quality protein in women.[84]

The calcium loss begins as early as 30 years in a woman, and the process accelerates for some 5 years around the time of the menopause. At some point, commonly 70 to 80 years, the bones become so weak that a mild fall, a bout of coughing, or even a vigorous muscle contraction can cause a

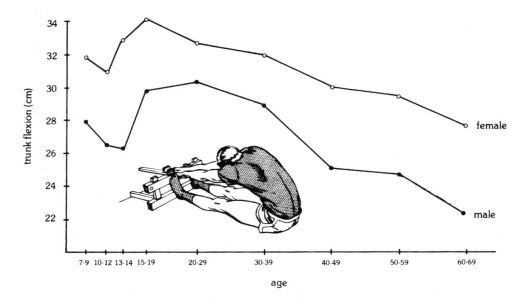

Figure 5   The influence of age upon flexibility of the lower back and hips, as measured by the "sit and reach" test. (Based on data from the Canada Fitness Survey of 1981, Fitness Canada, *Fitness and Lifestyle in Canada,* Ottawa, 1983.)

"pathological" fracture.[104] In the frail elderly, a fracture of the hip associated with a fall is quite commonly the event which initiates irreversible bed rest and death. Bone loss also contributes to vertebral collapse and senile kyphosis.

Controlled studies have shown that regular load-bearing exercise can halt the mineral loss, and in some instances it can even reverse this trend through the eighth decade of life.[105] Such a regimen is particularly effective when accompanied by a diet that provides an adequate quantity of calcium (a minimum of 1500 mg/day). In women, many authorities also recommend the administration of estrogens, although the risks of long-term estrogen administration have yet to be fully assessed.

E. AGING AND HORMONAL CHANGES

Aging is associated with an impairment of many hormonal control mechanisms. Sometimes, the problem arises from damage to and/or a decrease in the number of secreting cells (for instance, the pancreatic islets or the thyroid gland) and sometimes there may be a decrease in the number or the affinity of hormone receptors (for instance, the reduced ventricular response to catecholamines). Other possible changes with age are a reduced permeability of the target cell wall to the hormone or hormone/receptor complex, alterations in concentrations of the second messenger (cAMP), and a decreased responsiveness of the target cell nucleus to hormone/receptor complexes.[106] Perhaps the most common clinical disturbances of health arise from a decreased insulin sensitivity (with a resulting maturity-onset diabetes),[107] and a decreased output of thyroid hormone (with myxedema, obesity, poor cold tolerance, and depression).[106]

Diabetes mellitus presents the immediate risks of ketosis, hyperglycemia, and hypoglycemia. There are also long-term complications which can limit the subject's tolerance of exercise programs, including an increased risk of skin infections and ulceration, peripheral vascular arteriosclerosis, myocardial ischemia, peripheral neuropathy, retinopathies, and cataract formation.

Despite the formidable list of potential complications, there is good evidence that obesity is an important factor in the etiology of maturity-onset diabetes and that a combination of moderate exercise with some restriction of energy intake is an effective form of treatment for this condition. Given such a therapeutic regimen, many patients will be spared the complication of long-term insulin therapy and rigid control of food portions. Exercise may also be helpful to the hypothyroid patient, correcting both obesity and depression.

F. AGING AND ATHLETIC PERFORMANCE

The development of age-specific Master's competitions has allowed the study of peak athletic performance in many disciplines over a wide range of ages. As with comparisons between women and men, it is necessary to be cautious in drawing physiological inferences from such results, since the pool of potential competitors is still much smaller in the older age categories. Moreover, the motives governing participation of older individuals change from competitive success (winning at all costs) to social interaction, and indeed some participants in Masters events do not begin competing until they reach their late thirties.[108]

The age when performance peaks depends upon the key functional element required of the successful competitor. In events where flexibility is paramount (for example, gymnastics and brief swimming events) the top competitors are commonly adolescents. In aerobic events, performance usually peaks in the midtwenties, as gains from prolonged training, improved skills, and competitive experience are negated by decreases in maximal oxygen intake and flexibility. Further, the curve relating age to the time required to cover a given running distance closely matches the curve relating age to maximal oxygen intake.[109] Probably because of a longer plateauing of muscle strength, the performance in anaerobic events declines less steeply,[110] and in some pursuits such as golf and equitation, where experience is paramount, the best competitors are found in the age range 30 to 40 years.[111,112]

G. SAFETY OF EXERCISE PROGRAMS

There is now good evidence that the risk of a cardiac emergency is increased substantially during the period that a person is actually exercising.[113] In an attempt to minimize the risk of exercise-induced incidents, some physicians have thus argued that older people who intend to become involved in an exercise program should undergo an exhaustive preliminary medical clearance, including an exercise electrocardiogram.[114] This may indeed be desirable if the person concerned is intending to embark on a very strenuous training program with the objective of attaining a high level of competition. On the other hand, it seems undesirable on several counts if an older person merely desires to undertake a modest increase in their daily physical activity.

It is relatively difficult to motivate older people to engage in exercise on a regular basis. Insistence upon an extensive preliminary medical evaluation has the effect of suggesting that the proposed regimen is dangerous, and it also creates barriers of cost and time which reduce the likelihood that an intention to exercise will be translated into overt exercise behavior. In fact, the abnormal resting waveforms of the resting electrocardiogram make the interpretation of records very difficult in many elderly persons, and there is little evidence that either a clinical evaluation or a stress electrocardiogram is capable of detecting those individuals who will have an adverse outcome to exercise.[115] Moreover, the person who does initiate an exercise program is at a lower overall risk of sudden death than a sedentary peer,[116] and perhaps because of a less ambitious attitude toward exercise, the relative risks of physical activity decrease rather than increase as a person becomes older (Table 4).[117] Finally, it may be argued that even if a well-loved form of exercise does provoke a sudden cardiac death in an 80-year-old man, this offers a more pleasant end than many alternative causes of death.

Table 4 Risks of Sudden Death during Moderate and Strenuous Exercise, Relative to Sedentary State

Age (years)	Relative Risk of Sudden Death	
	Moderate Exercise	Strenuous Exercise
20–39	2.5	10.0
40–49	3.6	13.1
50–69	2.5	5.3

Table developed from data of Vuori et al.[117]

Certain recommendations can nevertheless be made to increase the safety of exercise programs for the older individual. The dose of exercise should not be enough to leave the participant more than pleasantly tired on the following day. Recovery processes proceed more slowly than in a younger person, and vigorous training is best pursued on alternate days rather than on a daily basis. Often there is preexisting articular disease, and it is preferable to substitute walking for jogging or running; fast walking offers an adequate intensity of exercise for the elderly person, there is less risk of slipping, and the impact stress on the knees is only one third to one sixth of that imposed by jogging.[118] Weight-supported activities such as swimming and aquabics are particularly helpful for those with joint problems. Vision, hearing, and balance are all poorer than in a younger person. The senior should thus avoid sports where there is a serious risk of collision with opponents or stationary objects such as goalposts. If the subject has a history of occasional, poorly explained falls, especial care is needed in pursuing activities that require a good sense of balance (whether climbing, skiing, and cycling, or merely walking on a slippery pool deck). Many older people are taking hypotensive medication, and there is a danger of a sudden loss of consciousness when standing at the end of a bout of exercise, particularly if the room is hot or the veins are relaxed by a period in a pool. An older person adapts less readily to environmental extremes, and if the weather is extremely hot or cold, it may be wise to opt for activity inside an air-conditioned facility (for example, rapid walking in an indoor shopping mall). For those who are extremely frail, some physical conditioning can be achieved using exercises taken from a sitting position.[119]

No program of exercise training can restore tissue that has already been destroyed. Nevertheless, regular physical activity protects the individual against a number of the chronic diseases of old age. More importantly, it maximizes the function of residual tissue. In some instances, biological age is reduced by as much as 20 years. Life expectancy is increased, partial and total disability are delayed, and perhaps most importantly there are major gains in the quality-adjusted life expectancy.

ACKNOWLEDGMENT

The studies of Dr. Shephard are supported in part by a research grant from Canadian Tire Acceptance Limited.

REFERENCES

1. Harris, D.V. Personality research: implications for women in sport. In *The Female Athlete. A Socio-Psychological and Kinanthropometric Approach*. J. Borms, M. Hebbelinck, and A. Venerando (eds.). S. Karger, Basel, 1980, pp. 49–57.
2. Ferris, E. Women and sport: a question of freedom. In: *Women and Sport. An Historical, Biological, Physiological and Sportsmedical Approach*. J. Borms, M. Hebbelinck, and A. Venerando (eds.). S. Karger, Basel, 1980, pp. 4–10.
3. Graydon, J.K. Psychological research and the sportswoman. In: *Sports Women*. M.J. Adrian (ed.). S. Karger, Basel, 1987, pp. 54–82.
4. Fasting, K. and Tangen, J.O. The influence of traditional sex roles on women's participation and engagement in sport. In: *The Female Athlete. A Socio-Psychological and Kinathropometric Approach*. J. Borms, M. Hebbelinck, and A. Venerando (eds.). S. Karger, Basel, 1980, pp. 41–48.
5. Wells, C.L. *Women, Sport and Performance*. Human Kinetics Publishers, Champaign, IL, 1985.
6. Murray, S.J., Shephard, R.J., Greaves, S., Allen, C., and Radomski, M. Effects of cold stress and exercise on fat loss in females. *Eur. J. Appl. Physiol.* 55, 610–618, 1986.
7. Hardman, A.E., Jones, P.R.M., Norgan, N.G., and Hudson, A. Brisk walking improves endurance fitness without changing body fatness in previously sedentary women. *Eur. J. Appl. Physiol.* 65, 354–359, 1992.
8. Wilmore, J.H., Brown, C.H., and Davis, J.A. Body physique and composition of the female distance runner. *Ann. NY Acad. Sci.* 301, 764–776, 1977.
9. Shephard, R.J. Assessment of occupational fitness in the context of Human Rights legislation. *Can. J. Sport Sci.* 15, 89–95, 1990.
10. Drinkwater, B. Women and exercise: physiological aspects. *Exercise Sport Sci. Rev.* 12, 21–52, 1984.
11. Costill, D.L., Daniels, D., Evans, W., Fink, W., Krahenbuhl, G., and Saltin, B. Skeletal muscle enzymes and fiber composition in male and female track athletes. *J. Appl. Physiol.* 40, 149–154, 1976.
12. Prince, F.P., Hikida, R.S., and Hagerman, F.C. Muscle fiber types in women athletes and non-athletes. *Pflügers Arch.* 371, 161–165, 1977.
13. Komi, P.V. Fundamental performance characteristics on females and males. In: *Women and Sport. An Historical, Biological, Physiological and Sportsmedical Approach*. J. Borms, M. Hebbelinck, and A. Venerando (eds.). S. Karger, Basel, 1980, pp. 102–108.
14. Fitness Canada. *Fitness and Lifestyle in Canada*. Directorate of Fitness and Amateur Sport, Ottawa, 1983.
15. Katch F.I. and Katch, V.L. Optimal health and body composition. In: *Women and Exercise. Physiology and Sports Medicine*. M. Shangold and G. Mirkin (eds.). F.A. Davis, Philadelphia, 1988, pp. 23–39.
16. Katch, V.L., Campaigne, B., Freedson, P., Sady, S., Katch, F.I., and Behnke, A.R. Contribution of breast volume and weight to body fat distribution in females. *Am. J. Phys. Anthropol.* 53, 93–100, 1980.
17. Beals, R.K. The normal carrying angle of the elbow. *Clin. Orthopaed.* 119, 194–196, 1976.

18. Hunter-Griffin, L.Y. Orthopedic concerns. In: *Women and Exercise. Physiology and Sports Medicine*. M. Shangold and G. Mirkin (eds.). F.A. Davis, Philadelphia, 1988, pp. 195–219.
19. Hoffman, K. Stride length and frequency of female sprinters. *Track Tech*. 48, 1522–1524, 1972.
20. Shephard, R.J. *Physical Activity and Growth*. Year Book Publishers, Chicago, 1981.
21. Von Döbeln, W. Kroppstorlek, Energieomsättning och Kondition. In: *Handbok i Ergonomi*. U. Aberg and N. Lundgren (eds.). Almqvist & Wiksell, Stockholm, 1966.
22. Shephard, R.J., Lavallée, H., LaBarre, R., Jéquier, J.-C., Volle, M., and Rajic, M. On the basis of data standardization in prepubescent children. In: *Kinanthropometry II*. M. Ostyn, G. Beunen, and J. Simons (eds.). S. Karger, Basel, 1980, pp. 306–316.
23. Scott, D.E. and Pritchard, J.A. Iron deficiency in healthy young college women. *J. Am. Med. Assoc*. 199, 897–900, 1967.
24. Kay, C. and Shephard, R.J. On muscle strength and the threshold of anaerobic work. *Int. Z. Angew. Physiol*. 27, 311–328.
25. Shephard, R.J., Vandewalle, H., Bouhlel, E., and Monod, H. Sex differences of physical work capacity in normoxia and hypoxia. *Ergonomics* 31, 1177–1192, 1988.
26. Shephard, R.J. *Health and Aerobic Fitness*. Human Kinetics Publishers, Champaign, IL, 1993.
27. Cureton, K. Matching of male and female subjects using V_{O2max}. *Res. Q*. 52, 264–268, 1981.
28. Karlsson, J. and Jacobs, I. Is the significance of muscle fibre types to muscle metabolism different in females than in males? In: *Women and Sport. An Historical, Biological, Physiological and Sportsmedical Approach*. J. Borms, M. Hebbelinck, and A. Venerando (eds.). S. Karger, Basel, 1980, pp. 97–101.
29. Haymes, E. Metabolism and performance. In: *Sports Science Perspectives for Women*. J. Puhl, C.H. Brown, and R.O. Voy (eds.). Human Kinetics Publishers, Champaign, IL, 1988, pp. 85–95.
30. Berg, A. and Keul, J. Physiological and metabolic responses of female athletes during laboratory and field exercise. In: *Women and Sport. An Historical, Biological, Physiological and Sportsmedical Approach*. J. Borms, M. Hebbelinck, and A. Venerando (eds.). S. Karger, Basel, 1980, pp. 77–96.
31. Shephard, R.J., Bouhlel, E., Vandewalle, H., and Monod, H. Anaerobic threshold, muscle volume and hypoxia. *Eur. J. Appl. Physiol*. 58, 826–832, 1989.
32. Wilmore, J.H. Alterations in strength, body composition and anthropometry measurements consequent to a 10-week training program. *Med. Sci. Sports* 6, 133–138, 1974.
33. Brown, C.H. and Wilmore, J.H. The effects of maximal resistance training on the strength and body composition of women athletes. *Med. Sci. Sports* 6, 174–177, 1974.
34. Oyster, N. Effects of heavy-resistance weight training program on college women athletes. *J. Sports Med. Phys. Fitness* 19, 79–83, 1979.
35. Greendorfer, S.L. and Brundage, C.L. Gender differences in children's motor skills. In: *Sports Women*. M.J. Adrian (ed.). S. Karger, Basel, 1987, pp. 125–137.
36. Wright, G.R. and Shephard, R.J. Brake reaction time — effects of age, sex and carbon monoxide. *Arch. Env. Health* 33, 141–150, 1978.
37. Yandell, K.M. and Spirduso, W.W. Sex and athletic status as factors in reaction latency and movement time. *Res. Q*. 52, 495–504, 1981.
38. Wyndham, C.H., Morrison, J.F., Williams, C.G., Bredell, G.A.G., Peter, J., von Rahden, M.J.E., Holdsworth, L.D., van Graan, C.H., van Rensburg, A.J., and Munro, A. Physiological reactions to cold of Caucasian females. *J. Appl. Physiol*. 19, 877–880, 1964.
39. Pugh, L.G.C.E., Edholm, O.G., Fox, R.H., Wolff, H.S., Harvey, G.R., Hammond, W.H., Tanner, J.M., and Whitehouse, R.H. A physiological study of channel swimming. *Clin. Sci*. 19, 257–273, 1960.
40. Kollias, J., Bartlett, L., Bergsteinova, V., Skinner, J.S., Buskirk, E.R., and Nicholas, W.C. Metabolic and thermal responses of women during cooling in water. *J. Appl. Physiol*. 36, 577–580, 1974.
41. Graham, T.E. Alcohol ingestion and sex differences on the thermal responses to mild exercise in a cold environment. *Hum. Biol*. 55, 463–476, 1983.
42. Sloan, R.E.G. and Keatinge, W.R. Cooling rates of young people swimming in cold water. *J. Appl. Physiol*. 35, 371–375, 1973.
43. Cunningham, D.J., Stolwijk, J.A.J., and Wenger, C.B. Comparative thermoregulatory responses of resting men and women. *J. Appl. Physiol*. 45, 908–915, 1978.
44. Shephard, R.J. Metabolic adaptations to exercise in the cold: an update. *Sports Med*. 16, 266–289, 1993.
45. Avellini, B.A., Kamon, E., and Krajewski, J.T. Physiological responses of physically fit men and women to acclimation to humid heat. *J. Appl. Physiol*. 49, 254–261, 1980.
46. Wells, C.L. Responses of physically active and acclimatized men and women to exercise in a desert environment. *Med. Sci. Sports Exercise* 12, 9–13, 1980.
47. Horstman, D.H. and Christensen, E. Acclimatization to dry heat: active men vs. active women. *J. Appl. Physiol*. 52, 825–831, 1982.
48. Horvath, S.M. and Drinkwater, B. Thermoregulation and the menstrual cycle. *Aviat. Space Environ. Med*. 53, 790–794, 1982.
49. Schoene, R.B., Robertson, H.T., Pierson, D.J., and Peterson, A.P. Respiratory drives and exercise in menstrual cycles of athletic and non–athletic women. *J. Appl. Physiol*. 50, 1300–1305, 1981.

50. Dalton, K. and Williams, J.G.P. Women in sport. In: *Sports Medicine* (2nd Ed.). J.G.P. Williams and P. Sperryn (eds.). Edward Arnold, London, 1976, pp. 200–225.

51. Zimmerman, E. and Parlee, M.B. Behavioural changes associated with the menstrual cycle; an experimental investigation. *J. Appl. Soc. Psychol.* 3, 335–344, 1973.

52. Anderson, J.L. Women's sports and fitness programs at the U.S. Military Academy. *Phys. Sportsmed.* 7(4), 72–80, 1979.

53. Frisch, R.E., Wyshak, G., and Vincent, L. Delayed menarche and amenorrhea in ballet dancers. *N. Engl. J. Med.* 303, 17–19, 1980.

54. Rippon, C., Nash, J., Myburgh, K.H., and Noakes, T.D. Abnormal eating attitude test scores predict menstrual dysfunction lean females. *Int. J. Eating Disorders* 7, 617–624, 1988.

55. Malina, R.M., Spirduso, W.W., Tate, C., and Baylor, A.M. Age at menarche and selected menstrual characteristics in athletes at different competitive levels and in different sports. *Med. Sci. Sports* 10, 218–222, 1978.

56. Prior, J.L. Reversible reproductive changes with endurance training. In: *Endurance in Sport.* R.J. Shephard and P.O. Åstrand (eds.). Blackwell Scientific Publications, Oxford, 1992, pp. 365–373.

57. Drinkwater, B.L., Bruemmer, B., and Chestnut, C.H. Menstrual history as a determinant of current bone density in young athletes. *J. Am. Med. Assoc.* 263, 545–548, 1990.

58. Wolffe, A., Brenner, I.K.M., and Mottola, M.F. Maternal exercise, fetal well-being and pregnancy outcome. *Ex. Sport Sci. Rev.* 22, 145–194, 1994.

59. Wong, S.C. and McKenzie, D.C. Cardiorespiratory fitness during pregnancy and its effect on outcome. *Int. J. Sports Med.* 8, 79–83, 1987.

60. Hall, D.C. and Kaufmann, D.A. Effects of aerobic and strength conditioning on pregnancy outcomes. *Am. J. Obstet. Gynecol.* 157, 1199–1203, 1987.

61. Clapp, J.F.I. and Dickstein, S. Endurance exercise and pregnancy outcome. *Med. Sci. Sports Exercise* 16, 556–562, 1984.

62. McKenzie, D.C. Pregnant women and endurance exercise. In: *Endurance in Sport.* R.J. Shephard and P.O. Åstrand (eds.). Blackwell Scientific Publications, Oxford, 1992, pp. 385–389.

63. Berry, M.J., McMurray, R.G., and Katz, V.L. Pulmonary and ventilatory responses in pregnancy, immersion and exercise. *J. Appl. Physiol.* 66, 857–862, 1989.

64. Leaf, D.A. Exercise during pregnancy: guidelines and controversies. *Postgrad. Med. J.* 85, 233–238, 1989.

65. Carpenter, M.W., Sady, S.P., Hoegsberg, B., Sady, M.A., Haydon, B., Cullinane, E.M., Coustan, D.R., and Thompson, P.D. Fetal heart rate response to maternal exertion. *J. Am. Med. Assoc.* 259, 3006–3009, 1988.

66. Lotgering, F.K., Gilbert, R.D., and Longo, L.D. The interactions of exercise and pregnancy. *Am. J. Obstet. Gynecol.* 149, 560–568, 1984.

67. Clapp, J.F., Wesley, M., and Sleamaker, R.H. Thermoregulatory and metabolic responses to jogging prior to and during pregnancy. *Med. Sci. Sports Exercise* 19, 124–130, 1987.

68. Lovelady, C.A., Lonnedal, B., and Dewey, K.G. Lactation performance of exercising women. *Am. J. Clin. Nutr.* 52, 103–109, 1990.

69. Shelkun, P.H. Exercise and breast-feeding mothers. *Phys. Sportsmed.* 19, 109–116, 1991.

70. Klaus, E.J. and Noack, H. *Frau und Sport.* Thieme, Stüttgart, 1971.

71. Shock, N.W. Physical activity and the rate of ageing. *Can. Med. Assoc. J.* 96, 836–842, 1967.

72. Gompertz, B. On the nature of the function expressive of the law of human mortality and a new method of determining the value of life contingencies. *Phil. Trans. R. Soc. Lond.* A115, 513–585, 1825.

73. Kenyon, G., Birren, J.E., and Schroots, J.J.F. *Metaphors of Aging in Science and the Humanities.* Springer Publishing, New York, 1991.

74. Comfort, A. *Ageing. The Biology of Senescence.* 2nd Ed. Holt, Rinehart, Winston, New York, 1979.

75. Shephard, R.J. *Physical Activity and Aging.* 2nd Ed. Croom Helm Publishing, London, 1987.

76. Health and Welfare Canada. *Health Promotion Survey.* Health and Welfare, Canada, Ottawa, 1988.

77. Shephard, R.J. Fitness and aging. In: *Aging into the Twenty First Century.* C. Blais (ed.). Captus University Publications, Downsview, Ont., 1991, pp. 22–35.

78. Spasoff, R.A., McDowell, I., Wright, P.A., and Dunkeley, G. Reviewing Health Hazard appraisal. *Chronic Dis. Can.* 1, 16–17, 1980.

79. Shephard, R.J., Corey, P., and Cox, M. Health hazard appraisal — the influence of an employee fitness programme. *Can. J. Publ. Health* 73, 183–187, 1982.

80. Heikkinen, E. Normal aging. Definition, problems and relation to physical activity. In: *Recent Advances in Gerontology.* H. Orimo, K. Shimada, M. Iriki, and D. Maeda (eds.). Excerpta Medica, Amsterdam, 1979, pp. 501–503.

81. National Academy of Sciences, Committee on Dietary Allowances, Food and Nutrition Board. *Recommended Dietary Allowances.* National Academy of Sciences, Washington, D.C., 1980.

82. Daderup, L., Opdam-Stockman, V.A., and Reichsteiner de Vos, H. Basal metabolic rate, anthropometric, electrocardiographic and dietary data relating to elderly persons. *J. Gerontol.* 21, 22–26, 1966.

83. Durnin, J.V.G.A. Nutrition. In: *Textbook of Geriatric Medicine and Gerontology.* 2nd Ed. J.C. Brocklehurst (ed.). Churchill-Livingstone, Edinburgh, 1978, pp. 417–432.

84. Tiidus, P., Shephard, R.J., and Montelpare, W. Overall intake of energy and key nutrients: data for middle-aged and older middle-class adults. *Can. J. Sports Sci.* 14, 173–177, 1989.

85. Kasch, F.W., Wallace, J.P., Van Camp, S.P., and Verity, L. A longitudinal study of cardiovascular stability in active men aged 45 to 65 years. *Phys. Sportsmed.* 16(1), 117–126, 1988.

86. Shephard, R.J. The aging of cardiovascular function. In: *Academy Papers. Physical Activity and Aging.* W.W. Spirduso and H.M. Eckert (eds.). Champaign, IL, 1988, pp. 175–185.

87. Asmussen, E. and Molbech, S.V. Methods and standards for evaluation of the physiological working capacity of patients. Hellerup, Denmark: *Commun. Testing Obs. Inst.* 4, 1–16, 1959.

88. Sidney, K.H. and Shephard, R.J. Maximum and submaximum exercise tests in men and women in the seventh, eighth and ninth decades of life. *J. Appl. Physiol.* 43, 280–287, 1977.

89. Londeree, B.R. and Moeschberger, M.L. Effect of age and other factors on maximal heart rate. *Res. Q.* 53, 297–304, 1982.

90. Weisfeldt, M.L., Gerstenblith, M.L., and Lakatta, E.G. Alterations in circulatory function. In: *Principles of Geriatric Medicine.* R. Andres, E.L. Bierman, and W.R. Hazzard (eds.). McGraw Hill, New York, 1985, pp. 248–279.

91. Niinimaa, V. and Shephard, R.J. Training and exercise conductance in the elderly. (2). The cardiovascular system. *J. Gerontol.* 35, 672–682, 1978.

92. Åstrand, I. Degree of strain during building work as related to individual aerobic work capacity. *Ergonomics* 10, 293–303, 1967.

93. Bonjer, F.H. Relationship between working time, physical working capacity and allowable caloric expenditure. In: *Muskelarbeit und Muskeltraining.* W. Rohmert (ed.). Gentner Verlag, Darmstadt, 1968, pp. 86–98.

94. Hughes, A.L. and Goldman, R.F. Energy cost of hard work. *J. Appl. Physiol.* 29, 570–572, 1970.

95. Sidney, K.H. and Shephard, R.J. Frequency and intensity of exercise training for elderly subjects. *Med. Sci. Sports* 10, 125–131, 1978.

96. Pekkanen, J., Marti, B., Nissinen, A., Tuomilheto, J., Punsar, S., and Karvonen, M.J. Reduction of premature mortality by high physical activity: a 20-year follow-up of middle-aged Finnish men. *Lancet* 1, 1473–1477, 1987.

97. Fries, J. Aging, natural death and the compression of morbidity. *N. Engl. J. Med.* 303, 130–135, 1980.

98. Shephard, R.J. and Montelpare, W. Geriatric benefits of exercise as an adult. *J. Gerontol. (Med. Sci.)* 43, M86–M90, 1988.

99. Davies, C.T.M. and White, M.J. Contractile properties of the elderly human triceps surae. Gerontology 29, 19–25, 1983.

100. Aoyagi, Y. and Shephard, R.J. Aging and muscle function. *Sports Med.* 14, 376–396, 1992.

101. McKelvey, R.S. and McCartney, N. Weightlifting training in cardiac patients: considerations. *Sports Med.* 10, 355–364, 1990.

102. Fiatarone, M.A., Marks, E.C., Ryan, N.D., Meredith, C.N., Lipsitz, L.A., and Evans, W.J. High intensity strength training in nonagenerians. Effects on skeletal muscle. *J. Am. Med. Assoc.* 263, 3029–3034, 1990.

103. Hall, D.A. Metabolic and structural aspects of aging. In: *Textbook of Geriatric Medicine and Gerontology.* 2nd Ed. J.C. Brocklehurst. Churchill-Livingstone, Edinburgh, 1978, pp. 452–461.

104. Smith, E.L., Smith, K.A., and Gilligan, C. Exercise, fitness, osteoarthritis and osteoporosis. In: *Exercise, Fitness and Health.* C. Bouchard, R.J. Shephard, T. Stephens, J. Sutton, and B. McPherson (eds.). Human Kinetics Publishers, Champaign, IL, 1990, pp. 517–528.

105. Chow, R., Harrison, J.E., and Notarius, C. Effect of two randomized exercise programmes on bone mass of healthy post-menopausal women. *Br. Med. J.* 295, 1441–1444, 1987.

106. Green, M.F. The endocrine system. In: *Principles and Practice of Geriatric Medicine.* M.S.J. Pathy (ed.). John Wiley, Chichester, 1985, pp. 909–973.

107. Vranic, M. and Wasserman, D. Exercise, fitness and diabetes. In: *Exercise, Fitness and Health.* C. Bouchard, R.J. Shephard, T. Stephens, J. Sutton, and B. McPherson (eds.). Human Kinetics Publishers, Champaign, IL, 1990, pp. 467–490.

108. Kavanagh, T., Lindley, L.J., Shephard, R.J., and Campbell, R. Health and socio-demographic characteristics of the Masters competitor. *Ann. Sports Med.* 4, 55–64, 1988.

109. Riegel, P.S. Athletic records and human endurance. *Am. Sci.* 69, 285–290, 1981.

110. Stones, M.J. and Kozma, A. Adult age trends in athletic performance. *Exp. Aging Res.* 6, 269–280, 1980.

111. Lehman, H.C. *Age and Achievement.* Oxford University Press, New York, 1953.

112. Hebbelinck, M. Kinanthropometry and aging: morphological, structural, body mechanics and motor fitness aspects of aging. In: *Physical Activity and Human Well-Being.* F. Landry and W.A.R. Orban (eds.). Symposia Specialists, Miami, 1978, pp. 95–110.

113. Shephard, R.J. Sudden death — a significant hazard of exercise? *Br. J. Sports Med.* 8, 101–110, 1974.

114. Cooper, K.H. Guidelines in the management of the exercising patient. *J. Am. Med. Assoc.* 211, 1663–1667, 1970.

115. Shephard, R.J. Can we identify those for whom exercise is hazardous? *Sports Med.* 1, 99–124, 1984.

116. Siscovick, D.S. Risks of exercising: sudden cardiac death and injuries. In: *Exercise, Fitness and Health.* C. Bouchard, R.J. Shephard, T. Stephens, J. Sutton, and R.B. McPherson. Human Kinetics Publishers, Champaign, IL, 1990, pp. 707–713.

117. Vuori, I., Suurnakki, L., and Suurnakki, T. Risks of sudden cardiovascular death (SCVD) in exercise. *Med. Sci. Sports Exercise.* 14, 114–115, 1982.

118. Pascale, M. and Grana, W.A. Does running cause osteoarthritis? *Phys. Sportsmed.* 17(3), 157–166, 1989.

119. McNamara, P.S., Otto, R.M., and Smith, T.K. The acute response to simulated bicycle and rowing exercise on the elderly population. *Med. Sci. Sports Exercise.* 17, 266, 1985.

Chapter 6

Cardiovascular Response to Exercise in Normal Persons and in Patients with Myocardial Ischemia

Ray W. Squires

CONTENTS

I. INTRODUCTION

A properly functioning cardiovascular system is crucial for the performance of exercise that persists for more than several seconds. The major functions of the cardiovascular system during exercise include:

1. Oxygen delivery to the active skeletal muscle at a rate necessary for the aerobic metabolic processes,
2. Carbon dioxide clearance from contracting skeletal muscle,
3. Transfer and dissipation of metabolic heat, and
4. Transport of endocrine substances used in the regulation of the various systems during exercise from sites of production to the target tissues.[1]

In health, the cardiovascular system responds to the complex demands of exercise in a coordinated and precise fashion and may greatly increase oxygen delivery to the exercising skeletal muscle. Oxygen

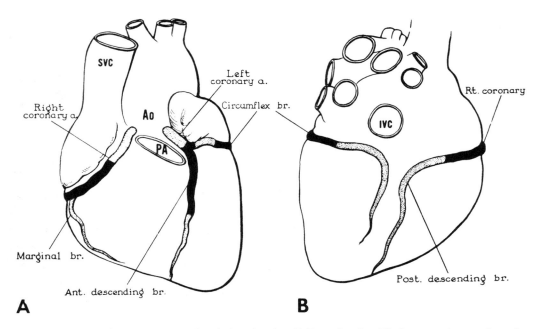

Figure 1   The epicardial coronary arteries. A. Anterior view. B. Posterior view. Black segments are prime sites for the development of obstructive atherosclerotic lesions. Ao = aorta, IVC = inferior vena cava, SVC = superior vena cava, PA = pulmonary artery. (From Lie, J. T., in Giuliani, E. R., Fuster, V., Gersh, B. J., McGoon, M. D., and McGoon, D. C., *Cardiology: Fundamentals and Practice*, 2nd ed., Mosby Yearbook, Chicago, 1991, ch. 34. With permission.)

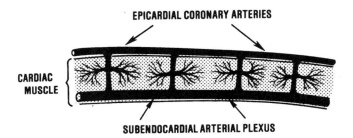

Figure 2   Structure of the intramyocardial and subendocardial coronary arteries in relation to the epicardial arteries. (From Guyton, A. C., *Textbook of Medical Physiology*, 7th ed., W.B. Saunders, Philadelphia, 1986, ch. 25. With permission.)

uptake at the mouth may increase 10 to 20 times the rate at rest during strenuous exercise. Exercise represents the greatest challenge to the capacity of the cardiovascular system.

In patients with coronary artery disease, insufficient blood flow (ischemia) to the myocardium may result in an abnormal response to acute and chronic exercise. The purpose of this chapter is to review the normal cardiovascular responses to exercise and highlight problems in cardiovascular function resulting from ischemia.

II. MYOCARDIAL BLOOD SUPPLY AND METABOLISM

The heart is a highly aerobic organ, under normal conditions, with an extensive circulatory system and an abundance of mitochondria.[2] The coronary arterial system is well developed and includes epicardial arteries (Figure 1) which bifurcate into intramyocardial and endocardial branches (Figure 2). Coronary blood flow is closely regulated to the need of the myocardium for oxygen. At rest, coronary blood flow averages 60 to 90 ml/min per 100 g of muscle and may increase five- to sixfold during exercise.[3] In normal persons, the proximal coronary arteries dilate during aerobic exercise.[4]

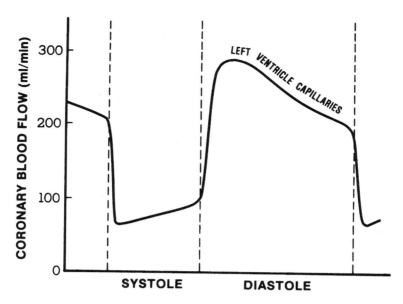

Figure 3 Left ventricular coronary artery blood flow during systole and diastole. (From Guyton, A. C., *Textbook of Medical Physiology*, 7th ed., W.B. Saunders, Philadelphia, 1986, ch. 25. With permission.)

Blood flow through any regional circulation is determined by arterial blood pressure and the resistance to the flow of blood offered by the vasculature, primarily the arterioles, which may change caliber and dramatically alter the resistance to flow. Coronary vascular resistance, and hence blood flow, is regulated by mechanical factors, the autonomic nervous system and local metabolic factors.[5]

During ventricular (systole) contraction, increased intramyocardial pressure (mechanical pressure from myocardial contraction) compresses the arterial tree and reduces forward flow. During ventricular relaxation (diastole), intramyocardial pressure is reduced, coronary vascular resistance is lower, and the majority of left ventricular coronary blood flow takes place (Figure 3).[6]

Myocardial oxygen needs are determined by the heart rate, the wall tension of the ventricles (wall tension is related to left ventricular pressure and volume of the ventricle at the end of diastole), and the degree of contractility (the forcefulness of the myocardial contraction).[2] Increased sympathetic nervous system activity during exercise leads to increased heart rate and contractility which augments the coronary blood flow in response to increased metabolic demand. The most powerful control of coronary blood flow comes from metabolic factors, such as the vasodilators adenosine, prostaglandins, and endothelium-derived relaxing factor, produced locally in the myocardium, the blood, or the endothelium (inner lining of cells found in blood vessels).[5]

Normal cardiac function depends on adequate concentrations of intramyocardial adenosine triphosphate (ATP). Under normal conditions at rest, the heart produces ATP aerobically (oxidative phosphorylation) and consumes 8 to 10 ml O_2 per 100 g of myocardium.[2] During exercise, the oxygen requirement may increase 200 to 300%. Free fatty acids are the predominant fuel (60 to 90% of energy production) with glucose, lactate, and amino acids serving as supplemental energy sources. Under aerobic conditions, the heart extracts lactate from the arterial blood for use in ATP regeneration.[2]

Unlike skeletal muscle, resting myocardium removes a very high percentage (70% extraction) of the available oxygen from arterial blood flowing through its capillary beds.[6] Because of this relative inability to further increase oxygen extraction, coronary blood flow must be closely regulated to the needs of the myocardium for oxygen. Thus, when the myocardial oxygen requirement is increased, as during exercise, coronary blood flow must rise to meet the demand.

III. CARDIOVASCULAR PHYSIOLOGY

Cardiac output ($\dot{Q}$) is the volume of blood ejected per minute by the left ventricle into the aorta.[6] The cardiac output is dependent on the amount of blood which flows from the great veins into the right atrium (venous return). Since the systemic and pulmonary circulations are in series, there exists interdependence between the left and right ventricles, and the output of the two ventricles is equal under

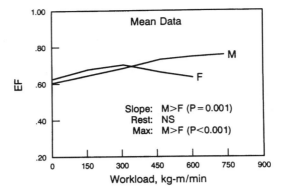

Figure 4 Gender differences in LVEF at rest and during supine exercise. (From Gibbons, R. J., *Circulation*, 84(Suppl. I), I93, 1991. With permission.)

normal circumstances.[7] At rest, cardiac output is approximately 4 to 6 l/min and may increase to 25 l/min or more during intense aerobic exercise. It is the product of stroke volume (SV, the volume of blood ejected by the left ventricle per beat) and heart rate (HR).

The cardiac cycle is composed of three events: diastasis — the period of time between beats when the heart is neither contracting nor relaxing; systole — atrial, then ventricular contraction; and diastole — atrial, then ventricular relaxation. During diastasis and most of diastole, the atrioventricular valves (mitral and tricuspid) are open and blood flows into the ventricles passively.[3,6] During atrial systole, an additional amount of blood enters the ventricles. The volume of blood in the left ventricle at the end of diastole, just prior to ventricular systole (the largest volume of blood in the ventricle), is the end-diastolic volume (EDV). At the end of systole, the blood volume of the ventricle is at its lowest and is called end-systolic volume (ESV). The difference between end-diastolic and end-systolic volume (EDV – ESV) is the stroke volume. Stroke volume is also the EDV multiplied by the left ventricular ejection fraction (LVEF, the percentage of the EDV ejected per beat) (LVEF × EDV). LVEF at rest is approximately 60% (normal range 55 to 70%) and usually increases or remains unchanged during exercise. Women generally have a flatter LVEF response to exercise than do men (Figure 4).[8]

Blood pressure changes occur in the cardiovascular system in response to systole and diastole and, aided by one-way valves in the heart and veins, cause forward flow of blood. Figure 5 describes the pressures in the aorta and in the left ventricle and atrium during the cardiac cycle under resting conditions. Peak systolic left ventricular and aortic pressures are approximately 120 mmHg at rest. The lowest diastolic pressures in the left ventricle and aorta are approximately 0 mmHg and 80 mmHg, respectively. Left atrial systolic pressure is less than 20 mmHg. Right heart pressures are much lower than for the left heart. Mean right atrial pressure is <5 mmHg. Right ventricular pressure is <25 mmHg during systole and <5 mmHg during diastole.[6,9] Figure 6 illustrates the changes in blood pressure during the cardiac cycle for the left ventricle, large and small arteries, capillaries, and the venous system. The pressure differences between systole and diastole gradually become dampened, and pressure gradually decreases as a result of resistance offered by the vasculature to the flow of blood. As noted, venous pressure is very low.

At the beginning of ventricular systole, the contraction of the left ventricle quickly increases ventricular pressure above that in the left atrium, and the mitral valve closes. (Figure 7 shows the heart valves: mitral, aortic, tricuspid, and pulmonic.) As systolic contraction continues, left ventricular pressure rises above the level in the aorta, the aortic valve opens, and blood is ejected from the heart into the aorta. At the beginning of ventricular diastole, pressure in the left ventricle decreases below that in the aorta and the aortic valve closes, ending the ejection phase of the cardiac cycle. As diastole continues, ventricular pressure falls below left atrial pressure and the mitral valve opens.

Cardiac output is dependent upon venous return. As mentioned previously, venous pressure is very low and venous return aids are critical in assisting with cardiac output regulation.[10] During inspiration, thoracic pressure decreases while intraabdominal pressure increases, and blood flow to the heart from the great veins is facilitated (respiratory pump). During rhythmic skeletal muscle contractions, venous pressure is increased and forward blood flow improved with the help of one-way venous valves (Figure 8, "muscle pump"). Finally, during exercise sympathetic nervous system activity is increased and causes

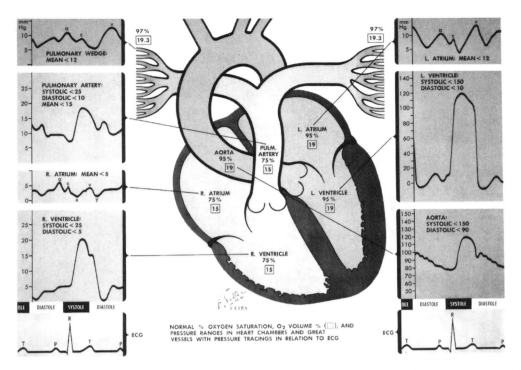

Figure 5 Pressures in the right (pulmonary artery, right atrium, right ventricle) and left (aorta, left atrium, left ventricle) heart during the cardiac cycle under resting conditions. Note the much lower pressures in the right heart. (From Netter, F. H. and Yonkman, F. F., *The Ciba Collection of Medical Illustrations, Volume 5: Heart,* Ciba, New York, 1978, 45. With permission.)

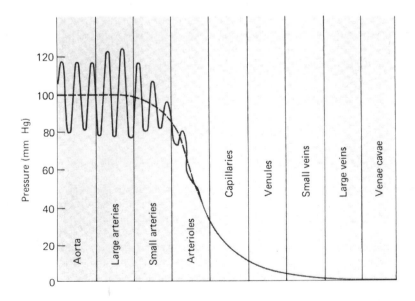

Figure 6 Blood pressures in various portions of the systemic circulation. Note the very low pressures found in the venous system. (From Guyton, A. C., *Textbook of Medical Physiology,* 7th ed., W.B. Saunders, Philadelphia, 1986, ch. 19. With permission.)

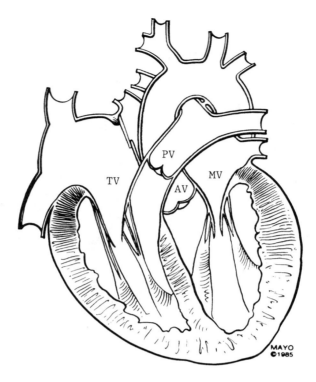

Figure 7   The cardiac valves. MV = mitral valve, AV = aortic valve, TV = tricuspid valve, PV = pulmonic valve. (From the Mayo Clinic Department of Medical Illustration. With permission.)

venoconstriction (venous vascular smooth muscle contraction) and a higher venous pressure which increases venous return.

Increased venous return results in a higher filling pressure in the ventricles which, in turn, results in a greater stroke volume.[11] The diastolic function of the left ventricle (the ability of the ventricle to accept venous blood) depends upon the compliance of the ventricle (the capacity to stretch and enlarge in response to a given filling pressure). In general, the higher the venous return and hence the EDV and end-diastolic pressure (termed preload), the greater the forcefulness of contraction (contractility). This is in accordance with the Frank–Starling mechanism whereby a greater amount of stretch on the myocytes (increased end-diastolic fiber length) results in a more forceful contraction and stroke volume.[6]

Another important factor determining cardiac output is the impedance or resistance offered by the circulation to the ejection of blood from the heart (afterload).[11] Total peripheral resistance, as reflected by aortic diastolic pressure, is an index of afterload.

IV. OXYGEN TRANSPORT DURING EXERCISE: NORMAL PERSONS

Oxygen transport is dependent on adequate gas exchange in the lungs, delivery of oxygen by the blood, and removal of oxygen by metabolically active tissues. Under normal conditions and in the absence of pulmonary disease, gas exchange in the lung (adequate lung function) does not limit oxygen transport.[10] For most persons, at maximal exercise a substantial breathing reserve is present (breathing reserve = difference between maximal voluntary ventilation and exercise minute ventilation).[12] Some athletic individuals do reach the capacity of their pulmonary system for gas exchange during intense aerobic exercise as indicated by a low breathing reserve and mild arterial desaturation.[13]

Maximal oxygen uptake ($\dot{V}O_2$max) (Figure 9) is the best single measure of the capacity of the cardiovascular system to respond to aerobic exercise. The Fick equation provides the components of the cardiovascular system which are crucial for proper oxygen delivery: oxygen uptake = cardiac output × arterial-mixed venous oxygen difference ($\dot{V}O_2 = HR \times SV \times a\text{-}\bar{v}O_2$ Diff).[14,15] Figure 10 provides estimates of the relative changes in the Fick equation variables during exercise in healthy persons. For an oxygen uptake of 10 times resting level, cardiac output doubles (increased heart rate and stroke volume), and

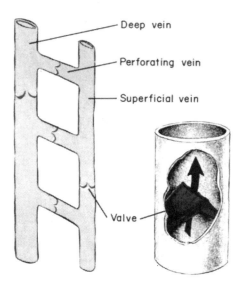

Figure 8 The venous valves of the lower extremity which aid in return of blood to the heart. (From Guyton, A. C., *Textbook of Medical Physiology*, 7th ed., W.B. Saunders, Philadelphia, 1986, ch. 19. With permission.)

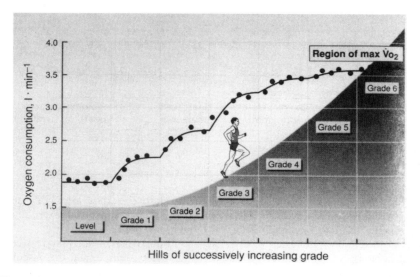

Figure 9 Plateau in oxygen uptake during incremental exercise indicating attainment of maximal oxygen uptake. (From McArdle, W. D., Katch, F. I., and Katch, V. L., *Exercise Physiology: Energy, Nutrition, and Human Performance*, 3rd ed., Lea and Febiger, Philadelphia, 1991, ch. 7. With permission.)

a-$\bar{v}O_2$ Diff increases by approximately 2.3 times. Table 1 gives typical values for oxygen transport system variables at rest and during maximal exercise for a normal man.

EDV increases during the early stages of graded aerobic exercise and may decrease slightly at higher intensities of exercise. LVEF increases during aerobic exercise resulting in a decrease in ESV (Figure 11).[16] As a result of these changes in ventricular volume and contractility, stroke volume changes during exercise. Stroke volume increases rapidly during the initial stages of upright graded exercise testing with a slower rate of increase at intensities requiring more than 50% of $\dot{V}O_2$max.[17] At higher exercise intensities, stroke volume may plateau or decrease slightly (Figure 12).[18]

Heart rate increases (chronotropic response) in a near linear fashion with increasing exercise intensity (Figure 13) with peak exercise heart rates dependent upon age.[1] A typical maximal heart rate is estimated by the equation 220 beats/min – age (years) with a standard deviation of approximately 10 beats/min. As a result of the increased stroke volume and heart rate, cardiac output climbs as exercise intensity

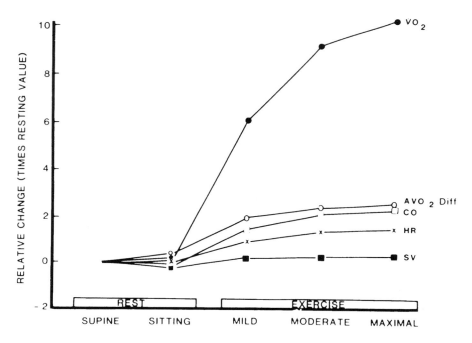

Figure 10 The relative changes in the Fick equation variables for an exercise intensity of 10 METs (multiples of resting metabolic rate). (From Hossack, K. F., *Cardiol. Clin.*, 251, H1101, 1986. With permission.)

Table 1 Oxygen Transport Variables at Rest and During Maximal Exercise in a Normal Male Subject

	Oxygen Uptake (ml/min)	Heart Rate (beats/min)	Stroke Volume (ml/beat)	a-$\bar{v}O_2$ Diff (ml/dl blood)
Sitting rest	300	75	75	5.2
Maximal upright exercise	3000	190	100	15.8

Source: From Sutton, J. R., *Sports Med.*, 13, 127, 1992. With permission.

increases (Figure 14). Cardiac output and oxygen uptake during exercise are highly correlated, and oxygen uptake during exercise serves as an index of cardiac output response to exercise (Figure 15).[19] Cardiac output is the "central" circulatory factor in oxygen transport.

Regulation of the cardiovascular response to exercise results from an interplay between the central and peripheral nervous systems and receptors located in skeletal muscle and the vasculature (Figure 16).[20] At the onset of exercise, motor cortex neural activity to the active skeletal musculature also irradiates the cardiovascular center in the brain stem. This parallel activation of both the skeletal muscle motor systems and the cardiovascular system is termed *central command*.[21]

At the same time, input from peripheral receptors (baroreceptors, chemoreceptors, stretch receptors) travels the spinal column to the cardiovascular center.[22] The net result is a change in the autonomic nervous system with a decrease in parasympathetic and an increase in sympathetic activity. Increased adrenal gland stimulation results in release of norepinephrine and epinephrine.

Neurohormonal control of heart rate and stroke volume is accomplished by the autonomic nervous system (parasympathetic and sympathetic divisions) and circulating catecholamines (epinephrine, nore-pinephrine).[23] At rest, parasympathetic nervous system activity is dominant and suppresses the heart rate below the inherent rate of the sinoatrial node. At the onset of exercise, heart rate increases because of withdrawal of parasympathetic tone and increased sympathetic nervous system activity mediated by beta receptors in the heart. After a few minutes of exercise, circulating catecholamines assist in elevating the exercise heart rate. Sympathetic nervous system activity and catecholamines increase myocardial contractility and enhance stroke volume.[10]

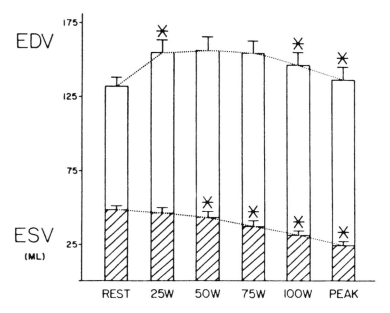

Figure 11 The changes in EDVs and ESVs during progressive cycle ergometer exercise. The difference between the EDV and ESV is the stroke volume. The percentage of the EDV ejected during systole is the LVEF. (From Plotnick, G. D. et al., *Am. J. Physiol.*, 251, H1101, 1986. With permission.)

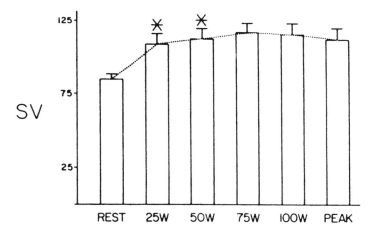

Figure 12 Stroke volume (SV) during progressive upright cycle ergometer exercise. (From Plotnick, G. D. et al., *Am. J. Physiol.*, 251, H1101, 1986. With permission.)

"Peripheral" circulatory function during exercise is represented by the a-$\bar{v}O_2$ Diff which indicates the amount of oxygen extracted from the blood by the metabolically active tissues.[1,24] The a-$\bar{v}O_2$ Diff is more "fixed" than cardiac output in that the differences from person to person in this variable are relatively small when compared with interindividual differences in cardiac output. As exercise becomes progressively more intense, a-$\bar{v}O_2$ Diff increases in a near linear fashion (Figure 17).

Arterial oxygen content (CaO_2) and mixed venous oxygen content ($C\bar{v}O_2$) are the determinants of a-$\bar{v}O_2$ Diff.[6,24] CaO_2 is determined by the hemoglobin (Hb) concentration (1.34 ml O_2 transported per gram Hb), and the saturation of Hb with oxygen which is a function of diffusion of oxygen into the capillary blood in the lung (dependent upon adequate ventilation of the lungs, diffusion capacity for O_2, and maintenance of the partial pressure of O_2 in the arterial blood). The relationship of arterial partial pressure of O_2 and Hb saturation with O_2 is given by the oxyhemoglobin dissociation curve (Figure 18). For

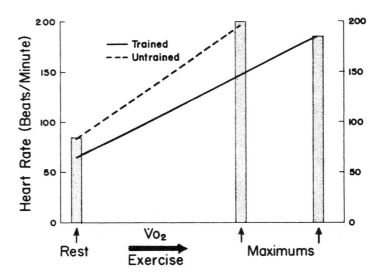

Figure 13 Heart rate during progressive exercise before and after an exercise training program. (From Mathews, D. K. and Fox, E. L., *The Physiological Basis of Physical Education and Athletics*, 2nd ed., W.B. Saunders, Philadelphia, 1976, ch. 10. With permission.)

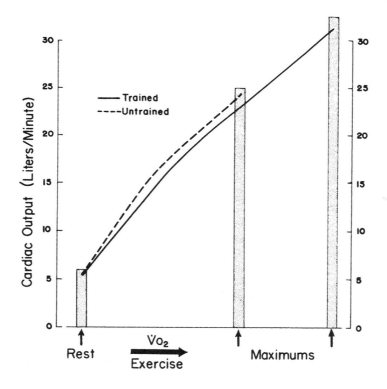

Figure 14 Cardiac output during graded exercise before and after an exercise training program. (From Mathews, D. K. and Fox, E. L., *The Physiological Basis of Physical Education and Athletics*, 2nd ed., W.B. Saunders, Philadelphia, 1976, ch. 10. With permission.)

normal Hb concentrations and arterial saturations with oxygen, CaO_2 ranges from 15 to 22 ml O_2 per 100 ml blood. During acute exercise, plasma volume decreases slightly while the total Hb amount remains stable. This "hemoconcentration" results in a slightly higher Hb concentration and CaO_2 during exercise than at rest (Figure 19).

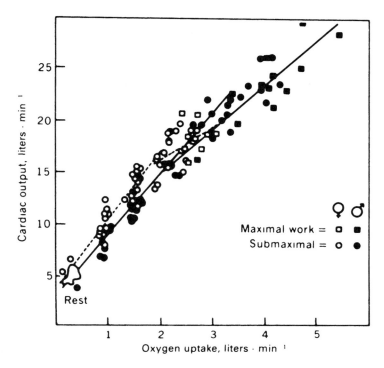

Figure 15 The relationship of cardiac output and oxygen uptake at rest, during submaximal exercise, and for maximal exercise. (From Åstrand, P. O. and Rodahl, K., *Textbook of Work Physiology: Physiological Bases of Exercise,* 3rd ed., McGraw Hill, New York, 1986, ch.4. With permission.)

$C\bar{v}O_2$ is determined by the amount of blood flowing through the metabolically active tissues and the capacity of the tissues to extract oxygen from the capillary blood.[10,24] During exercise, cardiac output increases, as discussed previously. There is also a redistribution of the cardiac output away from metabolically less-active (splanchnic, renal, hepatic, nonexercising skeletal muscle circulatory beds) to more-active tissues (exercising skeletal muscle, heart, skin). This is illustrated in Figure 20. Thus, systemic cardiac output is directed to the areas of greatest need for nutritive blood flow. For example, at rest approximately 18% of the cardiac output flows through leg musculature compared with 84% at peak cycle ergometer exercise.[15] The blood flow through active skeletal muscle is the "effective" blood flow. Blood flow is proportional to the mean arterial pressure divided by the vascular resistance. During progressively more intense aerobic exercise, sympathetic nervous system activity gradually increases resulting in norepinephrine-mediated vasoconstriction (increased vascular resistance) in the less metabolically active regional circulations. This effectively reduces flow in these regions. At the same time, local metabolic factors (low pH, increased carbon dioxide partial pressure, adenosine, potassium ions) and possibly sympathetic vasodilator fibers cause vasodilation in exercising skeletal muscle resulting in a large increase in muscle blood flow.[10,15,24] Total systemic vascular resistance decreases in an exponential pattern during exercise (Figure 21).

The capacity of the tissues to extract oxygen from the capillary blood is dependent upon the capillary density of the myofibers (the greater the capillary density, the larger the area for diffusion of oxygen into the skeletal muscle), and the amount and size of mitochondria in the myofibers (greater aerobic enzyme activity and capacity to utilize oxygen for the aerobic metabolic production of ATP). During exercise, a shift in the oxyhemoglobin dissociation curve due to increased muscle temperature, an increase in carbon dioxide partial pressure, and a decrease in pH (Bohr effect) enables more oxygen to be unloaded from Hb at a given partial pressure of oxygen (Figure 22).[10] $C\bar{v}O_2$ may reach 3 to 4 ml O_2 per 100 ml blood at peak exercise yielding a-$\bar{v}O_2$ Diff of 12 to 19 ml O_2 per 100 ml blood. Figure 19 shows the arterial oxygen-carrying capacity, arterial oxygen content, mixed venous oxygen content and a-$\bar{v}O_2$ Diff during progressive exercise for a typical man and woman. Note that arterial capacity increases slightly during exercise but arterial content remains almost constant. Hb saturation with oxygen decreases from approximately 98% at rest to 92% during maximal exercise. Table 2 gives typical values for oxygen

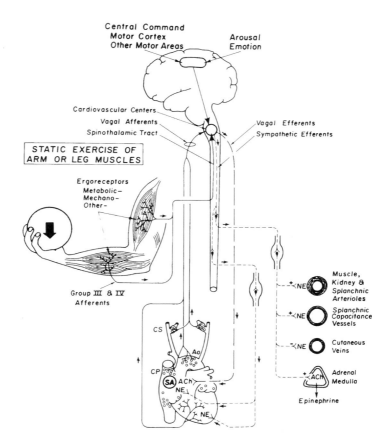

Figure 16 Nervous system pathways and factors involved in the control of the cardiovascular system during exercise. CS and Ao = baroreceptors of the carotid and aortic arch, SA = sinoatrial node, NE = norepinephrine, ACh = acetylcholine, CP = cardiopulmonary baroreceptors. (From Shepherd, J. T. et al., *Circ. Res.,* 48 (Suppl. I), I-179, 1981. With permission.)

transport variables for a normal individual, an athlete, and a patient with coronary artery disease during maximal exercise.

During progressive aerobic exercise, cardiac output increases in a near linear fashion as mentioned previously. Even though total peripheral vascular resistance decreases, systolic and mean blood pressure progressively increase while diastolic blood pressure does not change appreciably (Figure 23). However, diastolic blood pressure may increase during cycle ergometer exercise because of the isometric contraction of the forearms as the subject holds on to the handlebars. During exercise, baroreceptors are "reset" to a higher level to allow a higher blood pressure. [20,21] Table 3 provides average systolic and diastolic blood pressures for maximal treadmill exercise for men and women of various ages. If exercise intensity decreases, as during a cool-down period after a graded exercise test, systolic blood pressure decreases.

V. CORONARY ARTERY DISEASE AND ISCHEMIA

Atherosclerosis is a pathological phenomenon which may result in obstructive lesions in the coronary and other relatively large arteries.[25] The disease is a multifactorial process, and many risk factors have been identified, such as cigarette smoking, an adverse blood lipid profile, hypertension, genetic predisposition, diabetes mellitus, sedentary life-style, psychological disturbance, male gender, and obesity. Coronary atherosclerosis (coronary artery disease) tends to affect vessels in a diffuse manner with occasional discrete, localized areas of more–pronounced narrowing which may produce obstruction to blood flow.

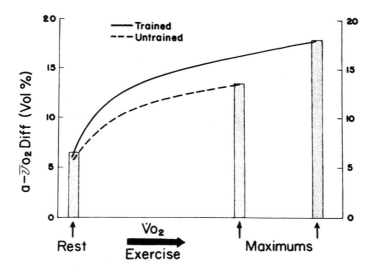

Figure 17 Arterial-mixed difference oxygen difference during progressive exercise before and after an exercise training program. (From Mathews, D. K. and Fox, E. L., *The Physiological Basis of Physical Education and Athletics*, 2nd ed., W.B. Saunders, Philadelphia, 1976, ch. 9. With permission.)

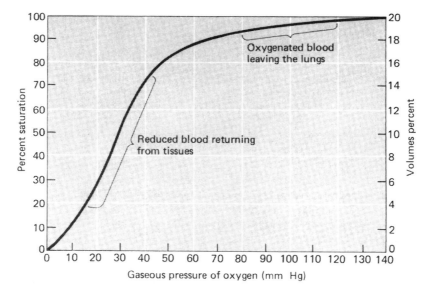

Figure 18 The oxyhemoglobin dissociation curve. (From Guyton, A. C., *Textbook of Medical Physiology*, 7th ed., W.B. Saunders, Philadelphia, 1986, ch. 41. With permission.)

A substantial reduction in vessel internal diameter may occur before a decrease in resting blood flow can be measured distal to the narrowed coronary artery segment. When the stenosis reduces the luminal cross-sectional area by 75% or more, blood flow through the artery will be reduced under resting conditions.[5] Beyond this level of critical stenosis, further small decreases in cross-sectional area will result in abrupt reductions in flow (Figure 24). The reduction in cross-sectional area of the artery may be caused by atherosclerosis alone or in concert with platelet aggregation leading to thrombus formation and/or vasospasm (contraction of vascular smooth muscle in the epicardial coronary arteries which decreases the cross-sectional area of the vessel).

Ischemia is defined as blood flow inadequate (decreased perfusion) to supply oxygen and nutrients for the metabolic needs of the myocardium.[2,3] It results in oxygen deprivation accompanied by inadequate removal of metabolites. Three physiological abnormalities result from ischemia:

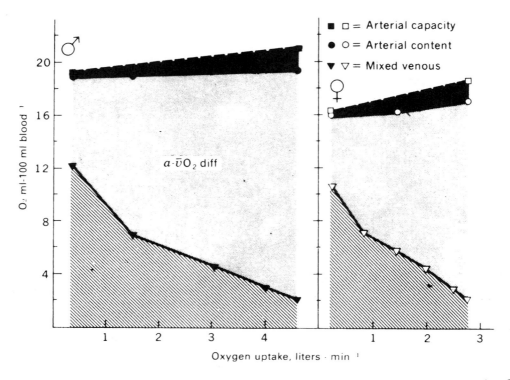

Figure 19 Arterial oxygen carrying capacity, arterial oxygen content, mixed venous oxygen content and a-vO$_2$ Diff during graded exercise to maximal levels for women and men. The arterial capacity and content increase during exercise because of a small reduction in plasma volume (hemoconcentration). (From Åstrand, P. O. and Rodahl, K., *Textbook of Work Physiology: Physiological Bases of Exercise*, 3rd ed., McGraw Hill, New York, 1986, ch. 4. With permission.)

1. Hypoxia-insufficient oxygen for the needs of aerobic metabolism,
2. Accumulation of toxic metabolites, and
3. Development of acidosis.

Hypoxia inhibits aerobic metabolism and the intracellular stores of ATP become depleted. This results in a shift from aerobic to anaerobic production of ATP with metabolism of carbohydrate as the predominant fuel with a marked increase in the production of lactic acid. Under ischemic conditions, the heart releases lactate into the venous blood.

Ischemia may result in progressive abnormalities in cardiac function referred to as the "ischemic cascade."[26] The first abnormality is a stiffening of the left ventricle, which decreases the ability of the chamber to fill with blood during diastole (diastolic dysfunction).[27] Second, systolic emptying of the left ventricle becomes impaired. Localized areas of the heart which are ischemic may develop asynergic contraction patterns such as hypokinesis (reduced systolic contraction), akinesis (absent contraction), or dyskinesis (paradoxical aneurysmic bulging of the segment of myocardium during contraction).[25] Under normal conditions, the ventricular myocytes shorten during systole and cause the walls to thicken and move inward as contraction continues. During ischemia, systolic functions may become abnormal with the development of segmental wall motion abnormalities, and reduction in left ventricular ejection fraction and stroke volume. Third, electrocardiographic changes associated with altered repolarization (ST segment elevation or depression, T wave inversion or pseudonormalization) occur as a result of nonuniform repolarization through the ischemic and surrounding normal tissue. Ischemia may initiate ventricular arrhythmias. Finally, the patient may develop symptoms such as angina pectoris.

Impairment of ventricular contraction and relaxation due to myocardial ischemia may result in elevated left ventricular filling pressures.[11] A back pressure in the pulmonary circulation leading to pulmonary congestion and dyspnea (air "hunger") may result.

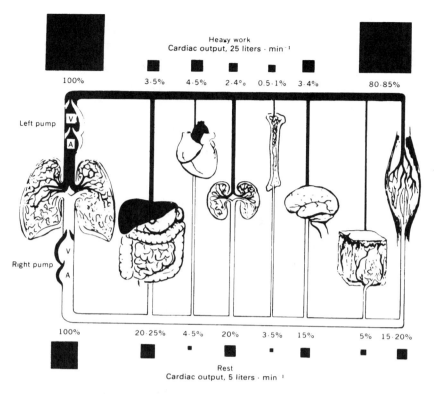

Figure 20 Schematic drawing showing the distribution of the cardiac output at rest and during intensive exercise. The cardiac output increased fivefold during exercise and the regional distribution of cardiac output favored the exercising skeletal muscle and skin at the expense of gastrointestinal and renal circulations. (From Åstrand, P. O. and Rodahl, K., *Textbook of Work Physiology: Physiological Bases of Exercise,* 3rd ed., McGraw Hill, New York, 1986, ch. 4. With permission.)

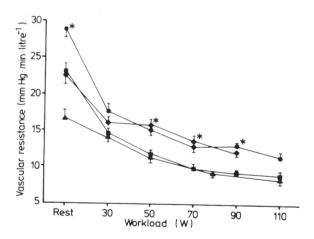

Figure 21 Total peripheral vascular resistance during graded upright cycle ergometer exercise in patients after myocardial infarction. (From Hetherington, M. et al., *Card. Res.,* 21, 399, 1987. With permission.)

If the episode of myocardial ischemia is brief, the abnormalities in cardiac function described above are reversible. With prolonged ischemia, myocyte necrosis (irreversible damage) may occur and is termed *myocardial infarction.*[2] If ischemia is prolonged but not severe enough to result in myocyte necrosis, chronic but reversible left ventricular contraction abnormalities may result (stunned or hybernating

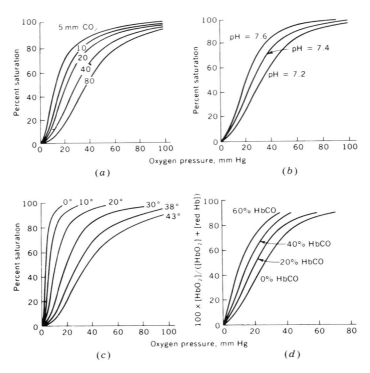

Figure 22 The effects of carbon dioxide (a), pH (b), temperature (c), and carbon monoxide (d) on the oxyhemoglobin dissociation curve. Percent saturation = percent hemoglobin saturation with oxygen. (From Åstrand, P. O. and Rodahl, K. *Textbook of Work Physiology: Physiological Bases of Exercise,* 3rd ed., McGraw Hill, New York, 1986, ch. 4. With permission.)

Table 2 Maximal Exercise Oxygen Transport Variables for a Patient with Significant Coronary Artery Disease, a Normal Untrained Subject, and a Well-Trained Endurance Athlete

	Oxygen Uptake (ml/min)	Heart Rate (beats/min)	Stroke Volume (ml/beat)	Cardiac Output (l/min)	a-$\bar{v}O_2$ Diff (ml/dl)
Patient	1500	175	50	8.8	17.0
Normal subject	3000	190	100	19.0	15.8
Endurance athlete	5600	180	180	32.5	17.0

Source: From Sutton, J. R., *Sports Med.,* 13, 127, 1992. With permission.

myocardium). More specific information regarding the effects of ischemia on myocardial performance during exercise will come later in the chapter.

VI. OXYGEN TRANSPORT SYSTEM IN PATIENTS WITH MYOCARDIAL ISCHEMIA

Myocardial ischemia may cause derangement in some or all of the components of the oxygen transport system. Not all patients with exercise-induced ischemia will have compromised oxygen transport, however. The amount of myocardium involved and the severity of the ischemia determine the effect on oxygen transport. In addition, some of the medications used in the treatment of coronary artery disease, such as beta and some calcium channel blockers, may reduce exercise heart rate and blood pressure.

The most apparent result of impaired oxygen transport is a reduction in aerobic capacity ($\dot{V}O_2$max). The magnitude of the impairment is highly variable. For patients with a history of myocardial infarction, infarct size does correlate positively with exercise capacity.[28] During incremental submaximal exercise, oxygen uptake may be lower for a given exercise intensity for patients with ischemia than for normal persons.[29] The time required for oxygen transport to increase to the level required by submaximal exercise may be prolonged.[30] Thus, these patients are more reliant on anaerobic energy production during exercise than are normal persons.

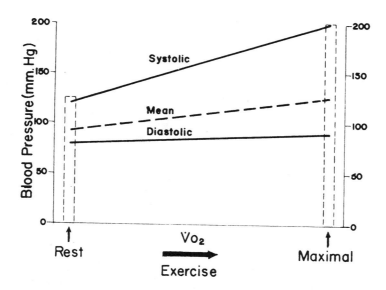

Figure 23 Blood pressure changes during progressive exercise. (From Mathews, D. K. and Fox, E. L., *The Physiological Basis of Physical Education and Athletics*, 2nd ed., W.B. Saunders, Philadelphia, 1976, ch. 10. With permission.)

Table 3 Mean Peak (±SD) Blood Pressures (mmHg) during Treadmill Exercise

Age Group (years)	Men Systolic	Men Diastolic	Women Systolic	Women Diastolic
18–29	182 ± 22	69 ± 13	155 ± 19	67 ± 12
30–39	182 ± 20	76 ± 12	158 ± 20	72 ± 12
40–49	186 ± 22	78 ± 12	165 ± 22	76 ± 12
50–59	192 ± 22	82 ± 12	175 ± 23	78 ± 11
60–69	195 ± 23	83 ± 12	181 ± 23	79 ± 11
70–79	191 ± 27	81 ± 13	196 ± 23	83 ± 11

Source: From Allison, T. G., Squires, R. W., and Gau, G. T., *Circulation*, 80, II-246, 1989. With permission.

In patients with coronary artery disease, exercise may cause constriction of stenotic coronary arterial segments, increasing the likelihood of exercise-related ischemia. The mechanism of this vasoconstriction is not well understood but may be related to elevated plasma catecholamine concentrations, a subnormal production of endothelium-derived vasorelaxing factor, or platelet aggregation with release of thromboxane A_2, a potent vasoconstrictor.[4] As discussed previously, ischemia may result in a reduction in the mechanical pump function of the heart.[25,26] Left and right ventricular ejection fractions may decrease during exercise, regional wall motion abnormalities may develop in ischemic portions of the myocardium, diastolic filling may be impaired due to a reduction in compliance of the ventricles (increased stiffness), and stroke volume may not increase normally during exercise. The heart rate response to exercise may be blunted, independent of medication effects.[15] In fact, for some patients with right coronary artery stenosis and exercise-induced ischemia, heart rate may actually decrease (sinus node deceleration) at some point during an incremental exercise test.[31] As a result of the impaired stroke volume and heart rate, cardiac output during exercise may not rise normally. In addition, skeletal muscle beds may not vasodilate normally, further reducing the effective muscle blood flow.[32]

Hossack[15] compared variables of the Fick equation during treadmill exercise with hemodynamic (arterial and right atrial catheters) and cardiopulmonary monitoring in patients (men and women) with coronary artery disease and in normal controls. Figure 25 shows the oxygen transport system for these subjects. Few of the patients took beta-blocking medications. The greatest difference between patients

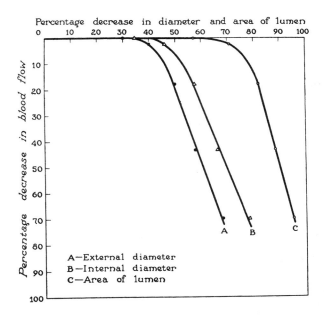

Figure 24   The relationship between coronary stenosis (area of coronary artery lumen obstruction) and coronary blood flow. (From Mann, F. C., Herrick, J. F., and Essex, H. E., *Surgery,* 4, 249, 1938. With permission.)

and controls was for oxygen uptake during exercise with a mean $\dot{V}O_2$max of 48% of age-matched normal for patients with coronary artery disease. Note the lower oxygen uptakes for patients compared with controls for submaximal exercise intensities, as well. The maximal cardiac output was 57% of age-adjusted normal. Both heart rate and stroke volume were lower for patients than for controls. In fact, mean stroke volume increased only slightly during exercise for the coronary patients. a-$\overline{v}O_2$ Diff was also lower for patients than for healthy controls. Thus, all variables of the oxygen transport (Fick) equation were subnormal for patients with coronary artery disease, on the average.

Severe, chronic left ventricular systolic dysfunction (LVEF < 35%) may result from extensive myocardial infarction and/or ischemia. If cardiac output during exercise does not increase normally in these patients, exercise capacity is reduced dramatically.[33] Skeletal muscle abnormalities, such as an impaired ability to vasodilate, reduced aerobic metabolic enzyme activity, and a conversion of slow-twitch muscle fibers to fast-twitch fibers may occur. However, resting LVEF does not correlate with aerobic exercise capacity in ambulatory patients[34] (Figure 26). Patients with reduced LVEFs may have relatively normal exercise responses or may be extremely debilitated. Patients with reduced LVEFs and well-preserved aerobic capacities generally have a near normal heart rate response to exercise, can enlarge EDV, and can adequately vasodilate skeletal muscle during exercise.

Most patients with coronary artery disease and exercise-induced ischemia have a normal blood pressure response to aerobic exercise. However, some patients exhibit hypotensive or hypertensive responses. The most serious abnormal blood pressure response to exercise is systolic hypotension, usually defined as a 20 mmHg or greater drop in systolic pressure or a lower than preexercise systolic blood pressure during graded exercise testing.[35] Patients with a hypotensive systolic blood pressure response during exercise are at higher risk for cardiac death or myocardial infarction. The mechanisms for the hypotensive response are speculative. However, cardiac output seldom decreases during exercise, even in patients with severe left ventricular dysfunction. Neurogenic reflex vasodilation involving activation of mechanoreceptors in the myocardium (Bezold–Jarisch reflex) may play a role.[35] Figure 27 shows the variety of systolic blood pressure responses to aerobic exercise in patients with ischemic heart disease. There are data to support the concept that exercise-induced (treadmill) diastolic hypertension (increase of 15 mmHg or more) is associated with worsening left ventricular function during exercise.[36] Some patients demonstrate an increase in systolic blood pressure during recovery from exercise, rather than the normal decline in systolic blood pressure seen with decreasing exercise intensity. This paradoxical blood pressure response is associated with severe myocardial ischemia and an increase in postexercise stroke volume.[37]

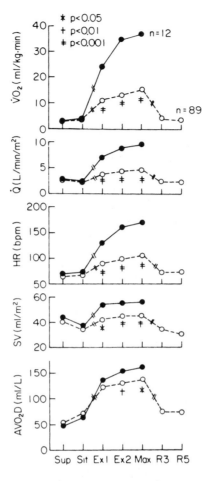

Figure 25 Mean values for oxygen uptake ($\dot{V}O_2$), cardiac index ($\dot{Q}$), heart rate (HR), stroke volume (SV), and arterial-mixed venous oxygen difference (AVO$_2$D) for normal male subjects (solid circles) and patients with coronary artery disease (open circles). (From Hossack, K. F. *Cardiol. Clin.,* 5, 147, 1987. With permission.)

VII. EXERCISE TRAINING AND THE CARDIOVASCULAR SYSTEM

A. NORMAL PERSONS

Regular exercise training (20 to 60 min, 50 to 85% of $\dot{V}O_2$max, three to five sessions per week) results in a predictable improvement in the oxygen transport function of the cardiovascular system.[38,39] The magnitude of the increase in $\dot{V}O_2$max is dependent upon the intensity and total amount of training, genetic potential for adaptation, and the initial aerobic capacity (greater improvements are expected for subjects with poorer initial aerobic capacities). $\dot{V}O_2$max increases by 10 to 30% after 2 or 3 months of training. Prolonged or very intense training may result in greater improvements in aerobic exercise capacity.[10] Once the cardiovascular system oxygen transport function has been improved by systematic training, cessation of regular exercise (detraining) will result in a loss of cardiovascular fitness.[40]

Habitual exercise will result in an increase in heart mass and chamber volume (physiological hypertrophy) yielding a higher cardiac output during exercise.[41,42] These cardiac adaptations to training have been observed in healthy persons of various ages, although the most impressive cardiac hypertrophy probably occurs in young persons.

During the past decade, several studies using echocardiography or radionuclide angiography have evaluated the effects of exercise training on left ventricular size and function. Table 4 shows selected echocardiographic findings before and after exercise training in previously sedentary persons.[43,44] Increased wall thickness was found for the interventricular septum as well as an increase in left ventricular

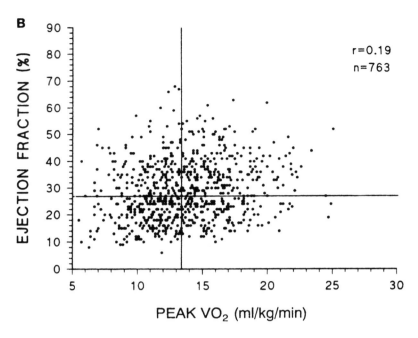

Figure 26   Plots of VO_2 peak and resting LVEF. (From Cohn, J. N. et al., *Circulation,* 87 (Suppl. VI), VI-5, 1993. With permission.)

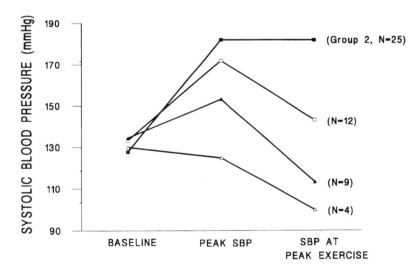

Figure 27   Various systolic blood pressure responses during graded exercise testing in patients with coronary artery disease. (From Iskandrian, A. S. et al., *Am. J. Cardiol.,* 69, 1517, 1992. With permission.)

mass of approximately 9%. Left ventricular internal diameter at end-diastole and end-systole was greater after training. Left ventricular EDV increased by approximately 8%. The contractile response of the left ventricle to beta adrenergic stimulation is enhanced by systematic exercise training as indicated by increased left ventricular fractional shortening measured by echocardiography in response to isoproterenol infusion.[45] LVEF at rest and during exercise may increase, although this is not a consistent finding. In healthy young subjects, cardiac hypertrophy occurs rapidly as a result of training. Figure 28 shows that after only 7 days of training left ventricular posterior wall thickness and end-diastolic dimension are increased and are associated with an improvement in $\dot{V}O_2$max.[42] Left ventricular mass increases dramatically during the first 3 weeks of training (Figure 29). Diastolic filling is also improved with

Table 4 Change in Left Ventricular (LV) Structure and Volumes after Exercise Training in Healthy Men

	Before	After	Δ%
LV end-diastolic dimension (mm)	45.8	49.6	8.3
LV end-diastolic volume (ml)	115.9	140.0	20.8
Stroke volume (ml)	71.4	92.1	29.0
Interventricular septal thickness at end systole (mm)	13.4	14.9	11.2
Left ventricular mass (g)	211.6	231.0	9.2

Source: Compiled from Adams, T. D. et al., *Circulation*, 64, 958, 1981; Cox, M. L. et al., *J. Appl. Physiol.*, 61, 926, 1986.

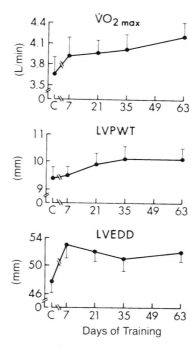

Figure 28 Adaptations of the cardiovascular system to endurance exercise training in young healthy subjects. Maximal oxygen uptake ($\dot{V}O_{2max}$) increased progressively while left ventricular end-diastolic diameter (LVEDD, measured by echocardiography) increased quickly, reaching maximum value in only 7 days. Left ventricular posterior wall thickness (LVPWT, by echocardiography) increased gradually over 5 weeks of training. (From Ehsani, A. A. et al., *Circulation*, 74, 350, 1986. With permission.)

training as indicated by an increase in peak exercise filling rate (Figure 30).[46] As a result of these changes in left ventricular morphology, stroke volume is increased.

For a given absolute exercise intensity, heart rate is lower (training bradycardia) although maximal heart rate is unchanged after a training program.[10,38,39] Table 5 provides information regarding the change at rest and during maximal exercise for heart rate, LVEF, EDV, cardiac output, and blood volume before and after a 6-month exercise training program.[47] Cardiac output at peak exercise improved by approximately 25%. Plasma volume increases rapidly as a result of systematic exercise training.[48-50] Total erythrocyte mass increases over a period of weeks.[50] Hemoglobin concentration either remains unchanged or may decrease slightly (training pseudoanemia).[49] Thus, while total blood volume (which augments cardiac output) and the total hemoglobin amount are higher after training, arterial oxygen content is usually not different.

Exercise training in animals has demonstrated structural adaptations in the coronary vasculature.[51] Proximal coronary arteries increase in cross-sectional area. In addition, the moderate cardiac hypertrophy with exercise training is associated with a maintenance or increase in capillary density and increase in arteriolar density (angiogenesis). The overall coronary tree size increases after training in animals.[52]

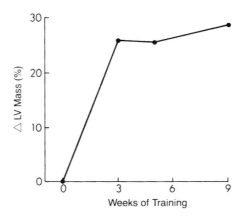

Figure 29 Rapid cardiac adaptation to vigorous endurance exercise training in young healthy subjects as evidenced by a dramatic increase in left ventricular mass after only 3 weeks. (From Ehsani, A. A. et al., *Circulation,* 74, 350, 1986. With permission.)

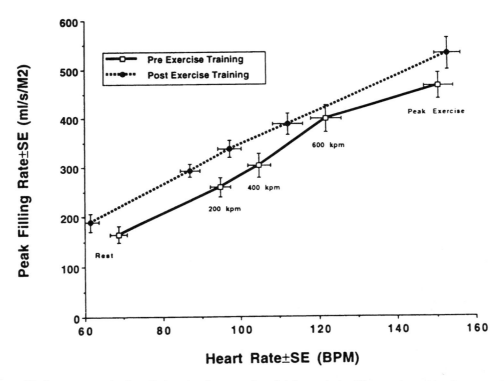

Figure 30 Improvement in diastolic function (increased peak left ventricular filling rate) resulting from exercise training in young and older subjects. (From Levy, W. C. et al., *Circulation,* 88, 116, 1993. With permission.)

Another method employed in studying cardiac adaptation to exercise training involves echocardiographic measurement of athletes in training and then making similar measurements after a period of inactivity (detraining).[40,42,53] Regression of cardiac hypertrophy occurs rapidly with cessation of training. Figure 31 shows that in the space of 3 weeks of detraining, left ventricular posterior wall thickness and left ventricular end-diastolic dimension decrease moderately. Left ventricular mass also regresses dramatically within 4 weeks of inactivity (Figure 32).[42] Maximal septal wall thickness decreases approximately 25% after 3 months of inactivity.[53] The training bradycardia discussed previously also disappears quickly with detraining.[40]

Table 5 Effects of Exercise Training on Left Ventricular Function and Blood Volume in Normal Subjects

	Heart Rate (beats/min)	Ejection Fraction (%)	EDV (ml)	Cardiac Output (l/min)	Body Blood Volume (l)
Rest					
Before training	74	73	133	6.9	8.7
After training	61	67	167	6.7	11.4
Maximal exercise					
Before training	185	87	166	25.5	8.0
After training	181	86	204	32.0	10.8

Source: From Rerych, S. K. et al., *Am. J. Cardiol.,* 45, 244, 1980. With permission.

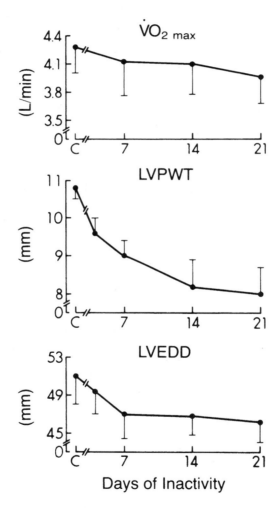

Figure 31 Loss of cardiovascular adaptations after 3 weeks of physical inactivity in previously exercise-trained young subjects. LVPWT = left ventricular posterior wall thickness, LVEDD = left ventricular end-diastolic diameter (both measured by echocardiography). (From Ehsani, A. A. et al., *Circulation,* 74, 350, 1986. With permission.)

Exercise training results in adaptation of the skeletal muscle vasculature. Capillary density is increased by up to 50% and vasodilatory capacity is improved.[54,55] Leg blood flow during maximal exercise is higher after training due to an increased cardiac output and to increased vascular conductance.[39,56]

Skeletal muscle adaptations to chronic exercise enhance the capacity for oxygen extraction from capillary blood. After 6 to 8 weeks of training, mitochondrial oxidative enzyme content of the active

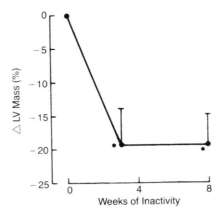

Figure 32 Rapid reduction in left ventricular mass after 3 weeks of detraining in previously well-conditioned young subjects. (From Martin, W. H. and Ehsani, A. A., *Circulation,* 76, 548, 1987. With permission.)

skeletal muscle increases by 40 to 50%.[54] Mitochondrial size increases, as well. The mixed venous oxygen content is lower at peak exercise after training (arterial oxygen content is unchanged) and the a-$\overline{v}O_2$ Diff is slightly greater.[10,19,39] Oxygen transport is improved by both an increase in cardiac output (increased stroke volume) and a widened a-$\overline{v}O_2$ Diff.

B. PATIENTS WITH ISCHEMIC HEART DISEASE

In general, exercise training improves the oxygen transport function of the cardiovascular system for patients with coronary artery disease. However, coronary patients are a heterogeneous group and do not always demonstrate a predictable and consistent response to exercise training. Patients may differ in respect to the extent of atherosclerotic disease, left ventricular systolic and diastolic function, and the extent and severity of exercise-related myocardial ischemia. Some patients with significant coronary obstructive lesions do not develop ischemia during exercise as a result of medical or surgical treatment, or extensive coronary collateralization.

As a result of exercise training, $\dot{V}O_2$max may increase 10 to 30% or more.[57,58] The rate of improvement is greatest during the first 3 months of training, but further increases in aerobic capacity may occur for 6 or more months.[59] Similar gains in $\dot{V}O_2$max have been documented for patients after myocardial infarction, coronary bypass surgery or for patients with angiographic disease without a cardiac event (Figure 33).[60] Properly screened patients with severe left ventricular dysfunction (LVEF < 30%) with well-compensated chronic heart failure usually exhibit a cardiovascular training effect.[33,61] There is no indication that moderate exercise training in patients with severe left ventricular dysfunction causes a further decline in cardiac pump function. Selected patients with left ventricular aneurysm after myocardial infarction have been shown to improve exercise capacity after training.[62] In general, patients with exercise-induced myocardial ischemia do not exhibit as much improvement in aerobic capacity as coronary patients without ischemia.[63,64]

Attention has been given to relatively low-intensity exercise training for cardiac patients with the goal of enhancing compliance with the program and minimizing the risks of training. Results from two investigations have demonstrated similar gains in aerobic capacity from exercise programs using an intensity of <45% of $\dot{V}O_2$max or a target heart rate of 20 beats/min above standing resting heart rate as more traditional programs (60 to 70% of $\dot{V}O_2$max).[65,66]

Some patients with coronary artery disease do not show much improvement in $\dot{V}O_2$max as a result of training, but do improve submaximal exercise performance. Such improvements include a lower heart rate and $\dot{V}O_2$ for a given submaximal exercise intensity and greatly prolonged endurance time at a given exercise pace.[68]

The improvement usually observed in oxygen transport after exercise training in patients with coronary artery disease has traditionally been assumed to be due primarily to an increase in a-$\overline{v}O_2$ Diff and not an increase in maximal exercise cardiac output. Mitochondrial enzyme activity of oxidative metabolism and regeneration of phosphocreatine have been shown to improve as a result of training in coronary patients.[69,70] Whether or not exercise cardiac output increases as a result of training has been

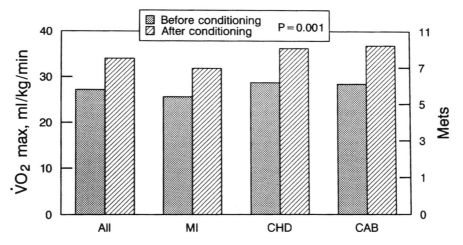

Figure 33 Increase in maximal oxygen uptake resulting from exercise training in patients with myocardial infarction, coronary artery bypass surgery, and angiographically documented disease. All = all coronary patients, MI = myocardial infarction, CHD = angiographically documented disease, CAB = coronary artery bypass surgery. (From Martin, W. H. and Ehsani, A. A., *Circulation,* 76, 548, 1987. With permission.)

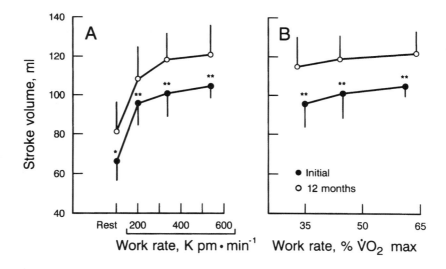

Figure 34 Stroke volume at rest and during exercise at the same absolute work intensity (A) and the same relative work intensity (B) before (●—●) and after (○—○) 12 months of exercise training. Differences from before vs. after training: *p < 0.05; **p < 0.01. (From Hagberg, J. M. et al., *Circulation,* 67, 1194, 1983. With permission.)

controversial. Some relatively early reports have demonstrated an increase in exercise cardiac output after training in some patients after myocardial infarction.[57,71]

Investigators at Washington University in St. Louis, Missouri have sought to answer the question regarding "central" circulatory adaptation to exercise training in coronary patients. They maximized the training stimulus by gradually increasing the training intensity and duration for highly motivated patients over the course of 1 year or more. The final training stimulus of their studies included 60 min of exercise, 5 days per week, at an intensity of 70 to 90% of $\dot{V}O_2$max.[72] In these studies, mean $\dot{V}O_2$max increased by approximately 40%, nearly twice the usual training effect of traditional exercise programs for cardiac patients. Evidence of improvement in exercise cardiac output was indicated by the following findings: echocardiographic evidence of improved left ventricular myocardial fractional shortening and mean velocity of shortening,[73] an average 18% increase in stroke volume measured during submaximal exercise

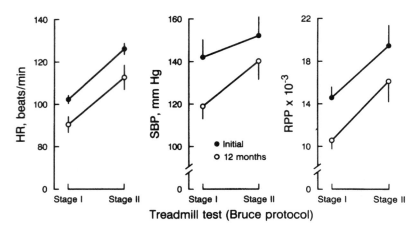

Figure 35 Effects of exercise training on heart rate (HR), systolic blood pressure (SBP), and rate–pressure product (RPP) at stages I and II of the Bruce treadmill protocol. All variables after 12 months of training (○—○) were significantly (p < 0.01) lower than before training (●—●). (From reference Ehsani, A. A. et al., *Am. J. Cardiol.*, 50, 246, 1982. With permission.)

(35 to 65% of $\dot{V}O_2$max) (Figure 34),[74] improvement in systolic time intervals after training,[75] increased exercise LVEF,[76] and reversal of exercise-related and ischemia-related drops in systolic blood pressure.[77] These data indicate that for at least some patients with coronary artery disease and myocardial infarction, improvement in exercise cardiac output is possible.

For patients with moderate-to-large size anterior wall myocardial infarctions, one investigation reported deterioration in left ventricular function after exercise training.[78] The authors felt that the exercise program had precipitated the decline in cardiac function and urged caution regarding exercise training for these patients. However, a recent randomized and controlled trial of the effects of exercise training after anterior wall myocardial infarction demonstrated an increase in aerobic capacity in the exercise group only. Subjects in both the exercise and control groups with LVEFs of less than 40% exhibited further left ventricular enlargement. Patients with poor left ventricular systolic function after anterior wall myocardial infarction experience adverse ventricular remodeling over time, and standard exercise training does not appear to influence the process.[79]

Exercise training may improve exercise-related myocardial ischemia. There is evidence that training may improve both the "demand" and "supply" sides of the ischemia equation. After training, for a specific submaximal exercise intensity the myocardial oxygen demand, as indicated by a reduction in heart rate and systolic blood pressure (rate–pressure product), is reduced (Figure 35).[80] This enables the patient to perform a higher intensity of physical activity before exceeding the "ischemic threshold" (the rate–pressure product which corresponds to the onset of measurable myocardial ischemia). Furthermore, some studies have determined that the rate–pressure product at the ischemic threshold is increased by exercise training, independent of changes in anti-ischemic drug therapy, suggesting that myocardial blood flow may be improved.[81,82] Thallium perfusion in conjunction with graded exercise testing before and after a period of exercise training has, in selected coronary patients, demonstrated improved myocardial perfusion. Reductions in exercise-induced ischemia measured by thallium perfusion of 54%[83] and 34%[84] have been recently reported. The reduction in ischemia after training cannot be explained on the basis of a lower rate–pressure product at peak exercise. Improved blood lipids or decreased blood viscosity are potential reasons for the reduction in ischemia although some investigators believe that enhanced coronary collateral flow is the cause for the improvement,[84] although no direct evidence for improvement in collateral flow exists. A recent review of investigations studying the question of coronary collateral development resulting from exercise training in patients with coronary artery disease emphasized the technical difficulty of visualizing small collateral vessel or vessels tunneled into the myocardium.[85] One study involved eight men with stable angina pectoris who participated in a 1-year supervised exercise training program with angiography performed at baseline and at completion of training.[86] Exercise capacity improved and two patients with pretraining ischemic electrocardiographic changes during treadmill exercise testing reverted to normal, although there was no direct evidence of enhanced coronary collateralization.

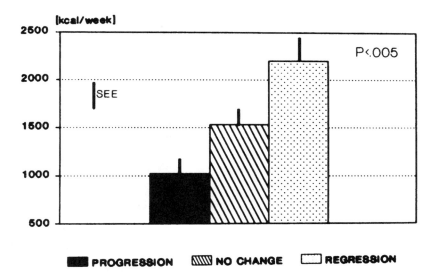

Figure 36 Effects of different levels of energy expenditure during exercise training on coronary atherosclerotic lesions measured 12 months apart using quantitative coronary angiography. Approximately 1500 kcal/week was required to halt measurable progression of disease while approximately 2200 kcal/week was needed to result in net regression of lesion size. (From Hambrecht, R. et al., *J. Am. Coll. Cardiol.*, 22, 468, 1993. With permission.)

Exercise training, in sufficient amounts, appears to retard or even reverse coronary atherosclerosis. A recent investigation studied the effects of 1 year of supervised, moderate-intensity exercise on the progression of coronary artery disease.[87] Approximately 60 cardiac patients were randomized into experimental or control groups. Both the control and experimental subjects were instructed in a low fat/cholesterol diet and received information regarding the benefits of regular aerobic exercise. The experimental subjects embarked on a supervised and home-based exercise program, and the control subjects were left to the usual care of their primary physicians. No medications to lower total or low-density lipoprotein cholesterol were used. Coronary angiography was performed before and after the 1-year study. Angiographic progression of coronary atherosclerosis occurred in 45% of controls and 10% of experimental subjects. No change in the appearance of coronary lesions occurred in 62% of experimental subjects compared with 49% of control subjects. Regression of lesions was observed 28% of exercising subjects vs. 6% of controls. Regression of coronary artery disease was observed only in patients who expended an average of 2200 kcal/week in physical activity (approximately 5 to 6 h of moderate-intensity exercise per week) (Figure 36).

VIII. CARDIOVASCULAR RESPONSES TO SUPINE POSTURE, UPPER–EXTREMITY, AND STATIC (ISOMETRIC) EXERCISE

Aerobic exercise performed in the supine position results in a characteristic cardiovascular response. Because the force of gravity is much less of a factor, venous return is higher in supine than in upright posture. EDV and stroke volume are maximal at rest and do not increase during exercise.[11] Submaximal exercise heart rate is lower due to the higher stroke volume although maximal heart rate is the same as for upright exercise.[88] Although $\dot{V}O_2$max (and peak work intensity during cycle ergometry) is lower for supine exercise, the linear relationship between cardiac output and $\dot{V}O_2$ is maintained.[11,88] Both systolic and diastolic exercise blood pressures are higher for supine than for upright exercise.

The responses of the cardiovascular system to upper-extremity exercise differ in some respects from leg exercise. The arms represent a much smaller muscle mass than the legs, although accessory muscle use (back, abdomen, etc.) may be important for some forms of upper-extremity exercise.[89] With progressive arm exercise, $\dot{V}O_2$ increases curvilinearly rather than linearly as with leg exercise. In comparing arm and leg exercise at a given submaximal absolute work intensity, $\dot{V}O_2$ is higher (arm exercise is less efficient than leg exercise), heart rate is higher, stroke volume is lower, cardiac output is higher, peripheral vascular resistance is higher (less vasodilation), both systolic and diastolic blood pressures are higher, and myocardial oxygen demand is higher (increased rate–pressure product).[10]

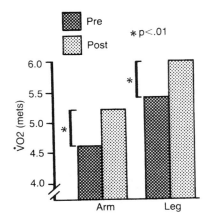

Figure 37 Change in maximal oxygen uptake resulting from arm and leg exercise training in patients with previous myocardial infarction. The magnitude of the training effect was similar for arm and leg training. (From Franklin, B. A. et al., *Chest,* 105, 262, 1994. With permission.)

For maximal exercise, $\dot{V}O_2$ peak for the arms is approximately 70% of the value for leg exercise, maximal heart rate is similar, maximal stroke volume is lower as is maximal cardiac output.[10] For patients with coronary artery disease, arm exercise usually results in less myocardial ischemia due to increased myocardial blood flow resulting from the increased exercise diastolic blood pressure (increased coronary perfusion pressure).

Exercise training responses include both a central circulatory improvement (increased cardiac output) and a peripheral circulatory improvement (increased aerobic metabolic capacity of tissue and better delivery of oxygen to skeletal muscle), as discussed previously. Training effects are thus somewhat specific to the muscle groups which have been involved in training. Figure 37 demonstrates that the relative magnitude of the increase in $\dot{V}O_2$ peak is similar for both arm and leg training programs.[90]

Static or isometric exercise results in a response of the cardiovascular system (increased blood pressure and heart rate, increased left ventricular contractility and wall tension) mediated by reflex afferent nervous system activity from contracting skeletal muscle and from impulses from the motor cortex to the cardiovascular center in the brain stem. The magnitude of the cardiovascular system response to static exercise is directly proportional to three factors:[89]

1. The intensity of the contraction relative to the maximal voluntary contraction (MVC, maximal isometric force development for a particular muscle group),
2. The size of the contracting muscle mass, and
3. The duration of the contraction.

As isometric contractions increase in intensity above 15% of MVC, increasing intramuscular pressure compresses the vasculature and results in a progressive impediment to skeletal muscle blood flow.[91] If the force of the isometric contraction exceeds 70% of MVC, blood flow through the contracting muscle group will be completely stopped.

Figure 38 compares the cardiovascular responses to graded aerobic cycle ergometer exercise to maximal effort and a moderate isometric contraction (2 min at 40% of MVC). Aerobic exercise is primarily a volume output demand for the heart as indicated by the large increase in cardiac index and oxygen uptake. Isometric exercise is primarily a pressure overload for the circulation as evidenced by the dramatic increase in blood pressure with only a modest increase in cardiac index and oxygen uptake.[91] Blood pressure can increase to extreme levels during isometric exercise (pressor response). Average intra-arterial pressure during maximal isometric deadlift exercise has been reported as 217/150.[92] During heavy weight-lifting exercise, which has a component of isometric contraction, intra-arterial pressures have been reported as high as 480/350.[93] The extremely elevated blood pressures measured during maximal isometric contractions and heavy weight lifting are related to performance of a Valsalva maneuver which is unavoidable with maximal or near maximal isometric force development.[94]

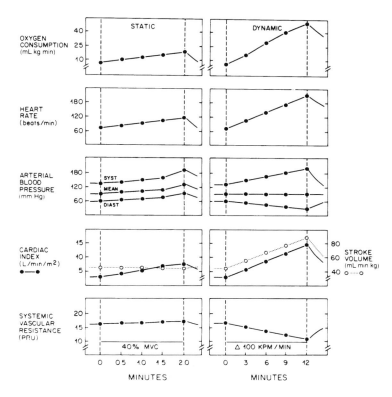

Figure 38 Cardiovascular response to static (40% of MVC for 2 min duration) and dynamic (12 min of cycle ergometry with periodic increases in exercise intensity of 100 kpm/min) exercise. Responses include total body oxygen uptake, heart rate, blood pressure, cardiac index, and systemic vascular resistance. (From Longhurst, J. C. and Stebbins, C. L., *Cardiol. Clin.*, 10, 281, 1992. With permission.)

Isometric deadlift exercise involves a large mass of contracting skeletal muscle. Figures 39 and 40 show the acute cardiovascular response to moderate (50% of MVC) and maximal isometric deadlift exercise.[95] Heart rate and mean arterial pressure increased more dramatically for the higher–intensity contraction. Continuous measurement of left ventricular systolic function during isometric exercise (echocardiography) demonstrated a transient decrease in LVEF and stroke volume at the beginning of the contraction. Cardiac volumes (end-diastolic and end-systolic) increased as well. Thus, left ventricular performance declines initially but improves later in the contraction due to the Frank–Starling mechanism. For isometric contractions involving small amounts of muscle mass, left ventricular function is not altered.[89]

Isometric exercise training results in skeletal muscle hypertrophy and an increase in MVC. For a given absolute intensity of static contraction, the heart rate and blood pressure response is attenuated as the contraction represents a smaller percentage of MVC.[89] The cardiac effects of isometric training are related to the increased afterload (increased diastolic blood pressure).[91] Left ventricular hypertrophy (increased left ventricular mass without an increase in ventricular volume) occurs in isometric athletes. Aerobic athletes experience a greater increase in left ventricular mass than in isometric athletes as well as an increase in ventricular volume. Cardiac hypertrophy resulting from systematic training (either aerobic or isometric) is less pronounced than for pathological states such as severe hypertension or valvular heart disease. No change in either systolic or diastolic left ventricular function results from isometric training. Resting blood pressure is not elevated by static exercise training in spite of the marked acute blood pressure elevation.

Moderate-intensity weight training (10 to 20 repetitions/set) has been demonstrated to be effective in improving skeletal muscle strength in selected patients with healed myocardial infarction or coronary bypass surgery.[96] Modest increases in heart rate and blood pressure occur with moderate weight-training exercise in cardiac patients, and no adverse cardiac effects have been reported for carefully selected patients.[97,98]

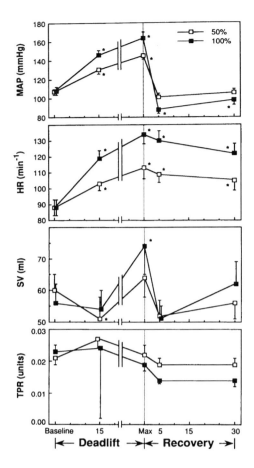

Figure 39 Cardiovascular responses to submaximal and maximal (50 and 100% MVC) isometric deadlift exercise. Times are in seconds. MAP = mean arterial pressure, HR = heart rate, SV = stroke volume, TPR = total peripheral resistance. * = significantly different from rest, p < 0.01. (From Sullivan, J. et al., *Circulation,* 85, 1406, 1992. With permission.)

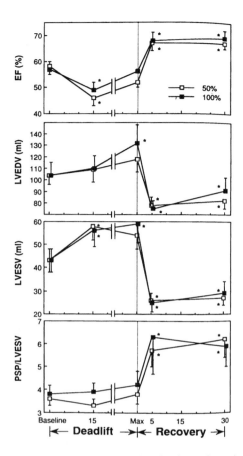

Figure 40 Left ventricular performance during and immediately after submaximal and maximal (50 and 100% MVC) isometric deadlift exercise. Times are in seconds. EF = left ventricular ejection fraction, LVEDV = left ventricular end-diastolic volume, LVESV = left ventricular end-systolic volume, PSP = peak systolic pressure. * = significantly different from rest, $p < 0.01$. (From Sullivan, J. et al., *Circulation,* 85, 1406, 1992. With permission.)

REFERENCES

1. Durstine, J. L., Pate, R. R., and Branch, J. D., Cardiorespiratory responses to acute exercise, in *ACSM's Resource Manual for Guidelines for Exercise Testing and Prescription*, 2nd ed., American College of Sports Medicine, Lea and Febiger, Philadelphia, 1993, ch. 7.

2. Garratt, K. N. and Morgan, J. P., Pathophysiology of myocardial ischemia and reperfusion, in *Cardiology: Fundamentals and Practice*, Giuliani, E. R., Fuster, V., Gersh, B. J., McGoon, M. D., and McGoon, D. C., Eds., Mosby Year Book, St. Louis, 1991, ch. 33 B.

3. Braunwald, E. and Sobel, B. E., Coronary blood flow and myocardial ischemia, in *Textbook of Cardiovascular Medicine*, 3rd ed., Braunwald, E., Ed., W.B. Saunders, Philadelphia, 1988, ch. 37.

4. Hess, O. M., Buchi, M., Kirkeeide, R., Niederer, P., Anliker, M., Gould, K. L., and Krayenbuhl, H. P., Potential role of coronary vasoconstriction in ischemic heart disease: effect of exercise, *Eur. Heart J.,* 11, 58, 1990.

5. Bove, A. A. and Santamore, W. P., Physiology of the coronary circulation, in *Cardiology: Fundamentals and Practice*, Giuliani, E. R., Fuster, V., Gersh, B. J., McGoon, M. D., and McGoon, D. C., Eds., Mosby Year Book, St. Louis, 1991, ch. 33 A.

6. Guyton, A. C., *Textbook of Medical Physiology*, W. B. Saunders, Philadelphia, 1986, ch. 25.

7. Bove, A. A. and Santamore, W. P., Mechanical performance of the heart, in *Cardiology: Fundamentals and Practice*, Giuliani, E. R., Fuster, V., Gersh, B. J., McGoon, M. D., and McGoon, D. C., Eds., Mosby Year Book, St. Louis, 1991, ch. 6.

8. Gibbons, R. J., Rest and exercise radionuclide angiography for diagnosis in chronic ischemic heart disease, *Circulation,* 84(Suppl. I), I93, 1991.

9. Netter, F. H. and Yonkman, F. F., *The Ciba Collection of Medical Illustrations, Volume 5: Heart*, Ciba, New York, 1978, 45.

10. Astrand, P. O. and Rodahl, K., *Textbook of Work Physiology: Physiological Bases of Exercise,* 3rd ed., McGraw Hill, New York, 1986, ch. 4.
11. Froelicher, V. F., Myers, J., Follansbee, W. P., and Labovitz, A. J., *Exercise and the Heart,* 3rd ed., Mosby, St. Louis, 1993, ch. 1, 15.
12. Wasserman, K., Hansen, J. E., Sue, D. Y., and Whip, B. J., *Principles of Exercise Testing and Interpretation,* Lea and Febiger, Philadelphia, 1987, p. 37.
13. Rowell, L. B., Taylor, H. L., Wang Y., and Carlson, W. S., Saturation of arterial blood with oxygen during maximal exercise, *J. Appl. Physiol.,* 19, 284, 1964.
14. Dehn, M. M., Blomqvist, C. G., and Mitchell, J. H., Clinical exercise performance, *Clin. Sports Med.,* 3, 319, 1984.
15. Hossack, K. F., Cardiovascular responses to dynamic exercise, *Cardiol. Clin.,* 5, 147, 1987.
16. Plotnick, G. D., Becker, L. C., Fisher, M. L., Gerstenblith, G., Renlund, D. G., Fleg, J. L., Weisfeldt, M. L., and Lakata, E. G., Use of the Frank–Starling mechanism during submaximal versus maximal upright exercise, *Am. J. Physiol.,* 251 (Heart Circ. Physiol. 20), H1101, 1986.
17. Sullivan, M. J., Cobb, F. R., and Higginbotham, M. B., Stroke volume increases by similar mechanisms during upright exercise in normal men and women, *Am. J. Cardiol.,* 67, 1405, 1991.
18. Spina, R. J., Ogawa, T., Martin, W. H., Coggan, A. R., Holloszy, J. O., and Ehsani, A. A., Exercise training prevents decline in stroke volume during exercise in young healthy subjects, *J. Appl. Physiol.,* 72, 2458, 1992.
19. Lowenthal, D. T. and Pollock, M. L., Cardiac response to exercise in health and disease, *Sem. Resp. Med.,* 14, 91, 1993.
20. Shepherd, J. T., Blomqvist, C. G., and Lind, A. R., Static (isometric) exercise: retrospection and introspection, *Circ. Res.,* 48 (Suppl. I), I-179, 1981.
21. Rowell, L. B., Reflex control of the circulation during exercise, *Int. J. Sports Med.,* 13, S25, 1992.
22. Joyner, M. J., Muscle chemoreflexes and exercise in humans, *Clin. Autonom. Res.,* 2, 201, 1992.
23. Blomqvist, C. G., Clinical exercise physiology, in *Rehabilitation of the Coronary Patient,* 2nd ed., Wenger, N. K. and Hellerstein, H. K., Eds., John Wiley, New York, 1984, ch. 9.
24. Sutton, J. R., Limitations to maximal oxygen uptake, *Sports Med.,* 13, 127, 1992.
25. Squires, R. W. and Williams, W. L., Coronary atherosclerosis and acute myocardial infarction, in *ACSM's Resource Manual for Guidelines for Exercise Testing and Prescription,* 2nd ed., American College of Sports Medicine, Lea and Febiger, Philadelphia, 1993, ch. 15.
26. Hurst, J. W., Coronary heart disease: the overview of the clinician, in *Rehabilitation of the Coronary Patient,* 3rd ed., Wenger, N. K. and Hellerstein, H. K., Eds, Churchill Livingstone, New York, 1992, ch. 1.
27. Perrone-Filardi, P., Bacharach, S. L., Dilsizian, V., and Bonow, R. O., Impaired left ventricular filling and regional diastolic asynchrony at rest in coronary artery disease and relation to exercise-induced myocardial ischemia, *Am. J. Cardiol.,* 67, 356, 1991.
28. Carter, C. L. and Amundsen, L. R., Infarct size and exercise capacity after myocardial infarction, *J. Appl. Physiol.,* 42, 782, 1977.
29. Hossack, K., Eldridge, J., Wolfel, E., Leddy, C., and Berger, N., Aerobic responses to low level exercise testing following an acute myocardial infarction, *Am. Heart J.,* 113, 694, 1987.
30. Zimmerman, P., Heigenhauser, G. J. F., McCartney, N., Sutton, J. R., and Jones, N. L., Impaired cardiac "acceleration" at the onset of exercise in patients with coronary disease, *J. Appl. Physiol.,* 52, 71, 1982.
31. Miller, T. D., Gibbons, R. J., Squires, R. W., Allison, T. G., and Gau, G. T., Sinus node deceleration during exercise as a marker of significant narrowing of the right coronary artery, *Am. J. Cardiol.,* 71, 371, 1993.
32. Hetherington, M., Teo, K. K., Haennel, R. G., Rossall, R. E., and Kappagoda, T., Response to upright exercise after myocardial infarction, *Cardiovasc. Res.,* 21, 399, 1987.
33. Sullivan, M. J., Higginbotham, M. B., and Cobb, F. R., Exercise training in patients with severe left ventricular dysfunction: hemodynamic and metabolic effects, *Circulation,* 78, 506, 1988.
34. Cohn, J. N., Johnson, G. R., Shabetai, R., Loeb, H., Tristani, F., Rector, T., Smith, R., and Fletcher, R., Ejection fraction, peak exercise oxygen consumption, cardiothoracic ratio, ventricular arrhythmias, and plasma norepinephrine as determinants of prognosis in heart failure, *Circulation,* 87(Suppl. VI), VI-5, 1993.
35. Iskandrian, A. S., Kegel, J. G., Lemlek, J., Heo, J., Cave, V., and Iskandrian, B., Mechanism of exercise-induced hypotension in coronary artery disease, *Am. J. Cardiol.,* 69, 1517, 1992.
36. Paraskevaidis, I. A., Kremastinos, D. T., Kassimatis, A. S., Karavolias, G. K., Kordosis, G. D., Kyriakides, Z. S., and Toutouzas, P. K., Increased response of diastolic blood pressure to exercise in patients with coronary artery disease: an index of latent ventricular dysfunction, *Br. Heart J.,* 69, 507, 1993.
37. Hashimoto, M., Okamoto, M., Yamagata, T., Yamane, T., Watanabe, M., Tsuchioka, Y., Matsuura, H., and Kajiyama, G., Abnormal systolic blood pressure response during exercise recovery in patients with angina pectoris, *J. Am. Coll. Cardiol.,* 22, 659, 1993.
38. American College of Sports Medicine, *Guidelines for Exercise Testing and Training,* 4th ed., Lea and Febiger, Philadelphia, 1991.
39. Crawford, M. H., Physiologic consequences of systematic training, *Cardiol. Clin.,* 10, 209, 1992.
40. Martin, W. H., Coyle, E. F., Bloomfield, S. A., and Ehsani, A. A., Effects of physical deconditioning after intense training on left ventricular dimensions and stroke volume, *J. Am. Coll. Cardiol.,* 7, 982, 1986.
41. Foster, C., Central circulatory adaptations to exercise training in health and disease, *Clin. Sports Med.,* 5, 589, 1986.
42. Ehsani, A. A., Loss of cardiovascular adaptations after cessation of training, *Cardiol. Clin.,* 10, 257, 1992.

43. Adams, T. D., Yanowitz, F. G., Fisher, A. G., Ridges, J. D., Lovell, K., and Pryor, T. A., Noninvasive evaluation of exercise training in college-age men, *Circulation*, 64, 958, 1981.
44. Cox, M. L., Bennett, J. B., and Dudley, G. A., Exercise training-induced alterations of cardiac morphology, *J. Appl. Physiol.*, 61, 926, 1986.
45. Spina, R. J., Ogawa, T., Coggan, A. R., Holloszy, J. O., and Ehsani, A. A., Exercise training improves left ventricular contractile response to β-adrenergic agonist, *J. Appl. Physiol.*, 72, 307, 1992.
46. Levy, W. C., Cerqueira, M. D., Abrass, I. B., Schwartz, R. S., and Stratton, J. R., Endurance exercise training augments diastolic filling at rest and during exercise in healthy young and older men, *Circulation*, 88, 116, 1993.
47. Rerych, S. K., Scholz, P. M., Sabiston, D. C., and Jones, R. H., Effects of exercise training on left ventricular function in normal subjects: a longitudinal study by radionuclide angiography, *Am. J. Cardiol.*, 45, 244, 1980.
48. Convertino, V. A., Keil, L. C., and Greenleaf, J. E., Plasma volume, renin, and vasopressin responses to graded exercise after training, *J. Appl. Physiol.*, 54, 508, 1983.
49. Green, H. J., Sutton, J. R., Coates, G., Alli, M., and Jones, S., Responses of red cell and plasma volume to prolonged training in humans, *J. Appl. Physiol.*, 70, 1810, 1991.
50. Schmidt, W., Maassen, N., Trost, F., and Boning, D., Training induced effects on blood volume, erythrocyte turnover and haemoglobin oxygen binding properties, *Eur. J. Appl. Physiol.*, 57, 490, 1988.
51. Laughlin, M. H. and McAllister, R. M., Exercise training-induced coronary vascular adaptation, *J. Appl. Physiol.*, 73, 2209, 1992.
52. Wyatt, H. L. and Mitchell, J., Influences of physical conditioning and deconditioning on coronary vasculature of dogs, *J. Appl. Physiol.*, 45, 619, 1978.
53. Maron, B. J., Pelliccia, A., Spataro, A., and Granata, M., Reduction in left ventricular wall thickness after deconditioning in highly trained Olympic athletes, *Br. Heart J.*, 69, 125, 1993.
54. Henriksson, J., Effects of physical training on the metabolism of skeletal muscle, *Diabetes Care*, 15 (Suppl. 4), 1701, 1992.
55. Martin, W. H., Montgomery, J., Snell, P. G., Corbett, J. R., Sokolov, J. J., Buckey, J. C., Maloney, D. A., and Blomqvist, C. G., Cardiovascular adaptations to intense swim training in sedentary middle-aged men and women, *Circulation*, 75, 323, 1987.
56. Roca, J., Agusti, A. G. N., Alonso, A., Poole, D. C., Viegas, C., Barbera, J. A., Rodriguez-Roisin, R., Ferrer, A., and Wagner, P. D., Effects of training on muscle O_2 transport at VO$_2$max, *J. Appl. Physiol.*, 73, 1067, 1992.
57. Clausen, J. P. and Trap-Jensen, J., Effects of training on the distribution of cardiac output in patients with coronary artery disease, *Circulation*, 42, 611, 1970.
58. Redwood, D. R., Rosing, D. R., and Epstein, S. E., Circulatory and symptomatic effects of physical training in patients with coronary-artery disease and angina pectoris, *N. Engl. J. Med.*, 286, 959, 1972.
59. Foster, C., Pollock, M. L., Anholm, J. D., Squires, R. W., Ward, A., Dymond, D. S., Rod, J. L., Saichek, R. P., and Schmidt, D. H., Work capacity and left ventricular function during rehabilitation after myocardial revascularization surgery, *Circulation*, 69, 748, 1984.
60. Hartung, G. H. and Rangel, R., Exercise training in post-myocardial infarction patients: comparison of results with high risk coronary and post-bypass patients, *Arch. Phys. Med. Rehab.*, 62, 147, 1981.
61. Coats, A. J. S., Adamopoulos, S., Meyer, T. E., Conway, J., and Sleight, P., Effects of physical training in chronic heart failure, *Lancet*, 335, 63, 1990.
62. Giordano, A., Giannuzzi, P, and Tavazzi, L., Feasibility of physical training in post-infarct patients with left ventricular aneurysm: a hemodynamic study, *Eur. Heart J.* (Suppl. F), 9, 11, 1988.
63. Fortini, A., Bonechi, F., Taddei, T., Gensini, G. F., Malfanti, P. L., and Serneri, G. G., Anaerobic threshold in patients with exercise-induced myocardial ischemia, *Circulation*, 83 (Suppl. III), III50, 1991.
64. Ades, P. A., Grunvald, M. H., Weiss, R. M., and Hanson, J. S., Usefulness of myocardial ischemia as predictor of training effect in cardiac rehabilitation after acute myocardial infarction or coronary bypass grafting, *Am. J. Cardiol.*, 63, 1032, 1989.
65. Blumenthal, J. A., Rejeski, W. J., Walsh-Riddle, M., Emery, C. F., Miller, H., Roark, S., Ribisl, P. M., Morris, P. B., Brubaker, P., and Williams, R. S., Comparison of high- and low-intensity exercise training after acute myocardial infarction, *Am. J. Cardiol.*, 61, 26, 1988.
66. Gobel, A. J., Hare, D. L., MacDonald, P. S., Oliver, R. G., Reid, M. A., and Worcester, M. C., Effects of early programmes of high and low intensity exercise on physical performance after transmural acute myocardial infarction, *Br. Heart J.*, 65, 126, 1991.
67. Dressendorfer, R. H., Smith, J. L., Amsterdam, E. A., and Mason, D. T., Reduction of submaximal exercise myocardial oxygen demand post-walk training program in coronary patients due to improved physical work efficiency, *Am. Heart J.*, 103, 358, 1982.
68. Ades, P. A., Waldman, M. L., Poehlman, E. T., Gray, P., Horton, E. D., Horton, E. S., and LeWinter, M. M., Exercise conditioning in older coronary patients: submaximal lactate response and endurance capacity, *Circulation*, 88, 572, 1993.
69. Ferguson, R. J., Taylor, A. W., Cote, P., Charlebois, J., Dinelle, Y., Perronet, F., DeChamplain, J., and Bourassa, M. G., Skeletal muscle and cardiac changes with training in patients with angina pectoris, *Am. J. Physiol.*, 243 (Heart Circ. Physiol. 12), H830, 1982.

70. Adamopoulos, S., Coats, A. J. S., Brunotte, F., Arnolda, L., Meyer, T., Thompson, C. H., Dunn, J. F., Stratton, J., Kemp, G. J., Radda, G. K., and Rajagopalan, B., Physical training improves skeletal muscle metabolism in patients with chronic heart failure, *J. Am. Coll. Cardiol.*, 21, 1101, 1993.

71. Paterson, D. H., Shephard, R. J., Cunningham, D., Jones, N. L., and Andrew, G., Effects of physical training on cardiovascular function following myocardial infarction, *J. Appl. Physiol.*, 47, 482, 1979.

72. Hagberg, J. M., Physiologic adaptations to prolonged high-intensity exercise training in patients with coronary artery disease, *Med. Sci. Sports Exercise*, 23, 661, 1991.

73. Ehsani, A. A., Martin, W. H., Heath, G. W., and Coyle, E. F., Cardiac effects of prolonged and intense exercise training in patients with coronary artery disease, *Am. J. Cardiol.*, 50, 246, 1982.

74. Hagberg, J. M., Ehsani, A. A., and Holloszy, J. O., Effect of 12 months of intense exercise training on stroke volume in patients with coronary artery disease, *Circulation*, 67, 1194, 1983.

75. Martin, W. H., Heath, G., Coyle, E. F., Bloomfield, S. A., Holloszy, J. O., and Ehsani, A. A., Effect of prolonged intense endurance training on systolic time intervals in patients with coronary artery disease, *Am. J. Cardiol.*, 107, 75, 1984.

76. Ehsani, A. A., Biello, D. R., Schultz, J. Sobel, B. E., and Holloszy, J. O., Improvement of left ventricular contractile function by exercise training in patients with coronary artery disease, *Circulation*, 74, 350, 1986.

77. Martin, W. H. and Ehsani, A. A., Reversal of exertional hypotension by prolonged exercise training in selected patients with ischemic heart disease, *Circulation*, 76, 548, 1987.

78. Jugdutt, B. I., Michorowski, B. L., and Kappagoda, C. T., Exercise training after anterior Q wave myocardial infarction: importance of regional left ventricular function and topography, *J. Am. Coll. Cardiol.*, 12, 362, 1988.

79. Giannuzzi, P., Tavazzi, L., Temporelli, P. L., Corra, U., Imparato, A., Gattone, M., Giordano, A., Sala, L., Schweiger, C., and Malinverni, C., Long-term physical training and left ventricular remodeling after anterior myocardial infarction: results of the exercise in anterior myocardial infarction (EAMI) trial, *J. Am. Coll. Cardiol.*, 22, 1821, 1993.

80. Clausen, J. P., Circulatory adjustments to dynamic exercise and effect of physical training in normal subjects and in patients with coronary disease, *Prog. Cardiovasc. Dis.*, 18, 459, 1976.

81. Raffo, J. A., Luksic, I. Y., Kappagoda, C. T., Mary, D. A. S. G., Whitaker, W., and Linden, R. J., Effects of physical training on myocardial ischemia in patients with coronary artery disease, *Br. Heart J.*, 43, 262, 1980.

82. Laslett, L. J., Paumer, L., and Amsterdam, E. A., Increase in myocardial oxygen consumption index by exercise training at the onset of ischemia in patients with coronary artery disease, *Circulation*, 71, 958, 1985.

83. Schuler, G., Schlierf, G., Wirth, A., Mautner, H. P., Scheurlen, H., Thumm, M., Roth, H., Scharz, F., Kohlmeier, M., Mehmel, H. C., and Kubler, W., Low-fat diet and regular, supervised physical exercise in patients with symptomatic coronary artery disease: reduction of stress-induced myocardial ischemia, *Circulation*, 77, 172, 1988.

84. Todd, I. C., Bradnam, M. S., Cooke, M. B. D., and Ballantyne, D., Effects of daily high-intensity exercise on myocardial perfusion in angina pectoris, *Am. J. Cardiol.*, 68, 1593, 1991.

85. Franklin, B. A., Exercise training and coronary collateral circulation, *Med. Sci. Sports Exercise*, 23, 648, 1991.

86. Kennedy, C. C., Spiekerman, R. E., Lindsay, M. I., Mankin, H. T., Frye, R. L., and McCallister, B. D., One-year graduated exercise program for men with angina pectoris: evaluation by physiologic studies and coronary angiography, *Mayo Clin. Proc.*, 51, 231, 1976.

87. Hambrecht, R., Niebauer, J., Marburger, C., Grunze, M., Kalberer, B., Hauer, K., Schlierf, G., Kubler, W., and Schuler, G., Various intensities of leisure time physical activity in patients with coronary artery disease: effects on cardiorespiratory fitness and progression of coronary atherosclerotic lesions, *J. Am. Coll. Cardiol.*, 22, 468, 1993.

88. Stenberg, J., Astrand, P. O., Ekblom, B., Royce, J., and Saltin, B., Hemodynamic response to work with different muscle groups, sitting and supine, *J. Appl. Physiol.*, 22, 61, 1967.

89. Balady, G. J., Types of exercise: arm–leg and static–dynamic, *Cardiol. Clin.*, 11, 297, 1993.

90. Franklin, B. A., Vander, L., Wrisley, D., and Rubenfire, M., Trainability of arms versus legs in men with previous myocardial infarction, *Chest*, 105, 262, 1994.

91. Longhurst, J. C. and Stebbins, C. L., The isometric athlete, *Cardiol. Clin.*, 10, 281, 1992.

92. Vitcenda, M., Hanson, P., Folts, J., and Besozzi, M., Impairment of left ventricular function during maximal isometric dead lifting, *J. Appl. Physiol.*, 69, 2062, 1990.

93. MacDougall, J. D., Tuxen, D., Sale, D. G., Moroz, J. R., and Sutton, J. R., Arterial blood pressure response to heavy resistance exercise, *J. Appl. Physiol.*, 58, 785, 1985.

94. MacDougall, J. D., McKelvie, R. S., Moroz, D. E., Sale, D. G., McCartney, N., and Buick, F., Factors affecting blood pressure during heavy weight lifting and static contractions, *J. Appl. Physiol.*, 73, 1590, 1992.

95. Sullivan, J., Hanson, P., Rahko, P. S., and Folts, J. D., Continuous measurement of left ventricular performance during and after maximal isometric deadlift exercise, *Circulation,* 85, 1406, 1992.

96. Kelemen, M. H. and Stewart, K. J., Circuit weight training: a new direction for cardiac rehabilitation, *Ann. Sports Med.*, 2, 385, 1985.

97. Squires, R. W., Muri, A. J., Anderson, L. J., Allison, T. G., Miller, T. D., and Gau, G. T., Weight training during phase II (early outpatient) cardiac rehabilitation: heart rate and blood pressure responses, *J. Cardiopulm. Rehabil.*, 11, 360, 1991.

98. Stewart, K. J., Mason, M., and Kelemen, M. H., Three-year participation in circuit weight training improves muscular strength and self-efficacy in cardiac patients, *J. Cardiopulm. Rehabil.*, 8, 292, 1988.

Chapter

7

Clinical Exercise Testing Procedures

Robert G. Holly and Karen E. Krstich

CONTENTS

0-8493-4593-6/97/$0.00+$.50

I. INTRODUCTION

Exercise may be the most natural physiological stressor. In a controlled setting, exercise testing can be used safely and progressively to increase the demands of the heart for oxygen up to maximal levels. When coronary artery disease (CAD) is present, its signs and symptoms may appear when the metabolic demands of the myocardium for oxygen exceed the ability of the diseased coronary arteries to deliver oxygen. In clinical cardiology, exercise testing may be used to assess function, diagnose CAD, evaluate CAD symptoms, evaluate the effects of procedures (e.g., bypass and valve surgery), assess prognosis, and screen older asymptomatic males at elevated risk for CAD.[1] In a cardiorespiratory laboratory, exercise testing may also be used to evaluate dyspnea and its causes.[2] Finally, in nonmedical settings, exercise testing may be used to assess fitness and prescribe exercise for athletes, public safety personnel, and the apparently healthy asymptomatic population.[3] Specific procedures, equipment, and concerns are dependent on the purpose of the exercise test and the population being tested. In this chapter we will review briefly the physiological basis of exercise testing and then describe in more detail the knowledge bases in exercise testing procedures and interpretation that are necessary to safely and effectively deliver exercise tests specific to the population being tested.

II. PHYSIOLOGICAL BASIS OF EXERCISE TESTING

Prior to administering any exercise test, the exercise technician must have a thorough grounding in the principles of exercise physiology relevant to exercise testing. These have been fully described in earlier chapters. Only the most important concepts will be reviewed here.

As illustrated in Figure 1, heart rate, cardiac output ($\dot{Q}$), and systolic blood pressure normally increase linearly with work rate up to near maximal effort, when all values may plateau in subjects approaching physiological limits.[4] In contrast, a too rapid or sudden increase in heart rate may indicate, among other things, paroxysmal tachycardia, inadequate increase in stroke volume secondary to heart disease, poor physical conditioning, vasoregulatory asthenia, or anxiety. Inadequate increases in heart rate or systolic blood pressure may indicate second- or third-degree heart block, sinus node disease, or significant cardiac disease, among other causes. A careful analysis of the exercise electrocardiogram (ECG) along with blood pressure responses and patient symptoms can help distinguish among these possibilities.

Oxygen consumption ($\dot{V}O_2$) increases in concert with $\dot{Q}$ and the arteriovenous oxygen (a-$\dot{v}o_2$) difference (Figure 1). This is to be expected since $\dot{V}O_2$ is the product of $\dot{Q}$ and a-$\dot{v}o_2$ difference. Because maximal a-$\dot{v}o_2$ difference tends to plateau between 0.15 to 0.17, the maximal value of $\dot{V}O_2$ ($\dot{V}O_2max$) becomes a good estimator of maximal $\dot{Q}$ (i.e., $\dot{Q}max \approx \dot{V}O_2max/0.16$).[5] Finally, since $\dot{V}O_2max$ is related to the primary function of the heart (i.e., to increase $\dot{Q}$ on demand), prognosis is linked to functional capacity as either measured by $\dot{V}O_2max$ or estimated by metabolic equivalents (METs) for the work rate performed (Table 1).[5]

The plateau in $\dot{V}O_2$ with increasing work rate has been used as the definition of $\dot{V}O_2max$ or maximal exertion.[6] Current thinking is that this is too restrictive a definition.[7] Other criteria for achievement of $\dot{V}O_2max$ in well-motivated subjects include a respiratory exchange ratio (R) of >1.0 and a blood lactate concentration >8 mmol/l.[2] In a clinical cardiology laboratory, $\dot{V}O_2$ and other respiratory variables will most likely not be measured, in which case maximal work rate should be reported in METs (1 MET = 3.5 ml/kg/min) to differentiate this measure of maximal exertion from measured oxygen consumption.

Finally, the distinction between $\dot{V}O_2$ and myocardial oxygen consumption ($m\dot{v}o_2$) is significant. $\dot{V}O_2$ is the measure of whole body oxygen uptake and is directly related to the body's caloric expenditure. In contrast, $m\dot{v}o_2$ is the measure of myocardial oxygen uptake and is linearly related to coronary blood flow.[5] During exercise coronary artery blood flow can increase fivefold in healthy coronary arteries. When the coronary arteries are obstructed by atherosclerosis as in CAD, the degree to which coronary blood flow can increase is limited. When coronary blood flow is insufficient to meet the needs of the myocardium for oxygen, myocardial ischemia occurs. Signs and symptoms of myocardial ischemia may present at levels of $\dot{V}O_2$ significantly below a physiologic $\dot{V}O_2max$. Quite often the exercise test is stopped at this time. The level of $\dot{V}O_2$ attained under these conditions is often referred to as the symptom limited or peak $\dot{V}O_2$ to differentiate it from a true physiologic maximal oxygen uptake. The relationship between $m\dot{v}o_2$ and $\dot{V}O_2$ is linear until the myocardium becomes ischemic. This relationship is a reproducible characteristic of each individual when tested under similar conditions. It may, however, be modified by physical conditioning and drugs such as the β blockers (Figure 2). Finally, $m\dot{v}o_2$ can be validly estimated by the rate pressure product (RPP), which is simply the product of heart rate and systolic blood pressure.[8]

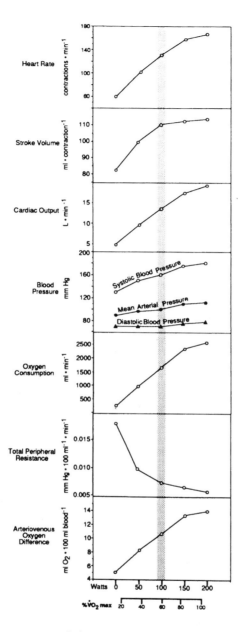

Figure 1 Cardiovascular responses to graded exercise for a typical sedentary individual plotted against work rates and % $\dot{V}O_2$max. The shaded area represents the lactate threshold. (From Durstine JL, Pate RR, Branch JD. In: *Resource Manual for Guidelines for Exercise Testing and Prescription.* Edited by American College of Sports Medicine. Lea and Febiger, Philadelphia, 1993, p. 68. With permission.)

Table 1 Clinically Significant METs for Maximum Exercise Capacity

<5 METs =	poor prognosis; usual limit of functional capacity immediately after myocardial infarction; peak cost of basic activities of daily living
10 METs =	prognosis with medical therapy as good as coronary bypass surgery
13 METS =	excellent prognosis regardless of other exercise responses
18 METs =	elite endurance athletes
20 METs =	world-class athletes

Note: 1 MET = 3.5 ml/kg/min oxygen uptake.

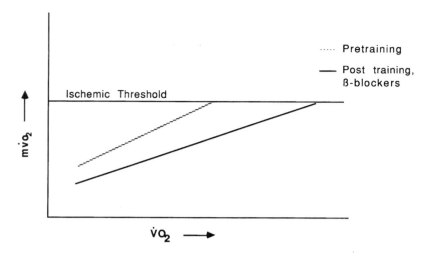

Figure 2   The relationship between myocardial oxygen demand ($m\dot{v}o_2$) and whole body oxygen uptake ($\dot{V}O_2$) in response to training and β-blocking medications.

III. EXERCISE TESTING PROCEDURES

A. EXERCISE TESTING LABORATORY

The exercise testing facility must be clean, safe, and nonthreatening. The atmosphere of the testing laboratory will have an effect upon the patient that can either be positive and comforting or negative and intimidating. Staff demeanor and professionalism are equally important in decreasing the patient's pretest anxiety.

There should be adequate room and privacy for the patient to change clothes for resting ECGs and for exercise testing and recovery. All rooms should be easily accessible to emergency equipment and personnel. Rooms should be well lit and have adequate access to electrical outlets. Avoid stringing electrical cords across the floor where patients or technicians may trip on them. Tables, desks, chairs, treadmills, ECG recorders, and other equipment and furniture should be arranged to provide easy access and a safe and comfortable environment.

Equipment and supplies should be available for all testing situations that will be encountered. At least one treadmill, leg ergometer, and arm ergometer should be present in the well-equipped laboratory. The ECG recorder should be capable of recording both rhythm strips and 12-lead ECGs and should contain adequate paper for an entire exercise test and recovery period. An oscilloscope for monitoring real–time ECGs during exercise is also required. A multichannel scope with freeze-frame capabilities is desirable. Emergency equipment, including a defibrillator/cardioverter, oxygen delivery system, and crash cart with drugs and supplies, should be readily available. Testing personnel should be familiar with the location and operation of all emergency equipment. All drugs and other dated or perishable supplies (e.g., intravenous solutions, laryngoscope batteries) should be current and regularly inventoried. Other equipment for testing include blood pressure cuffs of various sizes, sphygmomanometers (either mercury or aneroid), and stethoscopes. In some laboratories, a glucometer to measure blood glucose level prior to exercise or a pulse oximeter to monitor O_2 saturation during exercise is appropriate. Gas analysis equipment used to determine oxygen uptake during exercise may also be available. Supplies such as tape, razors, disposable electrodes, gauze, alcohol, and thermometers should be well stocked and conveniently located.

ECG equipment, exercise modes, emergency equipment, and ancillary equipment should be maintained and calibrated regularly. Equipment that is not properly calibrated will result in faulty measurements that may detract from patient safety, increase patient anxiety, and limit the value of the test. If you are unfamiliar with calibration procedures for any equipment in your laboratory, see the operator's manual for instruction or contact your service representative. Knowing what values to reasonably expect for a given patient before the start of the test may help you determine the validity of your results. For example, a patient who performs considerably more or less work than you expect might indicate that your mode is not properly calibrated. Furthermore, handrail-supported exercise on the treadmill invalidates standard estimates of oxygen consumption. If handrail-supported exercise is necessary, estimates of oxygen consumption either should not be made or should be corrected.[9]

The exercise testing staff must be professional and pleasant. Staff should be competent in exercise physiology, exercise test administration, and emergency procedures. Exercise technicians should have a good rapport with the patient and be able to communicate effectively in a nonthreatening manner. It should be obvious that the members of the exercise testing team, including both medical and nonmedical personnel, should also treat each other with professionalism and respect.

Every attempt should be made to answer all questions that patients may have and to alleviate their anxiety regarding the test. For most patients, the fear of the unknown is the most anxiety-provoking aspect of an exercise test. Provide them with explicit, step-by-step information regarding what is about to happen. Do not diminish their concerns, but rather be understanding and reassure them that they will be carefully monitored and that every effort will be made to ensure their comfort and safety.

B. EMERGENCY CONSIDERATIONS

Emergencies happen. However, primary attention should be focused on their prevention. Unfortunately, not all emergencies will be prevented, so all testing personnel must be prepared and trained to manage emergencies when they do occur.

1. Preventing the Cardiopulmonary Emergency

Appropriate screening and supervision along with an understanding of normal and abnormal responses to exercise are necessary to prevent cardiopulmonary emergencies. The American College of Sports Medicine (ACSM) presents recommendations for medical screening and supervision of exercise tests based on a person's age, gender, level of risk, and symptoms.[10] Physician clearance and supervision are recommended for patients with known disease or symptoms, for those with two or more major CAD risk factors, and for older apparently healthy persons (females >50 and males >40 years old). Good clinical judgment should always prevail. While pretest medical evaluation and physician supervision of the exercise test may be unnecessary in lower-risk, asymptomatic individuals, they are appropriate when testing higher-risk or symptomatic patients.

Prior to an exercise test, personnel should be thoroughly familiar with the patient's medical history and physical examination results. Particular attention should be paid to current and past cardiovascular diseases, symptoms, risk factors, procedures, and medications, as well as any other physical condition which may either contraindicate this test or alter its method of delivery. Prior ECGs should be compared with the current ECG, looking for changes that may also contraindicate the current test. Is this test indicated? Review the purpose of the test to ensure that the exercise test is the appropriate test to answer the question being asked. Look ahead to possible end points to each test so that the appropriate mode and protocol are selected, and testing personnel may be particularly vigilant for developing abnormalities that might indicate early test termination. For example, an active hypertensive patient who would ordinarily run on a treadmill protocol might be given a leg ergometer test so that blood pressure could be monitored more easily and accurately. Finally, it is well to remember that an exercise test is an elective, nonemergent procedure. It can always be postponed if there is any indication that it is currently unsafe to test a patient.

2. Preparing for the Cardiopulmonary Emergency

Despite our best efforts to prevent cardiopulmonary emergencies, they still occur. Thompson[11] has recently reviewed the literature concerning the incidence of cardiac complications during clinical exercise testing: approximately one death, four myocardial infarctions, and five hospitalizations (including the infarctions) can be expected per 10,000 exercise tests. For this reason all exercise testing personnel must be ready to respond to a cardiopulmonary emergency at any time. Each facility should have their own emergency/evacuation plan that deals with both cardiac and noncardiac emergencies. The mere presence of these plans, however, is insufficient. Emergency procedures *must* be practiced on a regular basis. Emergencies are stressful enough even to a highly experienced team. The less experienced the testing team is in responding to emergencies, the more important and frequent emergency practice should become. All exercise testing personnel should be certified at the level of Basic Life Support, while some staff should also be certified in Advanced Cardiac Life Support. Emergency supplies and equipment should be conveniently located. Drugs should be current, the defibrillator should be calibrated, supplies should be inventoried on a regular schedule, and the defibrillator should undergo a test discharge prior to each testing day to verify adequate battery charge and energy delivery. Tables 2 and 3 list emergency equipment, supplies, and drugs which should be readily available in any clinical exercise testing facility.

Table 2 Emergency Equipment and Supplies

Defibrillation/Cardioversion	Intubation/Oxygenation	Drug Management	Recording
Defibrillator	Airways	IV sets	Code sheets
Monitor	Oxygen mask	IV cannulas	Writing utensils
Electrode paste or gel pads	Pocket mask	IV stand	Stop watch
Electrodes	Nasal cannula	D_5W (5% dextrose solution)	
Monitoring leads	Endotracheal tube	Normal saline	
	Laryngoscope	Syringes	
	AMBU bag with O_2 reservoir	Needles	
	Oxygen	Adhesive tape	
	Suction equipment		

Table 3 Emergency Drugs

Positive ionotropics
    Epinephrine — ventricular fibrillation/pulseless ventricular tachycardia/asystole/electromechanical dissociation
    Digoxin — congestive heart failure
Antitachycardics — ventricular
    Lidocaine — ventricular fibrillation/ventricular tachycardia
    Bretylium — ventricular fibrillation/pulseless ventricular tachycardia
    Procainamide — ventricular tachycardia
Antitachycardics — supraventricular
    Verapamil — paroxysmal supraventricular tachycardia
    Digoxin — atrial fibrillation
Antibradycardics
    Atropine
    Isoproterenol
Antianginals
    Nitroglycerin — typical angina
    Verapamil — variant angina
Antihypertensive
    Nifedipine
Vasopressors
    Dopamine
    Metaraminol
Acid–base balance
    Sodium bicarbonate
Anticongestive heart failure
    Lasix
Antisyncope
    Aromatic ammonia
Miscellaneous
    D_5W — IV solution
    O_2 — blood oxygenation
    Morphine — sedation
    Valium — sedation

3. Managing the Cardiopulmonary Emergency

The American Heart Association publishes the *Textbook for Advanced Cardiac Life Support*.[12] Algorithms are provided to guide the emergency (code) team through various cardiac emergencies. Only personnel qualified to administer drugs, defibrillate, and supply oxygen to the patient should actually do so. However, all exercise testing personnel should be able to assist in advanced cardiac life support and perform cardiopulmonary resuscitation (CPR) during an emergency. It bears repeating that an exercise testing team's response to a cardiac emergency is in large measure dependent upon regular practice in emergency procedures. While practice may not necessarily make perfect, it does increase the probability of success.

C. MODE AND PROTOCOL SELECTION

The mode and protocol chosen for a particular exercise test can affect the outcome of the test. Matching the appropriate mode and protocol to the patient and the reason for doing the test is an important function of the exercise technician. There are many reasons for using a specific exercise mode for a test. Most have to do with the specificity of the test or the physical limitations of the patient. In some instances, a given mode may be chosen because of the particular physiological stress imposed upon the patient.

For example, in job-related exercise testing, it is important that the exercise mode relate to the job task as closely as possible. Using an arm ergometer test of arm power to assess a fire fighter's conditioning to extend a ladder would be more appropriate than using a measure of grip strength from a hand dynamometer. When developing an exercise prescription for fitness or rehabilitation, it is important to use the exercise mode which will allow the patient to give his or her best performance. Because most people are familiar and comfortable with walking, a treadmill exercise test is often the best choice of mode when an exercise prescription is desired. A patient who is unaccustomed to bicycling will often experience local fatigue and discomfort in the legs before adequate cardiovascular stress is attained when tested on a leg ergometer. In this case, the exercise prescription developed would be inadequate and inappropriate for the patient. There are a variety of patient-specific reasons to choose a particular exercise mode. These have to do with the health, age, and orthopedic limitations of the patient. A patient with severe arthritis in both legs may not be able to achieve adequate physiological stress using either a leg ergometer or treadmill to provide either diagnostic or functional information. This patient may benefit instead from an arm ergometer test. In some testing situations, the need to attain specific physiological data may dictate which mode to use. If determining accurate blood pressure measurements at high work rates is important, a leg ergometer may be a better choice of mode than a treadmill, even if the patient is a jogger. The characteristics, advantages, and disadvantages of several different exercise modes and protocols are considered below.

1. Modes

Numerous modes are available which can stress the cardiovascular system. These include steps, treadmills, arm and leg ergometers, swimming tethers and flumes, and recreational and work-related tasks. The utility, advantages, and disadvantages of each are discussed below.

An exercise step test may be useful when a submaximal exercise test is desired and minimal exercise equipment is available.[13] This mode is mostly of historical significance and is seldom used clinically today. There are various protocols for use with step tests. The step height is determined by the protocol used. The patient steps up and down on the step at a predetermined rate for a set number of minutes. Following the test, an ECG is recorded and/or a count of heart rate may be used to determine fitness level using a table or nomogram. Limitations of step tests include not being able to record or monitor an ECG during stepping because of movement artifact, not being able to grade work rate very easily, and the likelihood that patients may stumble on the step as they begin to fatigue. Many people are not able to maintain stepping cadence with a metronome, which is required to achieve valid results. As a result, step tests are not routinely used in the clinical setting.

The most common exercise testing mode is the motorized treadmill. Most people are able to walk comfortably on a treadmill, and, if given a short familiarization period, they can usually walk without holding on to handrails. This is extremely important when using speed and grade to estimate functional capacity.[9] The treadmill speed and/or grade are gradually increased to increase exercise intensity. One of the disadvantages of treadmill exercise is the difficulty in obtaining accurate blood pressure measurements at high work rates when a patient is jogging. For accurate blood pressure measurements in fit individuals, a leg ergometer may be the mode of choice. Other disadvantages to treadmill exercise testing include any orthopedic or neurological problem that precludes the patient from being able to safely and comfortably walk on the treadmill. For example, lower extremity injury, postural instability, neuromuscular disease, and stroke can all impair the patient's ability to safely and effectively perform a diagnostic or functional treadmill test.

A leg ergometer test may be useful if a patient is unable to walk safely on a treadmill, if the patient participates in cycling regularly, or if a treadmill is not available. There are different types of leg ergometers, including those with a mechanical flywheel against which resistance is applied (requiring constant-speed pedaling) and electronically braked ergometers which maintain a constant work rate regardless of pedaling speed. Leg ergometers allow for easier and more accurate blood pressure measurements, particularly at higher work rates, but may reduce the quality of ECG recordings because of tension in the muscles of the upper body. It may be necessary for the patient to let go of the handlebars periodically to obtain high-quality ECG recordings. The major disadvantage of the leg ergometer is that patients who do not participate in cycling on a regular basis may be limited by local muscular fatigue prior to adequately stressing the cardiovascular system.

Arm ergometry is an option for patients who are unable to use their legs for exercise. It is also useful to evaluate symptoms produced only by arm work or to measure functional capacity in a patient whose job requires a high level of arm power. An arm ergometer stress test requires that the patient crank the device at a given speed. Work rate is determined by the rate of cranking, the distance the flywheel travels per revolution, and the amount of resistance applied (similar to a mechanically braked leg ergometer).[10] While an arm ergometer may allow diagnostic or functional testing in patients who are unable to use their legs, it is difficult to obtain accurate blood pressure measurements and high-quality ECG recordings while the patient is cranking. Thus, it is necessary to interrupt the protocol periodically to obtain these data. Many patients are unable to reach a high enough work rate with arm ergometry to evoke an adequate cardiovascular stress to achieve a diagnostic test. However, many of these patients may be unlikely to do anything more strenuous than this test during their daily activities; thus, it would still be a valid test of exercise tolerance, despite its limitation in the diagnosis of ischemia.

It is possible to use swimming as a mode for exercise stress testing; however, this is rarely done outside of specialized laboratory settings. Swim stress testing requires either a tether, where the pull of the swimmer against a gauge can be measured as the swimmer swims increasingly hard, or a flume in which the speed of the water against which the patient swims can be varied to increase work rate. Swim stress testing is useful in obtaining an accurate measurement of functional capacity in elite swimmers. It is not, however, practical for diagnostic stress testing as it is very difficult to obtain accurate blood pressure or ECG measurements during swimming without costly specialized equipment.

When it is difficult to elicit a patient's exertional symptoms with conventional exercise modes, an ambulatory test such a Holter monitor may be used. A Holter monitor is a 24 to 48 h ECG monitor which the patient wears while going about his or her daily routine. A diary is kept by the patient, making notes of symptoms, time, physical activities, meals, medications, stressful situations, etc. A Holter monitor is especially helpful in detecting dysrhythmias, as these are not generally reproducible with exercise testing. Some disadvantages of Holter monitoring include the reliance on the patient to be a good diary keeper, the lack of an objective measure of exercise intensity, and the inconvenience to the patient of wearing the monitor for 24 or more hours.

Patients can also be monitored during regular exercise sessions with ECG telemetry. Telemetry allows the patient to move about in a large room without the problem of tangling or tripping over lead wires. The patient wears three disposable electrodes which are attached to a telemetry unit (about the size of a deck of cards). A small battery powers the telemetry unit which is worn around the neck or in a pocket. The ECG can then be monitored on a screen, and ECG tracings can be obtained as desired. Several patients can be monitored at one time, as in a group exercise session. Telemetry systems are relatively easy to use and they allow for direct monitoring of the ECG, heart rate, and rhythm during routine exercise sessions, occupational or recreational tasks, and exercise testing. The main drawback to telemetry is that usually only one lead can be monitored at a time. This makes detection of ischemic ECG changes difficult; however, accurate documentation of exercise-related dysrhythmias is easily accomplished.

Sometimes the exercise mode must be specifically designed to recreate patterns of activity which occur in the patient's daily life. The two most common indications for such task-specific exercise modes are to verify work capacity in job-related functions and to evaluate symptoms which occur only with specific types of exercise. Jobs that require an individual to carry heavy objects, climb stairs, or walk through water or mud can often be simulated well enough in a laboratory test. Patients can walk on a treadmill carrying weighted objects or wearing weight belts. They can perform arm or leg anaerobic power tests on ergometers, and specific movements can often be recreated in the laboratory setting. A second area in which using a task-specific exercise mode is useful is in evaluating reproducible exertional symptoms which are specific to one type of exercise (e.g., "I only pass out when I lift weights" or "I only get chest pain while shoveling snow"). Some work tasks are so complicated and unique, and some settings so private (e.g., symptoms during coitus), that rather than attempt to recreate the activity in the laboratory, monitoring of the actual activity in daily life is preferable. It is often possible to obtain accurate electrocardiographic records in these situations using either telemetry or Holter monitoring. It must be remembered, however, that the sensitivity of these devices in detecting ischemia may be decreased as a result of the lack of multilead monitoring.

2. Protocols

In an exercise test, one of the most important aspects of the test is how it progresses, that is, at what level of exertion does the test begin, and how is it advanced over time. There are many different protocols available for each mode of exercise. It is important to choose the protocol that most appropriately fits the ability of the patient and that will allow you to collect the physiological data desired. The initial load and the degree of increase in exertion with each subsequent stage should be determined as a function of the health, age, weight, and fitness level of the patient. Activity-related scoring systems exist that help estimate a patient's functional capacity.[14,15] Such scoring systems may be useful in determining an appropriate protocol for patients of unknown fitness levels. Older, frail, sedentary, obese, and diseased patients should be started at a relatively low work intensity, and the work rate should increase in increments of approximately $1/2$ to 1 MET/stage. A common error in exercise testing, particularly in obese and unfit individuals, is choosing a protocol (such as the Bruce treadmill protocol) that begins at too high a level of intensity and advances too quickly for the patient. In this case, a patient may only be able to complete a few minutes of the protocol, during which their heart rate increases inordinately for the level of exercise. The end result is that the test is terminated prematurely because of local muscle fatigue without a true measure of functional capacity. In these situations, allowing for a physiological warm-up by choosing a protocol which begins at a lower intensity and progresses more slowly will provide a longer and more physiological stress test. Conversely, a young, fit individual will need to have the test started at a higher intensity and the stages should advance in greater increments of 2 to 3 METs/stage. A good rule of thumb for both functional and diagnostic tests is to choose a protocol that will allow the patient to exercise for approximately 8 to 10 min, following a 5 to 6 min warm-up phase, before reaching fatigue.[16]

In some tests, there is a single load or stage of work to be performed. A step test is a good example of single load, or steady rate exercise testing. A single load test is typically performed for a set number of minutes, after which the patient's heart rate is monitored and a fitness level is estimated using a normative table. Although this type of testing is useful in estimating aerobic fitness, or determining the patient's ability to do a set work rate, it is rarely used in a clinical setting to evaluate functional capacity and has little diagnostic value.[13]

Another method of loading is to use discontinuous or interrupted stages. Discontinuous loading is useful when the patient is not able to tolerate continued exercise with increasing work intensities. Arm ergometer testing is a good example. Some patients may not be able to perform a very high work rate if the exercise continuously increases in intensity, but if they are allowed to rest briefly between stages, they can perform a much higher maximal work rate. Also in arm ergometry, it is difficult to obtain accurate blood pressures and ECG recordings during exercise. A discontinuous protocol allows for these measurements to be taken during the rest periods, although is should be noted that blood pressure drops off rapidly as soon as the exercise is stopped.[17]

The most common loading pattern in graded exercise testing is to use a stepped series of loads, or stages, that increase without interruption. These stages are typically 2 to 3 min each. If functional capacity is to be calculated from work rate, it is important to realize that it takes the cardiovascular system at least 2 to 3 min to "catch up" with a given work rate so that the heart rate and blood pressure measured are truly indicative of the level of exertion at that stage. Also, the higher the work intensity, and the lower the person's fitness level, the longer it takes the body to catch up. This same phenomenon holds true for diagnostic testing. If the exercise intensity is increased too rapidly, the heart may not be stressed sufficiently to exhibit ischemic changes before the patient fatigues; whereas, if the test had been increased more gradually, heart rate can reach higher values before the patient fatigues and ischemic changes may appear. In general, the larger the increase in work rate between stages, the longer each stage should be. For example, the Bruce protocol, which increases by 2 to 3 METs/stage, has 3-min stages. The Balke protocol, which increases by about 1 MET/stage, has 2-min stages. A modified Balke protocol (very low intensity) increases by about 1 MET/stage and has 3-min stages. This protocol would allow an ill, obese, or unfit individual more time to adjust to each increment in intensity and should allow better exercise performance for both functional and diagnostic testing.

Another type of loading is the continuous ramp which may be used with either the leg ergometer or the treadmill. On a treadmill, speed is held constant while the grade increases gradually over time, at about 1 to 3% per minute.[18] On a leg ergometer, work rate should increase by 5 to 30 W/min.[19] This type of loading is well tolerated by patients because there are no large jumps in work intensity. For this reason it is also an excellent protocol to elicit a plateau in $\dot{V}O_2max$. However, it is difficult to estimate functional capacity based on speed and grade or watts because of the physiological "lag time" discussed above. For this reason the continuous ramp protocol is best used when $\dot{V}O_2max$ is directly measured.

There is a variety of protocols available for every mode of exercise. It is important to understand how these protocols differ and to choose the protocol that best fits the characteristics of the patient and that will provide the desired physiological data. Although many protocols can be used for both diagnostic

Table 4   Modified Bruce Treadmill Protocol

Stage	Speed (mph)	Grade (%)	Duration (min)	METS
0	1.7	0	3	1.7
$^1/_2$	1.7	5	3	2.9
I	1.7	10	3	4.7
II	2.5	12	3	7.1
III	3.4	14	3	10.2
IV	4.2	16	3	13.5
V	5.0	18	3	17.3
VI	5.5	20	3	20.4
VII	6.0	22	3	23.8

and functional tests, sometimes a given protocol is better suited to one or the other. The health, weight, age, and fitness level of the patient should also be taken into account when choosing a protocol, just as in choosing an exercise mode. The exercise technician should be flexible and creative when choosing and/or customizing an exercise test protocol. The characteristics, advantages, and disadvantages of several different exercise protocols are discussed below.

The treadmill is the most common exercise mode for clinical testing. There are numerous protocols that have been published, some of which are designed for very specific patient populations. The protocol most commonly used in the clinical setting is the Bruce protocol.[20] However, it is seldom the most appropriate choice for a given patient. The Bruce protocol begins at a speed of 1.7 mph and a grade of 10% (stage 1 in Table 4). This is a high-intensity first stage, even for a fit individual. The modified Bruce adds two "pre-stages" where the grade is started at 0% (stage 0) and then advanced to 5% (stage $^1/_2$) (Table 4). This helps many patients to better adjust to stage 1. However, after that, the protocol advances at a rate of about 2 to 3 METs/stage which is too rapid and vigorous for many diseased or unfit individuals. As previously mentioned, these patients may exhibit early fatigue which may preclude detection of ischemic ECG changes and lead to misdiagnoses and erroneous exercise prescriptions. Highly trained patients may also have difficulty with some of the later stages of the Bruce protocol. For example, in stage 4, the patient is traveling at 4.2 mph up a 16% grade and often has difficulty deciding whether to walk or jog at this speed. It may be particularly difficult to do this without holding onto the railing which can invalidate the estimation of functional capacity based on speed and grade.[9]

For an obese, unfit, or cardiac patient, a low-level protocol such as Balke may be a better choice. The Balke protocol uses a constant walking speed of 3.0 mph and begins at a 2.5% grade (Table 5).[21] The MET level of this initial stage is about 4.3 METs, which is similar to stage 1 of the Bruce protocol. Each 2-min stage increases by 2.5% grade which translates into an increase of about 1 MET/stage. The modified Balke uses a constant speed of 2.0 mph (which may be a more comfortable pace for many patients) and begins with a grade of 0% or about 2.5 METs (Table 6). This protocol advances 3.5% grade every 3 min and also increases at about 1 MET/stage. With the modified Balke, a 12-min test would require a functional capacity of only 6.0 METs, which would allow for better physiological measurement than a Bruce protocol, in which 6 METs is required by the second stage.

The morbidly obese patient whose body fat exceeds 35 to 40% of body weight presents a particular problem. Due to their excess body weight, increasing grade during treadmill walking causes rapid increases in absolute oxygen consumption (liters per minute), and these subjects may fatigue early in the test without either sufficient warm-up or stress to the cardiovascular system. So that these individuals will not fatigue in the early minutes of a test, it has been our practice to halve all grade increases for whatever protocol we are using when testing a morbidly obese patient. This allows for both sufficient warm-up and test duration so that the cardiovascular system will be adequately stressed and the test will not be prematurely terminated because of local muscle fatigue. It should be appreciated that while these individuals will have low functional capacities when expressed relative to body weight (e.g., $\dot{V}O_2$max in ml/kg/min or estimated in METs), they may have normal levels of absolute oxygen consumption when $\dot{V}O_2$max is expressed in liters per minute.

For fit individuals, the challenge lies in finding a protocol that will adequately stress the cardiovascular system without causing limiting local leg fatigue. Many protocols, including Bruce and Balke protocols, require treadmill grades of 15 to 20% for those with a functional capacity greater than 10 METs. For most individuals, it is easier to walk or jog at a faster pace with a lower grade. Such a protocol would allow patients to reach higher maximal work rates prior to experiencing limiting muscular fatigue.[22]

Table 5 Balke Treadmill Protocol

Stage	Speed (mph)	Grade (%)	Duration (min)	METS
I	3.0	2.5	2	4.3
II	3.0	5.0	2	5.4
III	3.0	7.5	2	6.4
IV	3.0	10.0	2	7.4
V	3.0	12.5	2	8.5
VI	3.0	15.0	2	9.5
VII	3.0	17.5	2	10.5
VIII	3.0	20.0	2	11.6
IX	3.0	22.5	2	12.6

Table 6 Modified Balke Treadmill Protocol

Stage	Speed (mph)	Grade (%)	Duration (min)	METS
I	2.0	0	3	2.5
II	2.0	3.5	3	3.5
III	2.0	7.0	3	4.5
IV	2.0	10.5	3	5.4
V	2.0	14.0	3	6.4
VI	2.0	17.5	3	7.4
VII	3.0	12.5	3	8.5
VIII	3.0	15.0	3	9.5
IX	3.0	17.5	3	10.5
X	3.0	20.0	3	11.6
XI	3.0	22.5	3	12.6

Some protocols have a branching format that allows the technician to increase the speed or grade according to the patient's heart rate response (Figure 3).[22] This type of protocol is useful for sedentary, diseased, and fit individuals and demonstrates a very important aspect of exercise test administration: Each patient is different in ability and physiological response to exercise, and the protocol should be chosen and administered accordingly. It is much better to adjust and customize a protocol as a test progresses rather than stick to a predetermined and inappropriate advancement of speed and grade just because that is the established and accepted protocol. (However, it is better to have selected the appropriate protocol initially.) Modifying a protocol may make it more difficult to estimate oxygen consumption if $\dot{V}O_2$ is not measured. However, functional capacity in METs can be easily calculated from speed and grade (or ergometer wattage) using formulas in the ACSM Guidelines.[10]

Some treadmills can be set to increase continually in grade at a constant speed for a very gradual increase in work rate without discrete stages (Figure 4). This is called a continuous ramp protocol.[18] A continuous ramp treadmill protocol is also useful for a wide range of individuals. The speed can be increased and adjusted so that the patient can reach maximal exertion without using excessive grades. Again, the main disadvantage of the continuous ramp format is the difficulty in predicting functional capacity based on speed and grade if $\dot{V}O_2$ is not measured; however, it is an excellent protocol for diagnostic testing as it allows patients to gradually reach true maximal exertion levels. It can be easily modified to be appropriate for both low- and high-fit patients.

Because leg ergometry delivers absolute, external resistance, a larger individual with greater lean body mass is able to perform at higher absolute work rates than a smaller individual with less lean body mass. For this reason, leg ergometry protocols for smaller (<70 kg) and/or less-fit individuals should start at lower work rates (25 W) and increase in 2 to 3 min stages of approximately 25 W (1.0 to 1.5 MET/stage). In contrast, larger (>70 kg) and/or more-fit individuals should start at a higher initial work rate of 50 W and increase in 2 to 3 min stages of 50 W (2 to 3 MET/stage). As with treadmill testing, the protocol should be adjusted to the patient as the test progresses and the goal should be to have the patient perform approximately 8 to 10 min of exercise, after 5 to 6 min of warm-up, before reaching fatigue. Many electronically braked leg ergometers also allow for continuous ramp protocols. Wasserman et al.[19] propose continuous ramp leg ergometer protocols that advance at rates of 10 to 20 W/min for normal adult females and 15 to 25 W/min for normal adult males.

BRANCHING MULTISTAGE TREADMILL TEST PROTOCOL

STAGE	WALK TIME min	BRANCH I SPEED MPH	BRANCH I SPEED M/min	BRANCH I SLOPE %	BRANCH I $\dot{V}O_2$ ml/min·Kg	BRANCH II SPEED MPH	BRANCH II SPEED M/min	BRANCH II SLOPE %	BRANCH II $\dot{V}O_2$ ml/min·Kg	BRANCH III SPEED MPH	BRANCH III SPEED M/min	BRANCH III SLOPE %	BRANCH III $\dot{V}O_2$ ml/min·Kg	BRANCH IV SPEED MPH	BRANCH IV SPEED M/min	BRANCH IV SLOPE %	BRANCH IV $\dot{V}O_2$ ml/min·Kg	BRANCH V SPEED MPH	BRANCH V SPEED M/min	BRANCH V SLOPE %	BRANCH V $\dot{V}O_2$ ml/min·Kg
1	0-2	1.97	53	0	9.5																
2	2-4	2.62	70	0	12	If below 70% MHR* at 4 minutes, follow Branch II															
3	4-6	2.62	70	3	14	3.19	85	0	14.5												
4	6-8	2.62	70	6	17	3.19	85	3.5	18	If below 70% MHR* at 8 minutes, follow Branch III											
5	8-10	2.62	70	9	20	3.19	85	6	21	3.63	97	3.5	21								
6	10-12	2.62	70	12	23	3.19	85	9	24.5	3.63	97	7	25	If below 70% MHR* at 12 minutes, follow Branch IV							
7	12-14	2.62	70	15	26	3.19	85	12	28	3.63	97	10	29	4.01	107	7.5	30				
8	14-16	2.62	70	17.5	29	3.19	85	15	32	3.63	97	13	33.5	4.01	107	12	36.5	If below 70% MHR* at 16 minutes, follow Branch V			
9	16-18	2.62	70	20	32.5	3.19	85	17.5	36.5	3.63	97	16	38.5	4.01	107	15	42.5	5.21	139	12.0	47
10	18-20	2.62	70	22	36	3.19	85	20	41	3.63	97	19	44.5	4.01	107	18	49	5.21	139	16.0	57
11	20-22					3.19	85	22	44.5	3.63	97	22	51	4.01	107	20	54	5.21	139	19.5	66.5
12	22-24													4.01	107	22	60	5.21	139	22.0	77
13	24-26																	6.20	166	22.0	85

*MHR = Maximal Heart Rate

Figure 3 The branching multistage treadmill protocol begins with slow walking at 0% grade. After 4 min, if heart rate is above 70% of predicted maximal heart rate (MHR), the subject remains in Branch I for the entire test. However, if heart rate is less than 70% of MHR after 4 min, the protocol then moves into Branch II. The protocol keeps branching every 4 min until heart rate is greater than 70% MHR at a branch point. Then the protocol continues within the same branch until the test is terminated. (From Tonkin MJ, Garrett L, DeMaria AN, Miller RR, Mason DT. *Chest.* 1977; 72:714–718. With permission.)

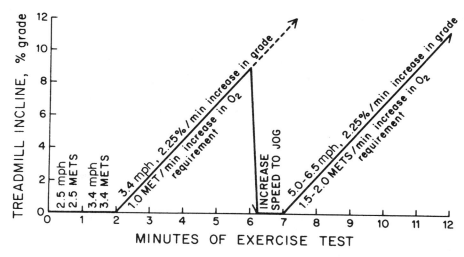

Figure 4 The continuous ramp treadmill protocol begins at 2.5 mph and 0% grade. Speed is increased to 3.4 mph after the first minute. At 2 min the ramp is turned on and grade increases at 2.25% per minute. After 6 min if heart rate is greater than 70% of predicted maximum, the protocol continues to ramp at 2.25% per minute, 3.4 mph, without further adjustment until the test is terminated. However, if heart rate is less than 70% of predicted maximum at minute 6, the grade is returned to 0% and speed is increased to a comfortable jog (5.0 to 6.5 mph). At minute 7 the ramp is turned back on and grade again increases at 2.25% per minute until the test is terminated. (From Dressendorfer RH, Amsterdam EA. *Cardiology.* 1980; 66:204–222. With permission.)

Arm ergometry protocols are very similar to leg ergometry protocols, again depending on body size and lean body mass. However, the muscle mass of the arms is markedly less than that of the legs, so these tests must start at even lower initial work rates and advance in smaller increments. For smaller (<70 kg) and/or less fit patients an initial work rate of 12.5 W with 2 to 3-min stages incrementing by 12.5 W/stage should be appropriate. Larger and/or more fit patients should be able to tolerate a higher-intensity initial stage of 25 W and perform 2 to 3-min stages with 25 W increments. Measured maximal functional capacity with arm exercise is usually only 60 to 70% of that determined for leg exercise, so it is advisable to use leg exercise for both functional and diagnostic testing whenever feasible.

D. INDICATIONS FOR EXERCISE TESTING

The American College of Cardiology/American Heart Association (ACC/AHA) Task Force on Cardio-vascular Procedures has published indications for exercise testing (Table 7).[1,16] Class I indications are those for which there is a consensus that testing is justified. Class II indications are those for which there is disagreement on its justification. Class III indications are those indications for which there is consensus that testing is not justified. These classifications are useful in guiding decisions in a clinical setting where exercise testing is attempting to answer questions relative to diagnosis and prognosis. However, when exercise testing is done for nonmedical purposes, such as evaluation of functional capacity in athletes, public safety workers, health club members, worksite wellness participants, and the like, these indications become too restrictive. Beyond establishing an individual's functional capacity, exercise testing may also be useful in exercise prescription, evaluating progress in a fitness program, and motivating individuals to become more physically active. It is also important to recognize the relationship between increased fitness and both improved prognosis (see Table 1) and decreased risk of cardiovascular disease.[23] Recently, Blair et al.[23] demonstrated in an apparently healthy, asymptomatic population that the relative risk for cardiovascular disease was approximately 8 for males and 9 for females when the lowest fit group within each gender was compared with the highest fit groups. Peak capacities around 9 METs (females) to 10 METs (males) were all that were needed to attain this level of protection. Furthermore, even in the presence of CAD risk factors, those with higher levels of fitness were still at lower risk for CAD than the less fit. Despite the clinicians' general consensus that exercise testing is not medically justified in the apparently healthy, asymptomatic population, functional tests may have real value in clarifying the risk of CAD in a given individual.

Table 7 ACC/AHA Task Force on Assessment of Cardiovascular Procedures: Guidelines for Indications for Exercise Testing

CLASS I	General consensus that exercise testing is justified
CLASS II	Frequently used but divergence of opinion regarding justification for exercise testing
CLASS III	General agreement that exercise testing is of little value, inappropriate, or contraindicated

Testing of Patients with Signs/Symptoms of CAD or with Known CAD

CLASS I	To assist in the diagnosis of male patients with atypical signs/symptoms of CAD
	To evaluate functional capacity
	To assess prognosis
	To evaluate patients with symptoms consistent with recurrent exercise-induced arrhythmias
CLASS II	To assist in the diagnosis of CAD in women with chest pain
	To assist in the diagnosis of patients on digoxin or with right bundle branch block
	To evaluate functional capacity and response to therapy with drugs in CAD or congestive heart failure
	To evaluate variant angina
	To serially follow (1 year or longer) patients with CAD
CLASS III	To evaluate patients with single premature ventricular contractions (PVCs)
	To serially evaluate functional capacity in patients in cardiac rehabilitation programs
	To diagnose CAD in patients with Wolff–Parkinson–White syndrome or left bundle branch block

Exercise Testing in the Screening of Apparently Healthy Individuals

CLASS I	None
CLASS II	To evaluate asymptomatic males over 40:
	In special occupations (e.g., pilots, fire fighters, police officers)
	With two or more risk factors (chol > 240, blood pressure ≥ 160/90, cigarette smoking, diabetes mellitus, family history of CAD < 55 years)
	Who are sedentary and plan to enter a vigorous exercise program
CLASS III	To evaluate asymptomatic men and women:
	With no risk factors
	With chest discomfort not thought to be cardiac

Exercise Testing Soon after Myocardial Infarction (MI)

CLASS I	To evaluate prognosis and functional capacity in uncomplicated MIs
CLASS II	To evaluate those with baseline ECGs or medical problems that affect responses
	To evaluate those with complicated MIs who have subsequently stabilized
CLASS III	To evaluate acute ischemia
	To evaluate patients who are unstable or have complicating illnesses

Exercise Testing after Specific Procedures

CLASS I	To evaluate coronary artery bypass graft (CABG) and percutaneous transluminal coronary angioplasty (PTCA) patients
CLASS II	To follow asymptomatic patients with CABG or PTCA yearly

Exercise Testing of Patients with Valvular Heart Disease

CLASS I	None
CLASS II	To evaluate functional capacity
CLASS III	To evaluate symptomatic critical aortic stenosis or hypertrophic obstructive cardiomyopathy

Exercise Testing in the Management of Patients with High Blood Pressure or Cardiac Pacemakers

CLASS I	None
CLASS II	To evaluate blood pressure response in patients treated for high blood pressure who wish to exercise vigorously
CLASS III	To evaluate patients with severe high blood pressure, to evaluate high blood pressure patients who do not plan to exercise, to evaluate pacemaker function

Exercise Testing in Children

CLASS I	To evaluate functional capacity in selected patients with congenital heart disease
CLASS II	To evaluate functional capacity in valvular or congenital heart disease

Adapted from McKirnan, M. D. and Froelicher, V. F., in *Exercise Testing and Prescription for Special Populations*. J. S. Skinner, Ed., Lea and Febiger, Philadelphia, 1993, 13. With permission.

Table 8 Contraindications to Exercise Testing

Absolute Contraindications

1. A recent significant change in the resting ECG suggesting infarction or other acute cardiac events
2. Recent complicated myocardial infarction
3. Unstable angina
4. Uncontrolled ventricular dysrhythmia
5. Uncontrolled atrial dysrhythmia that compromises cardiac function
6. Third-degree A-V block
7. Acute congestive heart failure
8. Severe aortic stenosis
9. Suspected or known dissecting aneurysm
10. Active or suspected myocarditis or pericarditis
11. Thrombophlebitis or intracardiac thrombi
12. Recent systemic or pulmonary embolus
13. Acute infection
14. Significant emotional distress (psychosis)

Relative Contraindications

1. Resting diastolic blood pressure > 120 mmHg or resting systolic blood pressure > 200 mmHg
2. Moderate valvular heart disease
3. Known electrolyte abnormalities (hypokalemia, hypomagnesemia)
4. Fixed-rate pacemaker
5. Frequent or complex ventricular ectopy
6. Ventricular aneurysm
7. Cardiomyopathy, including hypertrophic cardiomyopathy
8. Uncontrolled metabolic disease (e.g., diabetes, thyrotoxicosis, or myxedema)
9. Chronic infectious disease (e.g., mononucleosis, hepatitis, AIDS)
10. Neuromuscular, musculoskeletal, or rheumatoid disorders that are exacerbated by exercise
11. Advanced or complicated pregnancy

From American College of Sports Medicine. *Guidelines for Exercise Testing and Prescription.* Lea and Febiger, Philadelphia, 1991, 59. With permission.

E. CONTRAINDICATIONS TO EXERCISE TESTING

Table 8 lists absolute and relative contraindications to exercise testing according to the American College of Sports Medicine.[10] Absolute contraindications represent unstable conditions which should be corrected before exercise testing. Remember that exercise tests are not done on an emergent basis. It is far better to treat and correct an unstable condition before testing than to have to cope with a precipitous end to an exercise test. Relative contraindications are those for which the potential benefits and risks of exercise testing have to be carefully considered relative to a particular individual. When the information which may be obtained from the test outweighs the risks of the test in that individual, then the test may be considered appropriate when applied in a judicious manner.

F. TEST TERMINATION CRITERIA FOR EXERCISE TESTING

In the absence of calamitous signs and symptoms, exercise tests should be stopped for accumulating evidence of fatigue or exertional intolerance. They should not be stopped for an arbitrary criterion such as predicted maximal heart rate which is a notoriously inaccurate estimate of an individual's true maximal heart rate.[5] Criteria for test termination can be grouped according to clinical, hemodynamic, and ECG responses (Table 9).[10] Clinical responses encompass patient appearance (pallor, ataxia, cyanosis), symptoms (angina, claudication, dizziness, syncope, nausea, confusion, fatigue, dyspnea), and request to stop. While fatigue, breathlessness or dyspnea, and patient request to stop are normal responses to maximal exertion, the other clinical responses typically are not. Hemodynamic responses include inadequate or excessive blood pressure responses as well as an inadequate rise in heart rate (chronotropic incompetence). ECG responses include ventricular tachycardia, sustained supraventricular tachycardia (with or without aberrancy), increasing frequency and complexity of ventricular ectopy (sustained bi- or trigeminy, multiform premature ventricular contractions (PVCs), and R-on-T PVCs), rate-induced left bundle branch block, ≥4-mm ST segment depression, and failure of the ECG monitoring system. Another indication for stopping the test is ST elevation in leads which do not show significant Q waves. This may imply coronary artery spasm or an acute coronary thrombosis. It is always better to stop a test too soon and have to restart or repeat it, than to have stopped it too late in response to a cardiac catastrophe.

Table 9   Test Termination Criteria

1.	Subject requests to stop (including exertional fatigue)
2.	Symptoms of exertional intolerance
	Progressive angina (+3 on angina scale)
	Dizziness, confusion, ataxia, pallor, cyanosis, nausea
	Severe claudication
3.	Inadequate increase in heart rate
4.	Any significant drop (20 mmHg) of systolic blood pressure or a failure of the systolic blood pressure to rise with an increase in exercise load
5.	Excessive rise in blood pressure: systolic pressure: systolic pressure > 250 mmHg; diastolic pressure > 120 mmHg
6.	Early onset deep (>4 mm) horizontal or downsloping ST depression or elevation
6.	Complex or increasing ventricular ectopy, including ventricular tachycardia, multiform PVCs, and R-on-T PVCs
7.	Onset of second- or third-degree A-V block
8.	Sustained supraventricular tachycardia
9.	Exercise-induced left bundle branch block
10.	Failure of the monitoring system

G. PATIENT EVALUATION AND PREPARATION FOR EXERCISE TESTING

Important communications occur between the patient and the exercise testing staff prior to the patient's arrival at the laboratory. The patient should be told to dress comfortably for exercise (shorts and T-shirt or sweats) and to wear exercise or other comfortable shoes. Women may want to wear a shirt or blouse that buttons down the front and a sports bra or two-piece bathing suit top for comfort and modesty. Patients should be advised to eat lightly about 2 to 3 h before the test. If possible, they should not arrive for a morning test having fasted from the night before, especially if the test is anticipated to be a maximal functional test. A light meal of juice and toast is well tolerated by most patients. If patients must fast for a blood draw, they should be instructed to drink sufficient water to maintain hydration and avoid a possible hypotensive response during the test. Also, the patient should be advised to take all medications as scheduled, unless the patient's physician has specifically told the patient to stop taking medications. Very specific instructions about how to find the laboratory and what time to arrive are important to help alleviate some of the patient's pretest anxiety.

After greeting the patient and allowing him or her to change into appropriate clothing for the test, the exercise technician should obtain written informed consent. Informed consent requires that the patient understands what an exercise test is, consents to the procedure, and has had all questions answered. A signed paper, alone, is not adequate. The patient must understand the risks and benefits of the test and have had ample opportunity to ask questions. If patients do not ask questions, or do not appear to adequately read the consent form, the technician can question the patients to determine that they do, indeed, understand what is about to happen.

Once the patient arrives at the testing facility, all events related to evaluating and preparing the patient for the test are focused on either safety or information gathering. In terms of safety, there is a small but significant population for whom exercise testing is potentially harmful because of unstable disease states. It is important to screen all patients adequately to identify those patients who should not be tested, or who should have extra monitoring and medical supervision. To this end, a medical history, standard resting 12-lead ECG, resting blood pressure, oral temperature, and in some cases a physical examination should be obtained prior to a clinical exercise test. An elevated body temperature indicates an acute systemic illness which may not only decrease work capacity, but may also involve the heart (e.g., myocarditis which predisposes the heart to dysrhythmias). A previous 12-lead ECG (for comparison) is desirable if available. All patients should be interviewed regarding existing diagnosed diseases or injuries, exertional symptoms, medications, current medical problems, drug allergies, and recent food, caffeine, or alcohol intake. The patient's physical condition and the reason for performing the test will dictate the manner in which the test is administered as well as what information is gathered during the test. For example, a functional test on a 20-year-old male athlete may include only a single lead ECG for determining heart rate since 12-lead ECG monitoring is unnecessary. However, a diagnostic test on a 45-year-old sedentary male who complains of recent-onset chest pains should include 12-lead ECG monitoring, physician supervision, and perhaps more frequent and intensive physiological monitoring. The reason for the test and the physical condition of the patient will also determine the mode and protocol for the test and will suggest anticipated end points.

When preparing the patient for the exercise ECG, it is important to remember that the patient will be in motion during the test. The electrodes must be placed so as to give the best-quality tracing possible, and the lead wires must not get in the way or impede the patient's movement. Before placing electrodes, the skin should be clean and dry to increase the adhesion of the electrode and improve electrical conduction. After wiping each electrode site with an alcohol-soaked gauze pad to remove surface dirt and oils, a brisk rubbing with a dry gauze will dry the surface and remove any remaining dead skin that may decrease electrical conduction. For most exercise tests, a modified 12-lead system (Mason–Likar) is used.[24] The arm limb leads are moved to the subclavicular or deltopectoral fossae as close to the shoulder as possible without creating undue disturbance to the electrode during arm swing. The leg limb leads are placed directly below the arm limb leads between the umbilicus and the bottom rib. In obese patients, it may be advisable to place the leg limb leads directly over the lower rib as this tissue is likely to be more stable during activity. Very lean, athletic patients may need to have the leg limb leads placed closer to the umbilicus, as the skin over the ribs may move back and forth over the bone during heavy breathing, creating more artifact on the ECG. Secure the lead wires to the electrodes and attach the patient cable to the patient's waist so that it neither interferes with any of the electrodes nor impedes the patient during movement. Check for adequate electrode preparation by gently tapping or wiggling the lead wires near the electrode to simulate motion during exercise. If more than a small amount of artifact is seen on the ECG screen, a new electrode preparation or placement may be necessary to produce clear, high-quality ECG tracings.

It is much more difficult to obtain accurate blood pressure measurements in a moving patient than in one who is resting quietly. Resting blood pressure measurement should be taken according to the guidelines published by the AHA.[25] Systolic blood pressure is that level at which the first faint, clear tapping sounds are heard. This is the Korotkoff phase I. The phase IV sound is a distinct, abrupt muffling or softening of the sound. At phase V, the last sound is heard and then all sounds disappear. In adults, the phase V sound is thought to most closely reflect resting diastolic blood pressure. However, during exercise, it is often possible to hear the phase IV sounds all the way to 0 mmHg. For this reason, the beginning of the phase IV sound is often used to indicate diastolic blood pressure during exercise. To minimize confusion as to which sound was used to record diastolic pressure during exercise, both the phase IV and V values should be recorded following the phase I value (i.e., 170/80/0 mmHg). It is easier to get an accurate blood pressure measurement if the patient's arm is held straight, providing a flat space for the head of the stethoscope. Placing a mark on the brachial artery at the antecubital fossa or taping the stethoscope in position will expedite stethoscope placement and measurement during exercise. In some patients, particularly those with hypertension, the sounds heard over the brachial artery may disappear as the pressure in the cuff is released and may return again at a lower pressure. This temporary disappearance of sound is called an ausculatory gap. This gap may occur over a rather wide range (40 mmHg), making it possible to seriously underestimate systolic pressure if the cuff is not adequately inflated initially. To avoid missing an ausculatory gap, pump the cuff to 50 to 60 mmHg above suspected systolic pressure or palpate blood pressure at the radial artery as the cuff is pumped up. When the radial pulse is no longer felt, the pressure in the cuff has exceeded systolic pressure in the brachial artery.

Prior to exercise, the ECG and blood pressure measurements should be taken in all positions the patient is likely to be in during exercise and recovery (i.e., standing and sitting or supine for treadmill exercise). A post-hyperventilation ECG may also be recorded as some patients may have ST-T wave changes due to heavy ventilation that are not indicative of ischemic myocardium,[10] although some authorities recommend this only be done after a positive test is recorded.[16]

Immediately prior to the test, the patient should be instructed in the use of the Borg rating of perceived exertion (RPE) (Table 10) and pain scales (Table 11), and given another opportunity to ask questions.[10] The patient should be given an opportunity to practice on the exercise mode to ensure familiarity and comfort with the device.

Prior to beginning exercise, confirm that there are no contraindications to testing this patient and be sure that informed consent has been properly attained. Keeping in mind that this may be the last time your patient is conscious, do you need any further information that may be crucial in an emergency situation? The time to learn of an allergy to lidocaine is not during an episode of ventricular tachycardia. Consider and prepare for anticipated end points of the test. Notify the medical supervisor that the test is proceeding. Keep in mind that the patient may be very anxious and that it is not unusual for heart rate and blood pressure to actually decrease during the first few minutes of the test as the patient becomes more comfortable.

Table 10 Rating of Perceived Exertion

RPE SCALE	
6	
7	Very, very light
8	
9	Very light
10	
11	Fairly light
12	
13	Somewhat hard
14	
15	Hard
16	
17	Very hard
18	
19	Very, very hard
20	

Table 11 Angina Scale

+1	Light, barely noticeable
+2	Moderate, bothersome
+3	Severe, very uncomfortable
+4	Most severe pain ever experienced

H. EXERCISE TEST ADMINISTRATION

The test should begin with adequate warm-up time so that the patient adjusts to the exercise mode and the first stage of the protocol. If a patient appears unsteady on a treadmill, she or he should be given extra time at a slower speed to become more familiar and comfortable on the device. As previously discussed, some protocols provide for better and more thorough warm-up periods. This is important for sedentary, obese, and physically impaired patients and should be considered during protocol selection. As the patient progresses through the warm-up phase of the test, continually check the physiological responses to the work rate. Are the patient's vital signs adjusting as expected to the given work intensity? If the patient appears comfortable and willing to continue, advance the protocol throughout the predetermined stages. However, remember that you can adjust any protocol to better fit the patient's performance as the test proceeds, if this appears warranted.

As the test progresses, monitor the patient continuously. Visual contact and verbal inquiries as to the patient's state are vital. Physiological data should be collected at regular intervals, either every minute, or at least at the end of every stage. The ECG should be monitored continuously to assess for trends of ischemia or dysrhythmias. Whenever the patient reports any unusual symptoms (chest discomfort, dizziness, dyspnea, palpitations), an ECG should be recorded whether or not an ECG abnormality is present. Documentation of the absence of ECG changes in conjunction with symptoms is as important as documentation of their presence. Keep in mind that 12-lead ECGs are best used for determining ischemic changes (ST-segment depression) while rhythm strips are best used to identify dysrhythmias. A rhythm strip or 12-lead ECG should be recorded each minute of the test or at least once per stage. Each ECG recorded should be labeled with minute and/or stage of the test, heart rate, blood pressure, RPE, and symptoms. Keep in mind that it may be difficult to obtain clear, high-quality tracings during exercise. If this occurs, have the patient relax the muscles of the upper body (let go of handrail or handlebars if gripping tightly). It may be necessary to stop arm ergometry momentarily to obtain a clear ECG.

Blood pressure measurements should also be taken at regular intervals. Measurements should be taken more frequently if hypertensive or hypotensive responses are anticipated. Systolic blood pressure should increase proportionally with work at the rate of about 5 to 6 mmHg/MET, but may be less than this in the well-conditioned athlete. If it fails to increase with increasing work rate, the measurement should be repeated immediately and the patient's appearance, affect, and subjective experience should be evaluated. A blood pressure measurement should be recorded any time the patient reports lightheadedness, dizziness, chest discomfort, palpitations, or another change in physical status. The trends of heart rate and blood pressure during an exercise test provide information about progress toward test termination and, thus, should be followed closely by the exercise technician.

Subjective responses should also be monitored. These include reports from the RPE and pain scales as well as symptoms. As with heart rate and blood pressure, these subjective responses should be recorded regularly and assessed for trends indicating an abnormal response to exercise.

As the test advances, pay close attention to the patient and be alert for signs or symptoms indicating test termination. It is best to have several seconds warning before the end of the test. If possible, record an ECG rhythm strip through the end of the test to obtain an ECG at the patient's peak heart rate. Stop the test and begin the recovery period. Record peak heart rate, blood pressure, and RPE.

I. RECOVERY PROCEDURES

At the cessation of exercise, immediately obtain a clear 12-lead ECG. This "immediate post" 12-lead ECG combines a high rate pressure product with minimal motion artifact and is often the most valuable tracing obtained for the evaluation of exercise-induced ischemia. This tracing may be recorded in either the supine or upright position as described below.

There are two basic methods of recovery, active and supine. Supine recovery may be used preferentially in diagnostic exercise testing because it places an increased volume load on the heart. At the end of the exercise test, the patient lies down immediately, creating an increase in venous return to the heart and increasing preload. An ischemic heart may not be able to adapt to the increased volume load and may exhibit ischemic changes that were not present during exercise. During supine recovery, heart rate and blood pressure should be monitored and recorded regularly, as should subjective measures of chest pain, dyspnea, dizziness, or other symptoms. The ECG should be continuously monitored, assessed for trends, and recorded at regular intervals. Once the patient has returned to near baseline values of heart rate and blood pressure, the recovery period can be terminated. An exit 12-lead ECG and blood pressure measurement should be recorded. The patient should be assisted in slowly returning to a sitting and then standing position. Caution is warranted during this transition; the patient may become dizzy or light-headed.

Active recovery is used more often for functional tests. The purpose of an active recovery is to allow heart rate and blood pressure to be gradually reduced toward pretesting values. If the patient is allowed to simply stop exercising and stand or sit still, blood will pool in the legs, where blood vessels have dilated to accommodate the prior demands of exercise for increased blood flow. This pooling of blood may cause the patient to become hypotensive and light-headed. Many patients may also vomit if exercise was maximal or near maximal (particularly after leg ergometry). To avoid this, the patient is encouraged to continue exercising at very minimal work rates until heart rate and blood pressure approach pretest levels. This will typically take 3 to 6 min. Sedentary patients will require more time to recover from exercise. As the patient's heart rate and blood pressure approach pretest values, the patient may sit for the remainder of the recovery period. Keep in mind that during the warm-up and recovery periods of exercise, the patient's heart may be most vulnerable to dysrhythmias. The ECG should continue to be monitored closely. The patient can be released from the testing laboratory, usually after 6 to 10 min, when vital signs have returned to near baseline levels and the patient is no longer breathing hard or experiencing symptoms. An exit 12-lead ECG and blood pressure measurement should be recorded.

When the recovery period has been terminated, remove the blood pressure cuff and electrodes from the patient. Patients who shower at your facility should be instructed to use warm (not hot or cold) water to minimize the likelihood of syncope, arrhythmia, or ischemia following the recovery period. Patients should report back to you after showering to ensure that they are feeling well before leaving the testing facility.

IV. INTERPRETATION OF THE EXERCISE TEST

A. NORMAL VS. ABNORMAL EXERCISE TEST RESPONSES

The clinical context in which an exercise test occurs affects its interpretation beyond a simple dichotomous judgment based on whether the exercise ECG is positive or negative for ischemia. By looking for patterns in each subject's clinical, hemodynamic, and ECG responses, we seek to determine, first, the likelihood that disease is present and, secondly, its prognosis.[26] Not surprisingly, the test termination criteria discussed previously represent the end points for abnormal responses which may develop with progressively increasing work rate.

Table 12 Characteristics of Angina

1. Substernal pain
2. Precipitated by exertion
3. Promptly relieved by rest or nitroglycerin

Typical Angina	Patients with all three characteristics
Atypical Angina	Patients with two of three characteristics
Nonanginal Pain	Patients with one of three characteristics

Table 13 Normal Values of Maximum Oxygen Uptake in METs at Different Ages

Age	Men (METs)	Women (METs)
20–29	12	10
30–39	12	10
40–49	11	9
50–59	10	8
60–69	9	8
70–79	8	8

Note: 1 MET = 3.5 ml/kg/min oxygen uptake.

1. Normal and Abnormal Clinical Responses to Exercise Testing

The normal clinical response to maximal exercise is for the patient's skin to be flush and moist with perspiration. The patient is also short of breath and experiences either general or local muscular fatigue. In contrast, the patient with circulatory insufficiency (e.g., CAD, peripheral vascular disease, left ventricle dysfunction) may present with cool, clammy skin, peripheral cyanosis, and lack of blood return to the skin following skin compression (impaired capillary refill). Neurological symptoms such as dizziness, ataxia, nausea and confusion may also indicate insufficient cardiac output. Typical angina which appears and intensifies with increasing work and then disappears in recovery is highly suggestive of CAD. However, due to the nonspecific nature of chest pain that often brings patients to the exercise testing laboratory, nonspecific chest pain during exercise testing is not a reliable indicator of disease.[27] Every attempt should be made to specify any chest pain as either typical angina, atypical angina, or nonanginal chest pain (Table 12).[28] Excessive dyspnea and/or typical angina occurring at a low work rate and leading to poor functional capacity are indicators of either myocardial ischemia or left ventricle dysfunction. Normal values of exercise capacity for lean, healthy individuals adjusted for age are presented in Table 13.[5,18]

2. Normal and Abnormal Hemodynamic Responses to Exercise Testing

Figure 5 indicates the normal heart rate and blood pressure responses of healthy males (24 to 54 years of age) to submaximal ($^1/_3$ max and $^2/_3$ max) and maximal treadmill exercise.[26] Maximal rate pressure product varied from 25 to 40×10^3, for the 10th to the 90th percentiles, respectively. Abnormal heart rate responses include either too rapid or excessive increases or, conversely, inadequate increases in heart rate. While a rapid, but regular, rise in heart rate may be due to poor conditioning, an excessive or sudden increase is most likey due to a dysrhythmia. Inadequate increases in heart rate may be reflective of a conduction defect (e.g., 2° or 3° heart block) or, more likely, ischemia and/or left ventricular dysfunction. Examination of the ECG is often helpful in differentiating these possibilities.

While systolic blood pressure tends to increase between 5 to 6 mmHg/MET,[26] it normally does not exceed 225/90 at peak exercise. Blood pressures in excess of this may be considered a hypertensive response to exertion.[10] Preliminary evidence suggests that this response may be prognostic for the later development of resting hypertension.[29] There is some disagreement as to when the exercise test should be terminated in the presence of elevated blood pressure. For example, the AHA makes no recommendation in its *Exercise Standards*.[5] Herbert and Froelicher[30] recommend stopping the test at 280/115 mmHg, while ACSM[10] recommends stopping the test at 250/115 mmHg. Good clinical judgment is clearly warranted here. A young athlete may perhaps safely exercise to higher levels, while the exercise test of a diabetic, stroke, aortic aneurysm, or CAD patient might wisely be stopped at levels less than the above criteria.

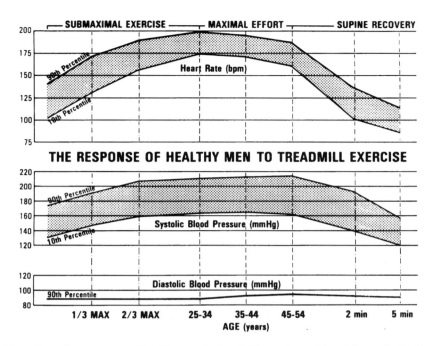

Figure 5 Hemodynamic responses of healthy men to treadmill exercise at $^1/_3$ and $^2/_3$ maximal effort, maximal effort (in three age groups) and recovery. The shaded areas represent the normal range between the 10th and 90th percentiles. (From Froelicher VF. *Exercise and the Heart.* Year Book Publishers, Chicago, 1987, p. 102. With permission.)

An inadequate increase in systolic blood pressure is cause for concern. This has been termed exercise-induced hypotension[31] and may be caused by valve disease or, more typically, by significant CAD or left ventricular dysfunction. Criteria for exercise-induced hypotension include less than a 20 mmHg increase from resting systolic blood pressure, a drop in systolic blood pressure below resting values, or a drop of ≥20 mmHg in systolic blood pressure below a previous reading.[10] Of particular concern is a drop below resting values.[26] If time and symptoms permit, recheck a dropping blood pressure; however, if a drop in systolic blood pressure occurs in the presence of symptoms, significant ST depression, dyspnea, and low work and heart rates, then stop the test immediately. These individuals appear at increased risk for ventricular fibrillation in the exercise laboratory.[26] Occasionally, anxious patients may present with a drop in systolic blood pressure in the first few minutes of the exercise test, followed by normal increases in systolic blood pressure as the test progresses. This is a normal response for an anxious person. Finally, two other less common findings that may be associated with cardiovascular disease are (1) an increase in systolic blood pressure early in recovery that is greater than peak exercise systolic blood pressure[5] and (2) a marked increase in diastolic blood pressure of ≥25 mmHg above resting values.[10]

3. Normal and Abnormal Electrocardiographic Responses to Exercise Testing

Heart rate (HR) normally increases during exercise as a result of sinus tachycardia. As the R-R interval shortens, both systole and diastole proceed more rapidly, and the P wave begins to encroach onto the T wave until they eventually fuse. The PR interval, QT interval, and TP segment all shorten. With increasing HR, the atrial repolarization wave (T_a wave) tends to pull down both the PR segment and the J point, particularly in the inferior leads. Near peak HR, R wave amplitude decreases and the S wave deepens. The ST segment slopes up rapidly from the J point into the T wave.[5] There is some disagreement among authorities about how much upsloping ST depression can be considered normal. For example, ACSM states that ≥1.0 mm of upsloping ST depression measured 0.08 s from the J point relative to the isoelectric line is abnormal.[10] Conversely, the AHA accepts only horizontal or downsloping ST depression (not upsloping) as abnormal.[5] In a recent survey of cardiologists,[32] only 24 of 88 responders considered upsloping ST depression as abnormal. Of those 24, 5 accepted 1.0 mm, 15 accepted 1.5 mm, and 4 accepted 2.0 mm of upsloping ST depression as abnormal. Thus, as an isolated finding it would appear that despite the position of ACSM, the majority of cardiologists are not impressed by upsloping ST depression. Herbert and Froelicher[30] suggest calling upsloping ST depression a borderline abnormal response if the ST integral is large (i.e., there is deep J point depression with slowly upsloping ST segments that persist for at least 80 ms). This finding obviously needs to be evaluated in conjunction with clinical and hemodynamic results and the individual's presenting symptoms and overall level of risk, since it is clear from prior studies that upsloping ST depression in a symptomatic population is predictive of disease.[33,34] Finally, T waves and U waves normally show minimal changes, and the mean QRS axis is unchanged or shifts slightly to the right.

Abnormal ECG responses include ST segment changes, dysrhythmias, U wave inversion, conduction abnormalities, and left axis shifts. It is worth noting that all these ECG changes, along with the clinical and hemodynamic responses, help us separate the normal from the abnormal exercise test. However, it is the response, of the ST segment alone which separates the "positive" from the "negative" test. During exercise the isoelectric line is defined by a line drawn through successive PQ junctions (Figure 6).[10] ST segment depression is measured relative to this isoelectric line at the J point. Thus, the ST segment is considered abnormally depressed if there is ≥1.0 mm of horizontal or downsloping ST segment depression measured at the J point relative to the isoelectic line.[5] The standard criterion states that this horizontal or downsloping ST depression should persist for ≥80 ms past the J point.[5] More recently, 60 ms persistence has been suggested due to the shortened R-R interval that occurs at the higher heart rates seen with exercise.[26] In our recent survey of standard practice,[32] nearly four times more cardiologists accept 80 ms than accept 60 ms. Thus, in general, clinicians prefer ≥1.0 mm of horizontal or downsloping ST depression which persists for 80 ms or more as the criterion measure of an abnormal ST segment response to exercise. This is the standard definition of the *positive* exercise ECG. ST segment depression less than this would constitute a *negative* test. Other criteria have also been proposed including the ST/HR index and ST integral. However, these and other criteria may be more specific to the population being studied. In general, they have not improved on the sensitivity and specificity attained from careful visual analysis.[5,35] Furthermore, while computer analysis of the ECG waveform is common on most modern exercise ECGs, a computer algorithm should never be depended on to interpret the exercise ECG. Averaging programs occasionally generate apparent ST depression which is artifactual.[36] Thus, careful visual inspection of the raw ECG tracing must always be used to confirm computer results. A noisy raw tracing with much artifact cannot be accurately analyzed by a computer (or a human). It is wise to remember the computer adage: garbage in, garbage out. A careful skin preparation is typically the best insurance against a noisy tracing. Finally, ST segment depression which occurs only during recovery appears to be as predictive of CAD as that which occurs during exercise.[37]

If there is ST depression in the resting ECG, then an additional 1.0 mm of ST depression during exercise or recovery is necessary for the exercise ECG to be considered positive, although many clinicians consider such a test to be non-diagnostic for ischemia. If ST elevation of early repolarization is present, the normal response is for the ST segment to return to the isoelectric line with exercise. Thus, an abnormal or positive response to exercise in an individual with early repolarization is the same as the standard criterion: ≥1.0 mm of horizontal or downsloping ST depression measured relative to the isoelectric line and persisting for ≥80 ms. ST segment depression in a few isolated beats is normal. A positive response requires that three or more successive beats or greater than 50% of the beats show ST depression. Finally, any ST elevation is abnormal. ST segment elevation that occurs in leads without significant $\dot{Q}$ waves is indicative of severe transmural ischemia (e.g., due to acute myocardial infarction or coronary artery spasm) and is also arrhythmogenic; this test should be terminated immediately.[5] ST segment elevation that occurs over significant $\dot{Q}$ waves (i.e., in leads with $\dot{Q}$ waves) is more likely indicative of left ventricular dysfunction from an aneurysm in the area of the existing old infarction. This is a common response, particularly in patients with prior large anterior infarctions;[5] this test may be continued safely in the absence of other criteria suggesting test termination.

Dysrhythmias are common and their prevalence increases with age in both healthy and diseased individuals during exercise testing.[5] Complex dysrhythmias like nonsustained ventricular tachycardia are infrequent (occurring in 1.2% of patients) and poorly reproducible (6.9% recurrence with repeat testing) with no effect on prognosis: in a clinical population of mostly CAD patients, mortality was 3.6% in those who experienced nonsustained ventricular tachycardia vs. 5.1% in those who did not.[38] Those with sustained ventricular tachycardia had a higher prevalence of prior infarction. While ST segment elevation is associated with an increased potential for dysrhythmia, ST segment depression is not.[26] Complex ventricular dysrhythmias tend to occur at lower heart rates in CAD patients compared with healthy patients. In our survey of cardiologists[32] we found that only 19% considered the presence

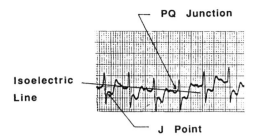

Figure 6 An ECG showing the J point and isoelectric line as defined by successive PQ junctions.

of complex ventricular dysrhythmias during the exercise test as a criterion for determining whether or not a test is indicative of ischemia. Other ECG abnormalities occurring during an exercise test which have been associated with the possible presence of ischemia are U wave inversion ,[26] left axis shifts,[38] and conduction defects.[5]

B. DIAGNOSIS, RISK ASSESSMENT, AND PROGNOSIS
In addition to functional information, the exercise test provides both diagnostic and prognostic information. Diagnosis deals with determining the presence of a disease while prognosis deals with determining the probable outcome of a disease.

1. Diagnosis
It is important to realize that the exercise test cannot answer a dichotomous question such as the presence or absence of CAD. Despite the fact that tests are termed either positve (for ischemia) or negative (for ischemia), it has been known for years that exercise test results only provide estimates of the probability that disease is present, and not a definitive diagnosis.[40] This is a consequence of Bayes's theorem which states that the posttest probability that a person has disease is the product of the pretest probability of disease presence and the probability that the test result is a true result.[26] Since no diagnostic test is perfect, results can be either truly positive (TP, i.e., a *positive* result in an individual *with CAD*), falsely positive (FP, i.e., a *positive* result in an individual *without CAD*), truly negative (TN, i.e., a *negative* result in an individual *without CAD*), or falsely negative (FN, i.e., a *negative* result in an individual *with CAD*). The ability of a test to distinguish diseased from nondiseased populations is measured by the sensitivity and specificity of the test. Sensitivity is the ability of the test to detect disease when it is present; i.e., it deals only with those who have CAD and is the proportion of CAD patients who have a positive test. The population with CAD can be defined as all the TP tests plus all the FN tests. Thus, sensitivity is equal to all those with TP tests divided by all those with disease, or

$$Sensitivity = TP/(TP + FN)$$

Specificity is the ability of the test to correctly exclude disease when it is absent; i.e., it deals only with those who do not have CAD and is the proportion of normal individuals who have a negative test. The population without CAD can be defined as all the TN tests plus all the FP tests. Thus, specificity is equal to all those with TN tests divided by all those without disease, or

$$Specificity = TN/(TN + FP)$$

Sensitivity and specificity are measures of test discrimination. As each approaches 100%, the ability of the test to discriminate diseased from nondiseased populations improves. The average sensitivity of the exercise test is 66%, meaning that 66% of those with disease will have a positive, TP, exercise ECG (and 34% will have a negative, FN, exercise ECG). However, sensitivity varies from around 40% for those with single-vessel disease to about 90% for those with three-vessel disease. The average specificity of the exercise ECG is 84%, meaning that 84% of those without disease will have a negative, TN, exercise ECG (and 16% will have a positive, FP, exercise ECG).[26] Unfortunately, sensitivity and specifity define population characteristics of the exercise test and provide little help in assessing the likelihood that any individual patient has CAD based on their test results. This information is provided by the predictive accuracy.

Table 14 Pretest Likelihood of Coronary Artery Disease in Symptomatic Patients According to Age and Gender

Age (yr)	Nonanginal Chest Pain		Atypical Angina		Typical Angina	
	Men	Women	Men	Women	Men	Women
30–39	5.2 ± 0.8	0.8 ± 0.3	21.8 ± 2.4	4.2 ± 1.3	69.7 ± 3.2	25.8 ± 6.6
40–49	14.1 ± 1.3	2.8 ± 0.7	46.1 ± 1.8	13.3 ± 2.9	87.3 ± 1.0	55.2 ± 6.5
50–59	21.5 ± 1.7	8.4 ± 1.2	58.9 ± 1.5	32.4 ± 3.0	92.0 ± 0.6	79.4 ± 2.4
60–69	28.1 ± 1.9	18.6 ± 1.9	67.1 ± 1.3	54.4 ± 2.4	94.3 ± 0.4	90.6 ± 1.0

Note: Each value represents the percent ± 1 standard error of the percent.

From Diamond, G. A. and Forrester, J. S., *N. Engl. J. Med.*, 300, 1352, 1979. With permission.

The predictive accuracy of a positive test is the probability that a positive test is a TP test. The population of all individuals with a positive test is defined as all those with TP tests plus all those with FP tests. Thus, predictive accuracy is equal to all the TP tests divided by all those with positive tests, or

$$\text{Predictive Accuracy} = TP/(TP + FP)$$

It can be readily appreciated that when testing a population in which CAD is very likely (e.g., patients with typical angina, Table 12) most of the positive tests will be TP and very few will be FP. As a consequence, the predictive accuracy of a positive test in such a population can be quite high, often in excess of 95% (as described below). However, since the pretest probability of CAD in this population may be in excess of 90% (Table 14), little new diagnostic information has been gained. Conversely, when testing a population in which CAD is very unlikely (e.g., asymptomatic or nonanginal chest pain, Table 12), it should be equally obvious that most of the positive tests will be FP and very few will be TP. In this case the predictive accuracy will be quite low (e.g., 5 to 10%) such that only 1 in 10 to 1 in 20 tests in this population will be TP. Thus, little useful information may be gained from the exercise test if the test result is viewed dichotomously, i.e., either positive or negative based on ≥1 mm of ST segment depression. A more appropriate approach is to use the seminal work of Diamond and Forrester[40] to assess the probabilty that disease is present by putting the exercise test result into the context of the larger clinical picture.

Table 14 presents pretest probabilities of CAD in symptomatic patients according to their age and gender.[40] Criteria for symptom characteristics are presented in Table 12. As a consequence of Bayes's theorem, we would expect that posttest probabilities of CAD in those with a positive test would be much higher in those with higher pretest probabilities. This expectation is confirmed by an examination of Table 15 which shows the posttest probabilities for CAD according to age, gender, pretest symptoms, and amount of ST depression.[40] The major problem with viewing the results of the exercise ECG dichotomously are well illustrated by examining the posttest probabilities for two hypothetical individuals, both of whom have a positive exercise ECG with 1.3 mm of ST depression. A 35-year-old asymptomatic female would have a posttest probability of CAD of only 0.6 ± 0.2%, while a 65-year-old male with typical angina would have a posttest probability of CAD of 97.2 ± 0.5%. This is essentially the difference between a 0% and a 100% probability of CAD; yet removed from the clinical context, each of these individuals has identically positive exercise ECGs. ST segment depression is a continuously distributed variable. The greater the amount of ST depression, the greater is the likelihood that disease is present. The more typical the anginal symptoms are, the greater is the risk that disease is present. These relationships should not be ignored in an effort to diagnose the presence of CAD. Instead, these relationships should be employed to assess the probability of the presence of CAD. Two caveats are appropriate here: First, these probabilities are population estimates and cannot be taken as exact measures of any individual's unique risk of CAD. Second, large standard errors are involved in some of these estimates, particularly in the middle groups (nonanginal and atypical chest pain), the two groups in which exercise testing is traditionally used in an effort to discriminate those with disease from those without disease.[26] It is quite likely, although not empirically established, that for a given amount of ST depression those with higher levels of conventional risk factors and more abnormal exercise test results would cluster at the higher probabilities predicted by the mean plus the standard error(s), while those at lower conventional risk and with an otherwise normal exercise test would cluster at lower probabilities predicted by the mean minus the standard error(s). Thus, a much fuller interpretation of the exercise test

Table 15 Posttest Likelihood of Coronary Artery Disease after an Electrocardiographic Exercise Test According to Age, Gender, Symptom, and Amount of ST Depression

Age (yr)	Asymptomatic		Nonanginal Chest Pain		Atypical Angina		Typical Angina	
	Men	Women	Men	Women	Men	Women	Men	Women
				>2.5 mm ST Depression				
30–39	43.0 ± 24.9	10.5 ± 9.9	68.1 ± 22.1	23.9 ± 19.5	91.8 ± 7.7	63.1 ± 24.5	98.9 ± 1.1	93.1 ± 6.8
40–49	69.4 ± 21.3	28.3 ± 20.8	86.5 ± 11.8	52.9 ± 25.8	97.1 ± 2.8	85.7 ± 12.7	99.6 ± 0.4	98.0 ± 2.1
50–59	80.7 ± 15.6	56.3 ± 24.9	91.4 ± 7.9	78.1 ± 17.3	98.2 ± 1.7	94.9 ± 4.9	99.8 ± 0.2	99.3 ± 0.7
60–69	84.5 ± 13.1	76.0 ± 18.4	93.8 ± 5.8	89.9 ± 9.2	98.8 ± 1.2	97.9 ± 2.1	99.8 ± 0.2	99.7 ± 0.3
				2.0–2.5 mm ST Depression				
30–39	17.7 ± 10.3	3.2 ± 2.4	37.8 ± 16.6	8.2 ± 5.9	76.0 ± 12.8	32.7 ± 16.7	96.2 ± 2.6	79.4 ± 12.6
40–49	39.2 ± 16.5	10.1 ± 6.5	64.5 ± 16.0	24.2 ± 13.5	90.5 ± 6.0	63.0 ± 17.1	98.7 ± 0.9	93.2 ± 4.7
50–59	54.3 ± 17.1	26.8 ± 13.8	75.2 ± 13.0	50.4 ± 17.7	94.1 ± 3.9	84.2 ± 9.4	99.2 ± 0.5	97.7 ± 1.6
60–69	60.9 ± 16.4	47.3 ± 17.3	81.2 ± 10.6	71.7 ± 14.2	95.8 ± 2.8	93.0 ± 4.5	99.5 ± 0.4	99.1 ± 0.6
				1.5–2.0 mm ST Depression				
30–39	7.5 ± 5.0	1.2 ± 1.0	18.7 ± 10.9	3.3 ± 2.5	54.5 ± 17.8	15.5 ± 10.1	90.6 ± 6.1	59.3 ± 18.9
40–49	19.6 ± 11.1	4.1 ± 2.8	40.8 ± 17.1	10.8 ± 7.2	78.2 ± 12.0	39.1 ± 17.7	96.6 ± 2.3	83.8 ± 10.2
50–59	31.0 ± 15.0	12.2 ± 7.6	53.4 ± 17.6	27.8 ± 14.4	85.7 ± 8.6	66.8 ± 15.9	98.0 ± 1.4	94.2 ± 3.9
60–69	37.0 ± 16.4	25.4 ± 13.4	62.1 ± 16.7	48.9 ± 17.8	89.5 ± 6.6	83.3 ± 9.8	98.6 ± 1.0	97.6 ± 1.7
				1.0–1.5 mm ST Depression				
30–39	3.9 ± 0.9	0.6 ± 0.2	10.4 ± 2.2	1.7 ± 0.7	37.7 ± 5.2	8.5 ± 2.8	83.0 ± 3.2	42.4 ± 9.4
40–49	11.0 ± 1.7	2.1 ± 0.5	25.8 ± 3.8	5.8 ± 1.7	64.4 ± 4.2	24.5 ± 5.6	93.6 ± 1.1	72.3 ± 6.2
50–59	18.5 ± 2.6	6.5 ± 1.3	36.7 ± 4.5	16.3 ± 3.1	75.2 ± 3.3	50.4 ± 5.4	96.1 ± 0.7	89.1 ± 2.2
60–69	22.9 ± 3.1	14.7 ± 2.3	45.3 ± 4.7	32.6 ± 4.6	81.2 ± 2.7	71.6 ± 3.9	97.2 ± 0.5	95.3 ± 0.9
				0.5–1.0 mm ST Depression				
30–39	1.7 ± 0.6	0.3 ± 0.1	4.8 ± 1.6	0.7 ± 0.4	20.7 ± 5.5	3.9 ± 1.6	67.8 ± 7.4	24.2 ± 8.4
40–49	5.1 ± 1.5	0.9 ± 0.3	13.1 ± 3.7	2.6 ± 1.0	43.9 ± 7.7	12.3 ± 4.3	86.3 ± 3.7	53.0 ± 10.0
50–59	9.0 ± 2.5	2.9 ± 0.9	20.1 ± 5.1	7.8 ± 2.4	56.8 ± 7.6	30.5 ± 7.1	91.3 ± 2.5	77.9 ± 5.8
60–69	11.4 ± 3.1	6.9 ± 2.0	26.4 ± 6.2	17.3 ± 4.7	65.1 ± 7.0	52.2 ± 7.9	93.8 ± 1.8	89.8 ± 2.9
				0.0–0.5 mm ST Depression				
30–39	0.4 ± 0.1	0.1 ± 0.0	1.2 ± 0.4	0.2 ± 0.1	6.1 ± 1.7	1.0 ± 0.4	24.5 ± 6.6	7.4 ± 2.9
40–49	1.3 ± 0.3	0.2 ± 0.1	3.6 ± 0.9	0.7 ± 0.2	16.4 ± 3.5	3.4 ± 1.2	61.1 ± 6.3	22.0 ± 6.2
50–59	2.4 ± 0.6	0.8 ± 0.2	5.9 ± 1.5	2.1 ± 0.6	24.7 ± 4.8	9.9 ± 2.5	72.5 ± 5.2	46.9 ± 7.2
60–69	3.1 ± 0.8	1.8 ± 0.6	8.2 ± 2.0	5.0 ± 1.3	31.8 ± 5.5	21.4 ± 4.5	79.1 ± 4.3	68.8 ± 5.9

Note: Each value represents the percent ± 1 standard error of the percent.

From Diamond, G. A. and Forrester, J. S., *N. Engl. J. Med.* 300, 1354, 1979. With permission.

is possible when we treat the results as probabilities that occur within the patient's larger clinical context rather than as a dichotomous, "positive–negative" result.

2. Risk Assessment in Asymptomatic Individuals

Although the joint ACC/AHA Guidelines (Table 7) recommends against exercise tests in asymptomatic individuals on clinical grounds, such tests clearly occur for other valid reasons as previously described. In low risk asymptomatic individuals it may be advisable to monitor a single transverse or lateral lead such as CC_5 which is a bipolar lead between the V_5 position on the right chest (negative terminal) and the V_5 position on the left chest (positive terminal).[5] Such a lead has the advantage of excluding the vertical component of atrial repolarization seen most prominently in the inferior leads and CM_5 which is, itself, largely an inferior lead. This has the effect of decreasing the influence of the negative wave of atrial repolarization on the J point and ST segment in the monitored lead and, thus, decreasing the probability of a FP response such as often occurs in the inferior leads.[41] If a positive response occurs on the exercise ECG, we recommend assessing the probability of CAD using Table 15. If the probability of CAD is high enough and the patient's individual situation warrants additional follow-up, sequential testing such as a myocardial perfusion study, exercise echocardiogram, or coronary angiography may be advisable.[42] Whatever the next level of testing, by Bayes's theorem, the patient now enters that next test at a higher pretest risk so that if that result is also abnormal, the risk of CAD may now be quite large. Conversely, if the subsequent test is normal, the risk of CAD is now substantially reduced, typically to values less than the original preexercise test risk. An excellent example of applying Bayes's theorem to an asymptomatic population is the study of Bruce et al.[43]

In our experience about 10 to 12% of asymptomatic men and women have positive tests. However, women will have more FP tests than men when corrected for age and symptoms. This is a direct consequence of Bayes's theorem since at any given age women are at lower risk for CAD than are men. This is nicely represented by the data in Table 15 which show that the posttest risk of CAD in women is between 10 and 20 years behind that of men at any given degree of ST depression (and at any level of symptoms). Thus, at any given age women will have a higher proportion of FP tests than men will.

3. Risk Assessment in Symptomatic Individuals

As individuals present with symptoms more characteristic of typical angina (Table 12), their pretest risk of CAD increases (Table 14). With higher pretest risk, by Bayes's theorem, their posttest probability of CAD with a positive test can be quite high (Table 15). Sequential testing may also be employed here for a further refinement of risk; however, this is often unnecessary as risk is already sufficiently high to confirm a diagnosis of CAD. Numerous studies have attempted to improve the diagnostic accuracy of the exercise test by employing several exercise test variables in a discriminant analysis.[27] One complicating factor in many of these studies has been test chest pain which, contrary to expectation, is not always a significant predictor of CAD. We have studied the effect of the interaction of chest pain that occurs during exercise testing with other exercise test variables and found that test chest pain is a significant predictor of disease only when it is associated with either a low maximum rate pressure product or a positive exercise ECG.[27] More-accurate characterization of the quality of chest pain may also improve the diagnostic value of test chest pain in predicting CAD.

4. Prognosis

In patients for whom the diagnosis of CAD has been made or is strongly suspected, prognostic information can be most valuable for both counseling the patient and selecting therapeutic interventions.[5] Considering both the difficulty in diagnosing CAD based on the exercise ECG and the ambiguity associated with the probability of CAD in a given patient, it might be most comforting to the patient to describe for them their prognosis, particularly if it is good when the "diagnosis" is equivocal.

Mark et al.[44] have proposed a treadmill score or nomogram for quantifying prognosis in outpatients suspected of CAD (Figure 7). Notice that duration of exercise or functional capacity in METs is an important component of this nomogram. Those with minimal ST depression and high functional capacity have an excellent prognosis. This is consistent with the information presented in Table 1 and again illustrates the importance of assessing functional capacity. It bears repeating that any handrail holding invalidates the estimation of functional capacity calculated by standard equations from treadmill speed and grade.[9] Additional signs and symptoms suggestive of more-severe disease and associated with a poorer prognosis include exertional hypotension; angina that limits the test; downsloping ST depression (particularly in recovery); and ST depression beginning at a low rate pressure product (<15,000), occurring in multiple leads and persisting late into recovery.[1,30]

It is important to note that not all ST depression is of ischemic origin. Most occurrences of ST depression in asymptomatic individuals are for unknown reasons. Known causes of nonischemic ST depression are left bundle branch block, left ventricular hypertrophy, Wolff–Parkinson–White syndrome (WPW), mitral valve prolapse, vasoregulatory asthenia, various drug (e.g., digitalis) and electrolyte (e.g., hypokalemia) abnormalities, and nonspecific repolarization abnormalities.[10] It is tempting to call a positive exercise ECG in individuals with these antecedent abnormalities FP tests; however, it must be appreciated that CAD may still be present. These ECGs are best described as nondiagnostic, and another test (e.g., myocardial stress scintigram) should be employed to rule out ischemia. Finally, with an average sensitivity of 66%,[5] about 34% of all tests in a diseased population will be FN tests. While lack of an ST response may be due to technical problems such as inadequate stress or an insufficient number of leads, it may also be due to various physiological mechanisms, such as cancellation effects from competing areas of ischemic myocardium, lack of residual ischemic tissue after a prior infarction, single-vessel disease, or good collateral circulation.[10] Regardless of the mechanism, lack of an ST response in a known CAD patient usually confers a better prognosis.[45]

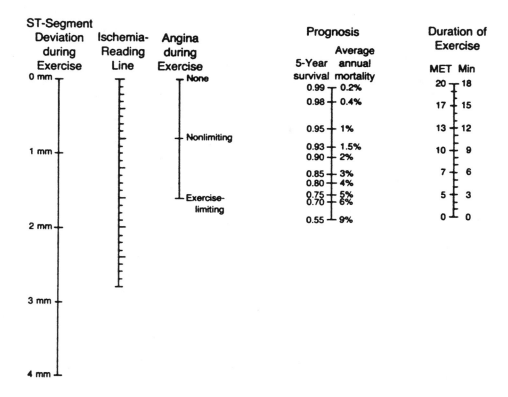

Figure 7 Prognosis as determined by functional capacity, and exercise induced angina and ST segment changes. Directions for use: (1) Connect amounts of exercise–induced angina and ST segment deviation with a ruler. (2) Mark the intersection of this line and the ischemia reading line. (3) Connect this point on the ischemia reading line to functional capacity (METs or minutes of the Bruce protocol) on the duration of exercise line. (4) Where this second line crosses the prognosis line indicates prognosis as 5-year survival or average annual mortality. (From Marks DB, Shaw L, Harrell FE et al. *N. Engl. J. Med.* 1991; 325, p. 850. With permission.)

V. CONCLUDING REMARKS

Clinical exercise tests as described in this chapter are a safe, inexpensive, and efficient means of assessing functional capacity, probability of CAD, and prognosis when performed in a thoughtful manner by competent and educated personnel. They are typically sufficient when evaluating symptoms suggestive of CAD. However, in the evaluation of dyspnea and poor work tolerance, the information obtained is most accurate and illuminating when obtained in a cardiorespiratory laboratory, in combination with expired gas analysis and measured $\dot{V}O_2$max. Such tests are termed cardiorespiratory or cardiopulmonary exercise tests.[2] These tests are described more fully in Chapter 11 and in the excellent text by Wasserman et al.[19]

ACKNOWLEDGMENT

The authors would like to thank James D. Shaffrath, M.D., and Ezra A. Amsterdam, M.D., for their careful and critical reading of this manuscript and for their many insightful and helpful comments.

REFERENCES

1. Subcommittee on Exercise Testing. Guidelines for exercise testing: a report of the American College of Cardiology/American Heart Association Task Force on Assessment of Cardiovascular Procedures. *J. Am. Coll. Cardiol.* 1986, 8:725–738.

2. Holly RG. Fundamentals of cardiorespiratory exercise testing. In: *Resource Manual for Guidelines for Exercise Testing and Prescription.* Edited by American College of Sports Medicine. Lea and Febiger, Philadelphia, 1993, pp. 247–257.

3. Skinner JS. General principles of exercise prescription. In: *Exercise Testing and Exercise Prescription for Special Cases.* Edited by JS Skinner. Lea and Febiger, Philadelphia, 1993, pp. 29–40.

4. Durstine JL, Pate RR, Branch JD. Cardiorespiratory responses to acute exercise. In: *Resource Manual for Guidelines for Exercise Testing and Prescription.* Edited by American College of Sports Medicine. Lea and Febiger, Philadelphia, 1993, pp. 66–74.

5. American Heart Association. *Exercise Standards. Circulation.* 1990; 82:2286–2322.

6. Taylor HL, Buskirk E, Henschel A. Maximal oxygen uptake as an objective measure of cardiorespiratory performance. *J. Appl. Physiol.* 1955; 8:73–80.

7. Davis JA. Direct determination of aerobic power. In: *Physiological Assessment of Human Fitness.* Edited by PJ Maud and C Foster. Human Kinetics. Champaign, IL, 1992.

8. Kitamura K, Jorgensen CR, Gobel FL, Taylor HL, Wang L. Hemodynamic correlates of myocardial oxygen consumption during upright exercise. *J. Appl. Physiol.* 1973; 32:516–522.

9. Beadle DH, Holly RG, Amsterdam EA. Metabolic equation for the estimation of oxygen consumption during handrail supported treadmill exercise. *Med. Sci. Sports Exercise.* 1991; 22:S89.

10. American College of Sports Medicine. *Guidelines for Exercise Testing and Prescription.* Lea and Febiger, Philadelphia, 1991.

11. Thompson PD. The safety of exercise testing and participation. In: *Resource Manual for Guidelines for Exercise Testing and Prescription.* Edited by American College of Sports Medicine. Lea and Febiger, Philadelphia, 1993, pp. 359–363.

12. American Heart Association. *Textbook of Advanced Cardiac Life Support.* American Heart Association, Dallas, 1990.

13. Weber KT, Janicki JS. Cardiopulmonary testing for the evaluation of chronic cardiac failure. *Am. J. Cardiol.* 1985; 55:22A–31A.

14. Goldman L, Hashimoto B, Cook E, Loscalzo A. Comparative reproducibility and validity of systems assessing cardiovascular functional class: Advantages of a new specific activity scale. *Circulation.* 1981; 64:1227–1234.

15. Hlatky MA, Boineau RE, Higginbotham MB et al. A brief self-administered questionnaire to determine functional capacity: the Duke activity status index. *Am. J. Cardiol.* 1989; 64:651–654.

16. McKirnan MD, Froelicher VF. General principles of exercise testing. In: *Exercise Testing and Prescription for Special Populations.* Edited by JS Skinner. Lea and Febiger, Philadelphia, 1993, pp. 3–27.

17. Featherstone JF, Holly RG, Amsterdam EA. Physiological responses to weight lifting in coronary artery disease. *Am. J. Cardiol.* 1993; 71:287–292.

18. Dressendorfer RH, Amsterdam EA. An approach to preventive cardiology in asymptomatic, sedentary adults. *Cardiology.* 1980; 66:204–222.

19. Wasserman K, Hansen JE, Sue DY, Whipp BJ. *Principles of Exercise Testing and Interpretation.* Lea and Febiger, Philadelphia, 1987.

20. Bruce RA. Exercise testing for ventricular function. *N. Engl. J. Med.* 1977; 296:671–675.

21. Balke B, Ware RW. An experimental study of physical fitness of Air Force personnel. *US Armed Forces Med. J.* 1959; 10:675.

22. Tonkin MJ, Garrett L, DeMaria AN, Miller RR, Mason DT. Effects of digitalis on the exercise electrocardiogram in normal adult subjects. *Chest.* 1977; 72:714–718.

23. Blair SN, Kohl HW, Paffenbarger RS et al. Physical fitness and all-cause mortality. A prospective study of healthy men and women. *JAMA.* 1989; 262:2395–2401.

24. Chaitman BR, Hanson JS. Comparative sensitivity and specificity of exercise electrocardiographic lead systems. *Am. J. Cardiol.* 1981; 47:1335–1349.

25. American Heart Association. Recommedations for human blood pressure determination by sphygmomanometers. *Circulation.* 1988; 77:501A–504A.

26. Froelicher VF, Marcondes GD. *Manual of Exercise Testing.* Year Book Medical Publishers, Chicago, 1989.

27. Richardson MT, Holly RG, Amsterdam EA, Miller MF. The value of chest pain during the exercise tolerance test in predicting coronary artery disease. *Cardiology.* 1992; 81:164–171.

28. Diamond GA. A clinically relevant classification of chest discomfort. *J. Am. Coll. Cardiol.* 1983; 1:574–575.

29. Tanji JL. Exercise and the hypertensive athlete. Clinic Sport Med. 1992; 11:291–302.

30. Herbert WG, Froelicher VF. Current status of exercise testing and prescription. *CVR&R.* 1979; (April):46–61.

31. Dubach P, Froelicher VF, Klein J et al. Exercise-induced hypotension in a male population. *Circulation.* 1988; 78:1380–1387.

32. Bursese-Taylor L, Holly RG, Krone RB, Amsterdam EA. A descriptive analysis of standard practice in clinical exercise testing. Manuscript in preparation.

33. Rijneke RB, Ascoop CA, Talmon JL. Clinical significance of upsloping ST segments in exercise electrocardiography. *Circulation.* 1980; 61:671–678.

34. Kurita A, Chaitman BR, Bourassa MG. Significance of exercise-induced junctional ST depression in evaluation of coronary artery disease. *Am. J. Cardiol.* 1977; 40:492–497.

35. Ribisl PM, Morris DK, Kawaguchi T, Ueshima K, Froelicher VF. Angiographic patterns and severe coronary artery disease. *Arch. Intern. Med.* 1992; 152:1618–1624.

36. Milliken JA, Abdollah H, Burygraf GW. False positive treadmill exercise tests due to computer signal averaging. *Am. J. Cardiol.* 1990; 65:946–948.

37. Lachterman B, Lehmann KG, Abrahamson D, Froelicher VF. "Recovery only" ST-segment depression and the predictive accuracy of the exercise test. *Ann. Intern. Med.* 1990; 112:11–16.

38. Yang JC, Wesley RC, Froelicher VF. Ventricular tachycardia during routine treadmill testing. *Arch. Intern. Med.* 1991; 151:349–353.

39. Peskoe S, McHenry PL, Richmond HW. Masking of exercise-induced ST-segment depression by rate-dependent left-axis deviation. *Heart Lung.* 1977; 6:1031–1034.

40. Diamond GA, Forrester JS. Analysis of probability as an aid in the clinical diagnosis of coronary artery disease. *N. Engl. J. Med.* 1979; 300:1350–1358.

41. Becker RC, Alpert JS. Electrocardiographic ST segment depression in coronary heart disease. *Am. Heart J.* 1988; 115:862–868.

42. Laslett LJ, Amsterdam EA. Management of the asymptomatic patient with an abnormal exercise ECG. *JAMA.* 1984; 1744–1746.

43. Bruce RA, DeRouen TA, Hossack KF. Value of maximal exercise tests in risk assessment of primary coronary heart disease events in healthy men. *Am. J. Cardiol.* 1980; 46:371–378.

44. Mark DB, Shaw L, Harrell FE et al. Prognostic value of a treadmill exercise score in outpatients with suspected coronary artery disease. *N. Engl. J. Med.* 1991; 325:849–853.

45. Ellestad MH. *Stress Testing.* F.A. Davis, Philadelphia, 1980.

Chapter 8

Exercise Electrocardiography

Carolyn I. Johns and Steven Ung

CONTENTS

I. INTRODUCTION

Analysis of the electrocardiographic (ECG) response to exercise was first performed in 1908 by Einthoven. In a postexercise ECG, he observed an increase in the amplitude of the P and T waves and depression of the J junction.[1] Feil and Siegal reported ST depression and T wave inversion after exercise in patients with angina.[2] In 1944, Master and colleagues[3] published a report in the *American Journal of Medical Science*, describing ECG response during "two-step" exercise.[3] This was the introduction of exercise ECG which has become a widely used test for detecting coronary artery disease.

Optimal usefulness of the exercise test requires that the exercise test evaluator use multiple responses to exercise to evaluate the subject, with the ECG response being only one of those responses. Analysis of all responses in conjunction with the clinical history and findings provides the most accurate diagnostic and prognostic data. The purpose of analyzing the ECG during exercise is to assess for coronary artery

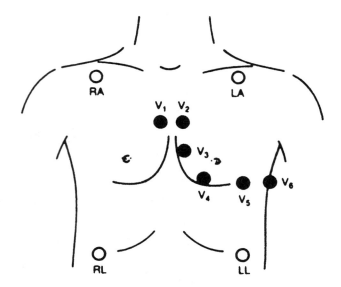

Figure 1   Mason-Likar 12-Lead ECG placement for exercise testing.

disease, as well as to make a prognosis of the likelihood of cardiac events in the future. The ECG response to exercise also provides information concerning the severity of coronary artery disease.

An ECG combined with exercise is sometimes used for analysis of exercise-induced arrhythmias. The use of an ECG during exercise to identify supraventricular arrhythmias is occurring with greater frequency because of advances in the mechanical treatment of such arrythmias. Analysis of exercise-induced ventricular arrhythmias is more difficult, with the significance of these arrhythmias with exercise depending on the complexity of the arrhythmia and the presence and severity of coronary artery disease.

A. LEAD SYSTEMS

During ECG analysis of exercise, the use of multiple lead systems has been shown to be more sensitive than the use of single lead systems in accurately detecting evidence of coronary artery disease.[4] Optimal lead systems are those that include 12 leads. Bipolar leads in single or multiple combination (CM5, CC5) are less sensitive for diagnostic testing, but may be useful for routine ECG monitoring during functional capacity testing.

During exercise, because of significant limb movement, a 12-lead ECG cannot be obtained accurately if electrodes are placed on wrists and ankles during exercise. Mason and Likar[5] developed a system with 12 leads where limb leads were placed at the base of the limbs on the torso, thereby avoiding placement of electrodes on exercising limbs. The Mason–Likar simulated standard 12-lead ECG electrode placement is represented in Figure 1. The ankle and wrist electrodes are replaced by electrodes mounted on the torso at the base of the limbs. The standard precordial leads use Wilson's central terminal as their negative reference, which is formed by connecting the right arm, left arm, and left leg. The triangular configuration around the heart results in a zero voltage reference through the cardiac cycle.

The Mason–Likar arrangement is the electrode system most commonly used today for exercise testing. There is evidence that the Mason–Likar placement of electrodes alters the QRS amplitude frontal plane axis when compared with standard placement of ECG electrodes. Thus 12-lead ECG recordings obtained using the Mason–Likar system are not fully comparable with standard resting ECG tracings. Changes seen using modified lead placement with the Mason–Likar system can be kept to a minimum by keeping the arm electrodes on the shoulders instead of the chest. A baseline ECG recording with the subject supine and/or in a standing position with standard electrode placement will provide an accurate baseline recording prior to the exercise test.

Standing and hyperventilation can change the configuration of the baseline ECG. Axis shifts, Q wave formation, and ST and T wave changes may occur as a result of these maneuvers. Many exercise testing laboratories record a standing and hyperventilation ECG prior to beginning the exercise test. If standing and/or hyperventilation produce significant changes, especially in the ST segment, the specificity of the test can be reduced.

A study by Miranda and colleagues[6] found that monitoring of the inferior leads alone during exercise is of little value. It was demonstrated, with angiographic data of coronary arteries, that ST segment depression in the inferior leads alone was a poor marker for coronary artery disease. It was also found that lead V_5 was markedly superior to Lead II in reliably identifying true ischemia.[6] Approximately 70 to 89% of abnormal ST segment changes can be detected by V_5 alone.[7]

B. ELECTRODES AND SKIN PREPARATION

Disposable electrodes with gel-filled caps and a silver chloride element are recommended to decrease motion artifact and to improve the accuracy of the recording.[8] The importance of skin preparation prior to electrode placement cannot be overemphasized. All of the sophisticated computerized equipment in use today is of little value, if a clear recording with minimal artifact is not maintained during the stress test. Good electrode contact is the key to a high-quality recording. Skin oils should be removed with alcohol or acetone at the sites of electrode placement. Male patients may have to have hair shaved in the appropriate locations. This is followed by removal of the superficial layer of skin with light abrasion with a fine-grained emery paper or other abrasive pad. Dead skin cells act as an insulator, increasing the skin resistance. The goal is to reduce skin resistance to less than 5000 Ω. After placement, each electrode should be tapped with a finger to ensure that there is a minimum of "noise" on the recorder with this maneuver. A well-prepared electrode should display no artifacts.

C. COMPUTERIZED ECG ANALYSIS

Despite careful skin preparation with electrode placement, muscular artifact on the ECG recording during exercise can make tracings uninterpretable. Computer analysis of tracings is used in most modern exercise laboratories to minimize muscular artifact (Figure 2) and 60-cycle interference (Figure 3). There are other benefits of computerized analysis, with reduction of "noise" being the major benefit.

The computer processor converts the continuous analog ECG signal into a digital signal of voltages sampled at regular fixed intervals. Signal averaging is used to reduce noise by storing consecutive beats in a memory to produce a representative complex. The normal complexes are stored in the memory so that the computer will recognize an ectopic complex and not include that complex in the signal-averaging process. Most computers keep track of the number of ectopic complexes generated during a test.[8]

Waveform recognition and measurement of ST segment depression are important computer functions in today's ECG analysis. Algorithms have been written to identify important points on the QRS-T complex. The J point is identified and the ST segment is measured at 80 ms from the J point.[8,9] Computer technology is constantly being updated to produce more-accurate ECG tracings. However, there can be great differences between computerized tracings and "raw" tracings. The practitioner should never rely totally on computerized data for accurate analysis and diagnosis. A review of raw tracings and careful inspection of real-time tracings as well as recorded tracings is essential for comprehensive analysis of the exercise ECG.

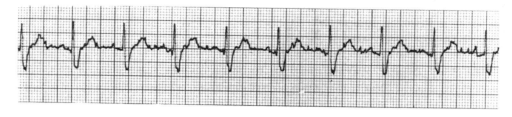

Figure 2 Artifact from muscular activity.

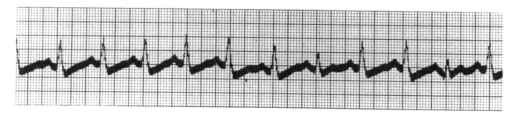

Figure 3 60-cycle interference.

Table 1 Eight Conditions That Prevent Reliable Diagnostic ECG Analysis during Exercise Testing

1. Left bundle branch block
2. WPW pre-excitation
3. Physiological rate-responsive pacing
4. Left ventricular hypertrophy
5. Extensive anterior wall infarction
6. Resting ST and/or T wave abnormalities
7. Drug effects (i.e., digoxin)
8. Electrolyte abnormalities

D. BASELINE ECG ANALYSIS

There are eight conditions that can prevent reliable diagnostic ECG analysis during exercise testing. These include left bundle branch block, Wolff–Parkinson–White (WPW) preexcitation, physiological rate-responsive pacing, left ventricular hypertrophy, extensive anterior wall infarction, resting ST and/or T wave abnormalities, drug effects (i.e., digoxin), and electrolyte abnormalities (Table 1). In the presence of these conditions, exercise testing can provide information about hemodynamic response to exercise and aerobic capacity, but ECG analysis will most likely be unreliable. All exercise subjects should be screened for these conditions with a resting ECG prior to initiating the exercise test.

II. THE ECG DURING EXERCISE TESTING

A. NORMAL ECG RESPONSE TO EXERCISE

Predictable changes occur in a normal ECG tracing during exercise. As the heart rate increases with exercise, the PR interval shortens. There is a progressive rate-related shortening of the QT interval and superposition of the P and T waves. The amplitude of the R wave decreases and amplitudes of septal Q waves and T waves increase. The ST segment is noted to have a progressively positive upsloping, beginning from the J point, which is usually displaced below the isoelectric line. The ST segment then returns to above the baseline within 60 to 80 ms from the J point.[11]

B. EXERCISE-INDUCED ARRHYTHMIAS

Exercise-induced arrhythmias occur as a result of enhanced sympathetic tone, increased myocardial oxygen demand, or both. The increased sympathetic tone in the myocardium may stimulate ectopic foci in the Purkinje fibers, initiating spontaneous discharge and leading to increased automaticity. Some arrhythmias such as premature ventricular complexes (PVCs) or premature atrial complexes are common during exercise testing, occurring in as many as 40% of normal subjects, and are due to reentry or abnormal automaticity in the ventricles.[12]

Since exercise increases myocardial oxygen demand, in the presence of coronary artery disease, myocardial ischemia during exercise could predispose a subject to ectopic activity. The immediate postexercise period is especially dangerous because of high catecholamine levels and generalized vasodilation. Peripheral arterial dilation induced by exercise and reduced cardiac output resulting from reduced venous return following abrupt termination of large muscle activity, may result in diminished coronary artery perfusion. Exercise may also induce cardiac arrhythmias under conditions including digitalis or diuretic therapy and recent ingestion of alcohol, caffeine, or other stimulants. Metabolic acidosis can also potentiate cardiac arrhythmias.

Sinus arrhythmias, such as isolated premature contractions, are fairly common during exercise and recovery phases. Sustained supraventricular tachycardia (SVT) can be induced by exercise and may require immediate medical attention to revert it. First-degree Atrio-ventricular (A-V) block may occur in the late exercise phase and recovery phase in those who are predisposed by condition or drug therapy. This may include persons on digitalis or beta blockers. The occurrence of second-degree A-V block in the form of Wenckebach or Mobitz Type I A-V block and Mobitz Type II A-V block is relatively rare, and the clinical significance is uncertain. The occurrence of complete or third-degree A-V block at rest or with exercise is considered a contraindication to exercise testing.

The occurrence of intraventricular blocks with exercise is relatively rare. Left or right bundle branch blocks and fascicular blocks may occur with exercise, and usually precede the appearance of chronic bundle branch block at rest. Exercise may provoke, suppress, or not affect accessory pathway conduction

Examples of Arrhythmias with Exercise

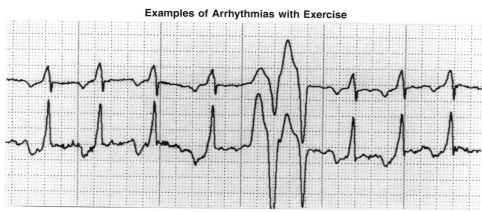

Ventricular couplet

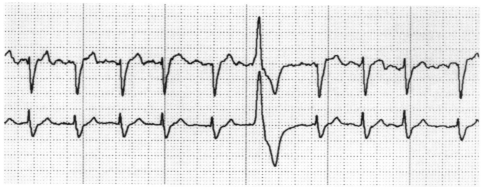

Isolated premature ventricular contractions

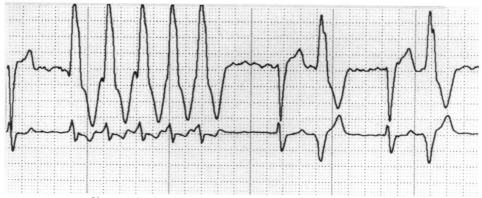

Nonsustained ventricular tachycardia and ventricular bigeminy

in persons with known WPW pre-excitation. When pre-excitation conduction is present, marked ST segment depression may occur with exercise testing, and may be secondary to ischemia, but is most likely a false positive response. Exercise is considered to be a stimulus for developing tachyarrhythmias in WPW syndrome, although their occurrence is not common. Approximately 20 to 50% of individuals with pre-excitation present on the ECG will develop normal conduction with exercise.[13]

Exercise-induced atrial premature beats and nonsustained SVT may occur in normal or diseased hearts. Exercise-induced atrial flutter or atrial fibrillation which is transient may occur in those with normal hearts or in conditions including ischemic heart disease, pulmonary disease, rheumatic heart disease, hyperthyroidism, WPW accessory conduction, cardiomyopathy, or recent caffeine or alcohol ingestion. The occurrence of exercise-induced supraventricular arrhythmias is not diagnostic for ischemic heart disease.[1]

Approximately one third of subjects develop ventricular ectopy in response to exercise testing. The appearance of frequent premature ventricular complexes as well as three to six beats of nonsustained ventricular tachycardia is not a reliable diagnostic indicator for ischemic or other forms of heart disease, in the absence of ischemic ECG changes. Approximately 50% of subjects with coronary artery disease develop ventricular arrhythmias with exercise. The prognostic significance of exercise-induced ventricular arrhythmias in persons with coronary artery disease remains controversial. Suppression of ventricular ectopy with exercise is a nonspecific finding and can occur in normal subjects as well as in those with coronary artery disease.

Using the exercise test to evaluate subjects with arrhythmias is an important part of the total evaluation, along with ambulatory monitoring and electrophysiological studies. Exercise testing provokes repetitive ventricular beats in most subjects with a history of sustained ventricular arrhythmia. In those subjects with a recent myocardial infarction, the presence of exercise-induced repetitive ventricular complexes is associated with an increased risk of future cardiac events including sudden death.

The exercise test is also valuable in the assessment of the effects of antiarrhythmic medications and in the management of subjects with chronic atrial fibrillation. Exercise testing can be indicated in subjects who have symptoms consistent with arrhythmias (e.g., syncope, palpitations). The testing may be used to reveal complex ventricular arrhythmias, to provoke supraventricular arrhythmias, to determine the relationship between arrhythmias and activity, to aid in determining optimal antiarrhythmic therapy, and to reveal proarrhythmic responses to antiarrhythmic drugs. However, sole reliance on exercise testing results may be misleading.

C. ST SEGMENT DEPRESSION

Correct interpretation of the ECG response during exercise testing is crucial to the safe performance of the examination and accurate diagnosis of abnormalities suggesting the presence of ischemic heart disease. As previously noted, during exercise normal changes occur to the ECG consisting of minor shortening of the P-R and QRS durations and progressive shortening of the Q-T interval. Isolated J point (see Figure 6 in Chapter 7) or junctional depression is a normal finding due to the effect of atrial T wave repolarization changes during exercise. The principal ischemic ECG abnormalities during exercise that should concern the individual supervising the treadmill test center on the ST segment. During exercise an abnormal ST segment response will consist of depression, elevation, or "normalization." Analysis of the ST segment provides the best evidence for the presence of myocardial ischemia.

ST segment depression occurs in three general varieties: horizontal, downsloping, or upsloping. The J point serves as a reference point for the analysis of the ST segment. Upsloping ST segment depression is defined as an ST segment that is depressed greater than 0.7 mm but less than 1.5 mm by 80 ms past the J point. In this case, it may be suggestive of myocardial ischemia. Where it is greater than 1.5 mm, the response is suggestive of myocardial ischemia.[11]

Horizontal ST depression is defined as 1 mm or more of J point depression and that ST depression then continues for 80 ms after the J point. Due to motion artifact during exercise, one usually prefers to see this depression in three consecutive complexes with a reasonably stable isoelectric baseline.

Downsloping ST depression occurs when the ST segment measured 80 ms from the J point is greater than 1 mm, resulting in a negative slope of the ST segment. In patients with a normal, isoelectric ST segment at baseline, the presence of either horizontal or downsloping ST depression is abnormal and suggests exercise-induced myocardial ischemia. With worsening ischemia the depth of ST depression may increase; occasionally it can worsen during the recovery phase and in about 10% of patients the ST depression occurs only during the recovery phase.[14]

The reason ST segment depression occurs with ischemia relates to the ST segment being "isoelectric" (i.e., at baseline) under normal conditions. During exercise, induced subendocardial ischemia creates an electrical gradient between normal epicardial cells and the lower-potential ischemic cells. This results in an ST segment shift which, for subendocardial ischemia, produces ST depression relative to the ECG baseline. The surface lead location of this ST depression does not anatomically locate the site of ischemia, nor does it identify which coronary artery is involved.[15] However, the severity of ST depression (greater than 2 mm), a downsloping character, early time of onset, the number of ECG leads involved, and persistence of the ST depression late into recovery are all associated with the severity of myocardial ischemia and the extent of the coronary artery disease (see Figure 7 in Chapter 7).

Although J point depression is a normal finding during exercise, it is often seen with either a rapid or "slow upsloping" ST depression following the J point. A rapid upsloping ST segment (>1 mV/s with <1.5 mm ST depression) is likely to be normal whereas a "slow upsloping" ST segment (>1.5 mm ST

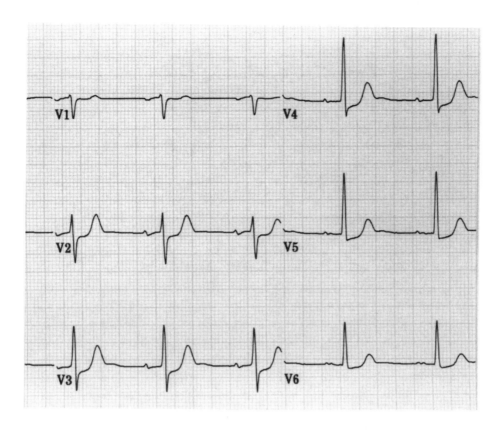

depression 80 ms from the J point) is more likely to be abnormal in individuals with a high pretest likelihood of coronary artery disease. In other words, the probability and severity of coronary artery disease are inversely related to the slope of the ST segment.

D. ST SEGMENT ELEVATION

Exercise-induced ST segment elevation is a relatively rare finding during treadmill testing. ST segment elevation is defined as 1 mm or more of J point elevation which persists during the ST segment for 80 ms in three consecutive beats. This finding is usually considered to be abnormal, representing some form of abnormal cardiac pathology. The nature of this pathology depends upon the clinical setting in which the exercise is performed. In evaluating the significance of ST elevation, it is important to determine if Q waves are present in the same or adjacent leads. Without prior Q wave myocardial infarction, ST elevation and its location (inferior, anterior, lateral, etc.) identify a site of severe transient ischemia, often involving a proximal coronary artery stenosis in the territory surrounded by the lead changes. Dunn and colleagues[16] have reported this finding to be associated with a reversible thallium defect.

In subjects with a prior Q wave myocardial infarction, the ST segment elevation may represent abnormal wall motion (e.g., left ventricular aneurysm), per-infarction ischemia, or both.[8] Several retrospective studies[17,18] have suggested that patients having ST segment elevation with associated q waves on a resting ECG have multivessel disease, whereas ST segment elevation in the absence of q waves is associated with single-vessel disease at catheterization.

E. PSEUDONORMALIZATION OF ST SEGMENTS

Occasionally, baseline ST-T abnormalities such as ST depression and/or T wave inversion will become "normal" with exercise (i.e., with exercise the baseline resting ST depression returns to the isoelectric line and/or the resting T wave inversion becomes upright). Relatively small studies of groups of patients exhibiting these findings have noted that these changes are often associated with wall motion abnormalities by radionuclide angiography or the clinical association of coronary artery disease.

Although the theoretical mechanisms of pseudonormalization are thought to be due to cancellation of rest ST segment vectors by new ischemic ST vectors, the precise mechanism is unknown. The most

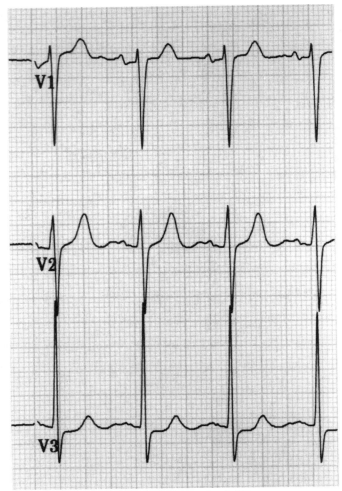

Horizontal ST depression in V3

prudent means to interpret the clinical significance of pseudonormalization is by carefully evaluating the clinical company it keeps. In the setting of prior myocardial infarction, pseudonormalization during exercise would be suggestive of additional ischemia.

F. FALSE POSITIVE ECG CHANGES DURING EXERCISE

There is a variety of preexisting conditions which can result in false positive responses during exercise stress testing. Although an in-depth discussion can be found elsewhere, these conditions can be classified by (1) intrinsic cardiac disease — cardiomyopathy, valvular heart disease, hypertensive heart disease, mitral valve prolapse, pericardial disease; (2) metabolic disturbances — electrolytes, nonfasting state, anemia, hyperventilation; (3) baseline ECG abnormalities — left and right bundle branch block, WPW syndrome, left ventricular hypertrophy; (4) drugs — digitalis; and (5) miscellaneous causes — excessive double product, female gender (Table 3).

III. PREDICTIVE VALUE OF CLINICAL EXERCISE TESTING

The predictive value of exercise testing is a measure of how accurately an exercise test correctly identifies an individual with coronary artery disease (positive test) or without coronary artery disease (negative test) . Establishing the predictive value of exercise testing is based on Bayes's theorem, which is a mathematical rule relating the interpretation of present observations in light of past experience.[19] Bayes's theorem helps to increase the accuracy of a test to predict coronary artery disease by incorporating the pretest probability of disease with the test result to determine the posttest probability of disease.

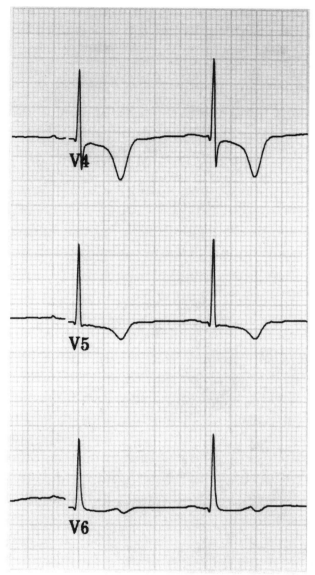

T wave inversions

Table 2 Diagnostic ST Segment Criteria for Myocardial Ischemia

1. Horizontal or downsloping ST segment depression that is equal to or greater than 1 mm at 80 ms past the J point
2. ST segment elevation of greater than or equal to 1 mm at 80 ms past the J point
3. Upsloping ST depression that is equal to or greater than 1.5 mm at 80 ms past the J point

The probability of a subject having coronary artery disease is determined from the test result, the diagnostic features of the test, and the pretest likelihood of the patient having disease prior to administration of the test. Bayes's theorem determines that the probability of disease after a test is performed is the product of disease probability before the test and the probability that the test was a true positive.[19] More simply stated:

Past Experience + Present Observations = Future Interpretation

Table 3 Causes of False Positive
Test Results

1.	A preexisting abnormal resting ECG
2.	Cardiac hypertrophy
3.	WPW and other conduction defects
4.	Hypertension
5.	Drugs (i.e., digitalis)
6.	Cardiomyopathy
7.	Hypokalemia
8.	Vasoregulatory abnormalities
9.	Sudden intense exercise
10.	Mitral valve prolapse
12.	Pectus excavatum
13.	Technical or observer error
14.	Coronary spasm
15.	Anemia
16.	Female gender

With Bayes's theorem it is easy to understand that the ability of a given test result to predict the presence or absence of disease is related to the presence of disease in that population of subjects being tested. For example, a teenage female with a positive ST segment depression during a stress test has a low posttest likelihood of coronary disease compared with a 65-year-old male with typical chest pain and multiple risk factors who would have a very high posttest likelihood of coronary artery disease. This difference is due to the significant difference in the pretest likelihood of disease in these two different populations, in spite of similar ST segment displacement during exercise.

The accuracy of diagnosing coronary artery disease based on ischemic ST changes during treadmill testing comes from studies which compared exercise ECG data with coronary angiography findings, because coronary artery angiography is the gold standard of detecting the extent and severity of coronary artery disease.

A. SENSITIVITY

The predictive accuracy of exercise testing is determined by the sensitivity and specificity of the test and the prevalence of coronary artery disease in the population tested. *Sensitivity* refers to the percentage of individuals being tested who will have an abnormal test.

$$\text{Sensitivity} = \frac{\text{True Positive Tests}^*}{\text{True Positive} + \text{False Negatives Tests}^\dagger} \times 100$$

The sensitivity of clinical exercise testing varies from 50 to 90%, or approximately 71%.[20] There is a 71% pretest likelihood of correctly identifying an individual with coronary artery disease, based on a true positive exercise test (ST depression of at least 1.0 mm at 0.08 s past the J point). The sensitivity of exercise testing can be enhanced (increase in the likelihood of a true positive test) by (1) administering a true maximal exercise test, (2) using multiple-lead ECG monitoring, and (3) monitoring additional data, such as abnormal blood pressure responses. It can also be decreased (increase in the likelihood of a false negative test) by (1) administering a submaximal exercise test, (2) insufficient ECG monitoring, and (3) certain cardiac drugs (beta blockers and nitrates).

The sensitivity of stress tests is affected not only by the prevalence of disease, but also by the criteria used to determine what constitutes a "positive" or "negative" result. The magnitude of stress demanded during exercise, liberalizing the ST criteria for "abnormal" results, and applying more ECG leads will increase the identification of disease. However, as will be soon identified, this increase in sensitivity will be at the expense of its specificity. Likewise, a reduction in the sensitivity can be made by increasing the false negative rate by increasing the magnitude of ST depression required for a positive test or reducing the magnitude of stress during exercise.

* True Positive Test = individuals who had both abnormal stress tests and abnormal angiograms.

† False Negative Test = individuals who had abnormal stress tests, but normal angiograms.

B. SPECIFICITY

Specificity refers to the percentage of individuals being tested who will have a normal exercise stress test. Thus, a true negative stress test correctly identifies a person without coronary artery disease. Specificity of exercise stress testing varies from 60 to 98%, or approximately 73%.[20]

$$\text{Specificity} = \frac{\text{True Negative Tests}^*}{\text{True Negative} + \text{False Positive Tests}^\dagger} \times 100$$

The specificity of exercise testing (increase in the likelihood of a false positive test) is reduced by (1) preexisting abnormal resting ECG abnormalities, (2) hypertrophy of the left ventricle, (3) certain medications (e.g., digitalis), (4) mitral valve prolapse, and (5) anemia.

The *predictive value* of exercise stress testing is a measure of how accurately the results from an exercise stress test correctly identify the presence or absence of coronary artery disease in individuals being tested (positive test = disease, negative test = no disease).

$$\text{Predictive Value} = (\text{positive test}) \frac{\text{True Positive Tests}}{\text{True Positive} + \text{False Positive Tests}} \times 100$$

$$\text{Predictive Value} = (\text{negative test}) \frac{\text{True Negative Tests}}{\text{True Negative} + \text{False Negative Tests}} \times 100$$

When an individual comes to a physician's office to have an exercise stress test and he or she has multiple risk factors (smoking, hypertension, diabetes, family history, etc.) and symptoms, the pretest likelihood of disease is high (predictive value for a positive test is high). On the other hand, if a young, active, healthy individual with perhaps only one or two risk factors for coronary artery disease has an exercise stress test, the pretest likelihood of disease is low (predictive value for a positive test is low). In addition to ECG recordings, the predictive value of exercise stress testing is enhanced by recording additional data such as the total exercise time; maximal metabolic equivalent (MET) level obtained; blood pressure responses before, during, and following exercise; and symptoms of angina or shortness of breath.

* True Negative Test = individuals with normal stress tests who have normal angiograms.
† False Positive Test = individuals with normal stress tests who have abnormal angiograms.

IV. REVIEW OF CLINICAL CASE STUDIES

A. CLINICAL CASE STUDY #1
DOB: 7/10/26
SEX: M
REASON FOR REFERRAL: Angina
CURRENT MEDICATIONS: Copoten, Mevacor
BASELINE: ECG: T wave abnormality in anterior leads.
RESTING HR: 55
RESTING BP: 165/85
TESTING PROTOCOL: Bruce

STAGE	STAGE TIME	HR(bpm)	BP	
Supine		55	165/85	
Standing		56		
Posthyperventilation		59		
I	1:00	89		
	2:00	98		
	3:00	106	150/70	
II	4:00	123		
	4:15	129		Termination
Recovery	1:00	112		
	2:00	91	160/80	
	3:00	76		
	3:48	73	150/80	
	4:00	71	150/80	pain gone
	5:00	73		
	6:00	71	140/80	

TREADMILL RESULTS:
    TOTAL EXERCISE TIME: 4:15 min.   TOTAL METS: 5.7
    MAX HR: 130   MAX BP: 165/85
    MAX HR ACHIEVED/MAX HR PREDICTED: 73%
    PREDICTED MAX HR/TARGET HR: 178/151
    DOUBLE PRODUCT: 21.4 (thousands)
    PREDICTED AGE/SEX EXERCISE DURATION (minutes): 8
PHYSIOLOGICAL RESPONSE TO EXERCISE:
    Blood pressure response was blunted. Normal heart rate response.
TEST STOPPED FOR
    ST depression
ARRHYTHMIAS
    None noted.
ST SEGMENT RESPONSE
    RESTING ECG — T wave abnormality in anterior leads.
    HYPERVENTILATION ECG — No change from baseline.
    EXERCISE ECG — Downsloping ST depression 1–1.5 mm V_5–V_6 and 2 mm in inferior
    leads. ST elevation in V_1–V_4.
IMPRESSION
    TMT:
    Positive for ischemic changes.
    Positive for angina.
OTHER COMMENTS: Strongly positive treadmill suggestive of multivessel CAD,
    including LAD involvement.

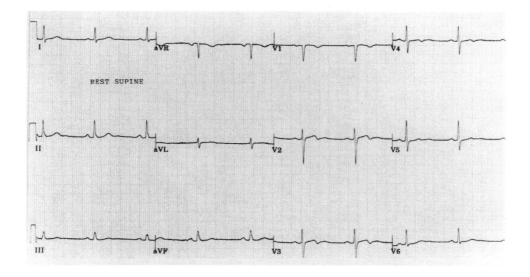

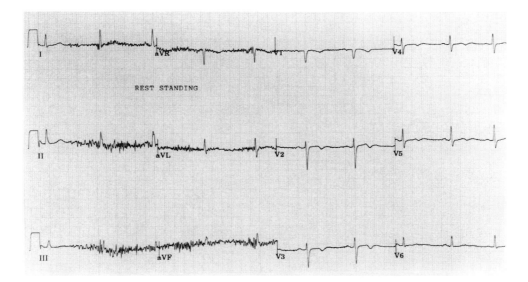

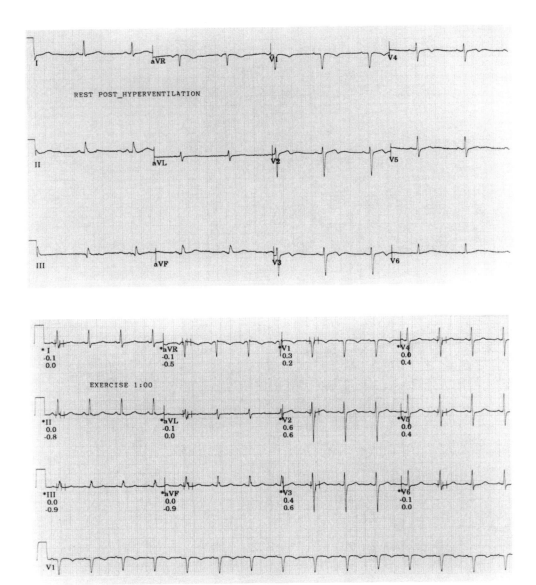

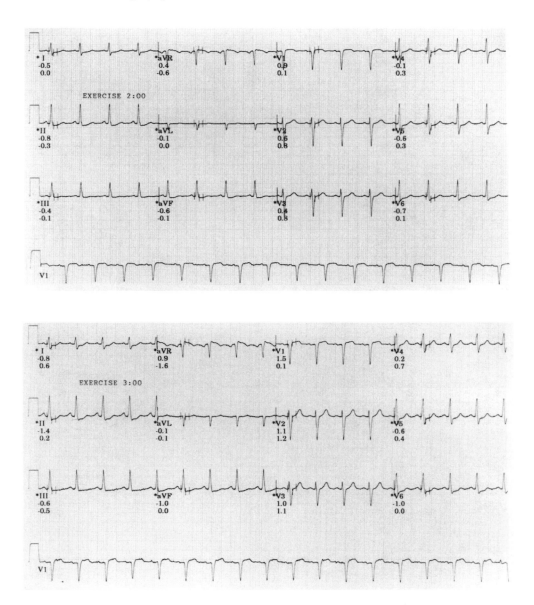

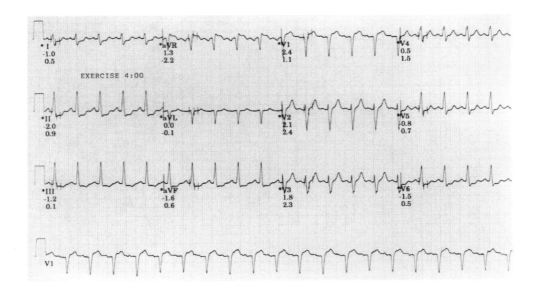

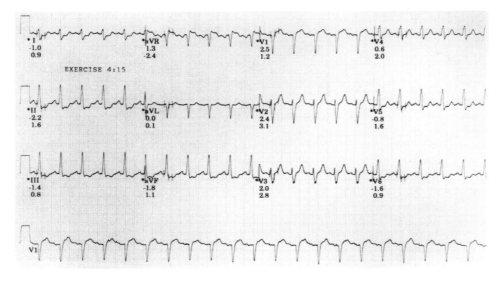

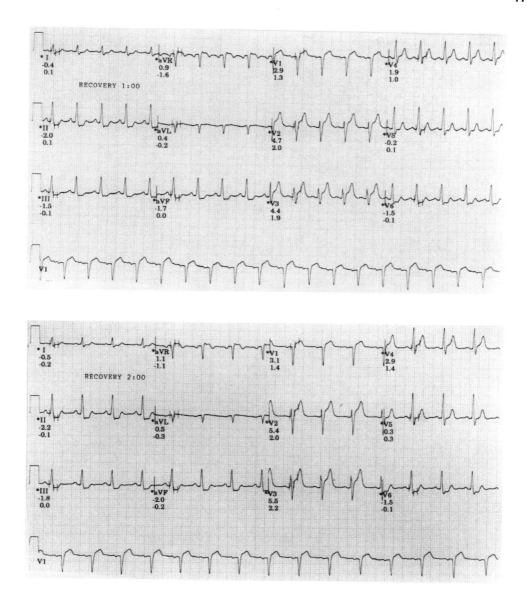

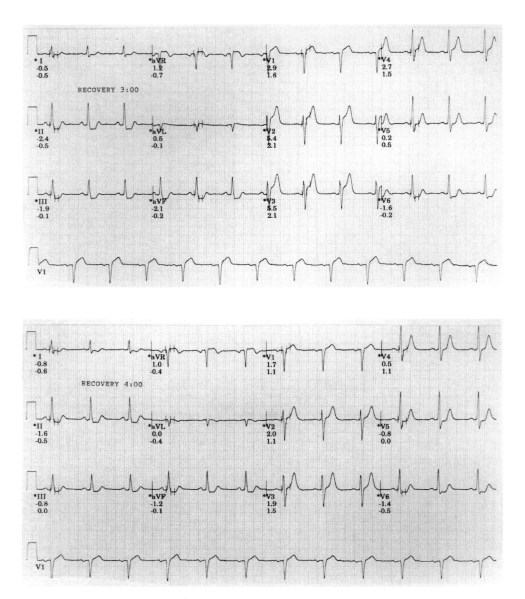

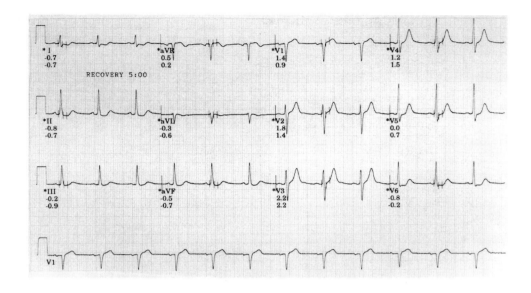

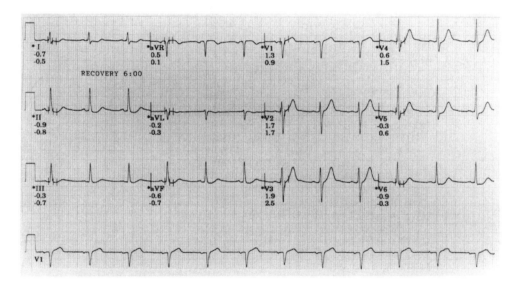

B. CLINICAL CASE STUDY #2

DOB: 3/9/32
SEX: M
REASON FOR REFERRAL: Dyspnea
CURRENT MEDICATIONS: Questran, ASA
BASELINE ECG: Poor R wave progression.
BASELINE HR: 73
RESTING BP: 135/80
TESTING PROTOCOL: Bruce

STAGE	STAGE TIME	HR(bpm)	BP
Supine		73	135/80
Standing		80	
Posthyperventilation		99	
I	1:00	98	
	2:00	98	142/70
	3:00	98	
II	4:00	107	
	5:00	115	155/80
	6:00	116	
III	7:00	127	
	8:00	135	
	9:00	142	160/80
IV	10:00	156	
	11:00	164	Termination
Recovery	1:00	131	
	2:00	117	170/85
	3:00	108	
	4:00	105	160/80
	5:00	103	138/70

TREADMILL RESULTS:
 TOTAL EXERCISE TIME: 11:05 min.   TOTAL METS: 13.4
 MAX HR: 166   MAX BP: 165/80
 MAX HR ACHIEVED/MAX HR PREDICTED: 92%
 PREDICTED MAX HR/TARGET HR: 180/153
 DOUBLE PRODUCT: 27.4 (thousands)
 PREDICTED AGE/SEX EXERCISE DURATION (minutes): 8.5
PHYSIOLOGICAL RESPONSE TO EXERCISE:
 Normal for age and sex. Normal heart rate and blood pressure response.
TEST STOPPED FOR
 Leg pain/fatigue. No chest pain reported.
ST SEGMENT RESPONSE
 RESTING ECG — Poor R wave progression.
 HYPERVENTILATION ECG — No change from baseline.
 EXERCISE ECG — Abnormal. Horizontal ST depression 1 mm L, I.
 ST segment returns to baseline in recovery after 5 min.
IMPRESSION
 TMT:
 Positive for ischemic ECG changes.
 Aerobic capacity is normal.
COMMENT
 In the setting of excellent exercise capacity and no exercise-induced chest pain,
 the isolated finding of positive ischemic ECG changes should be questioned as
 possibly being a false positive finding. If clinically indicated would recommend
 stress imaging study.

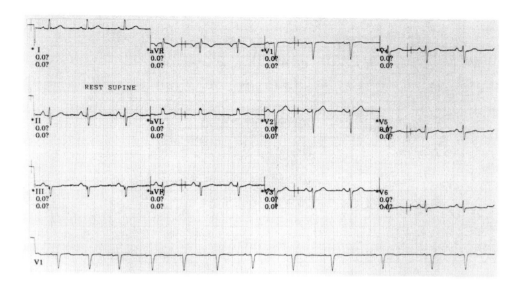

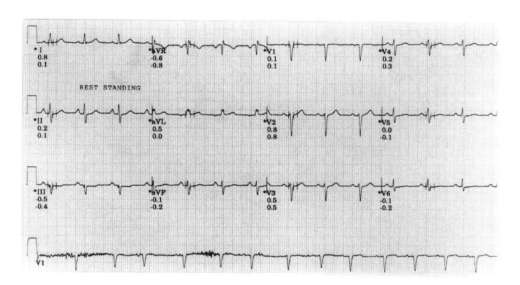

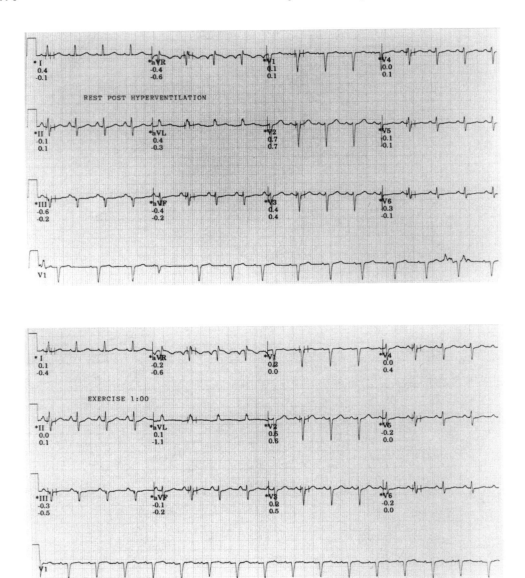

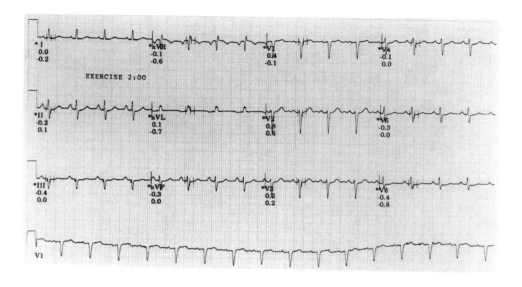

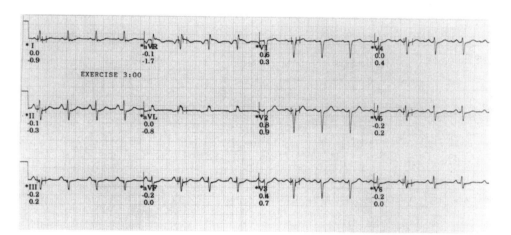

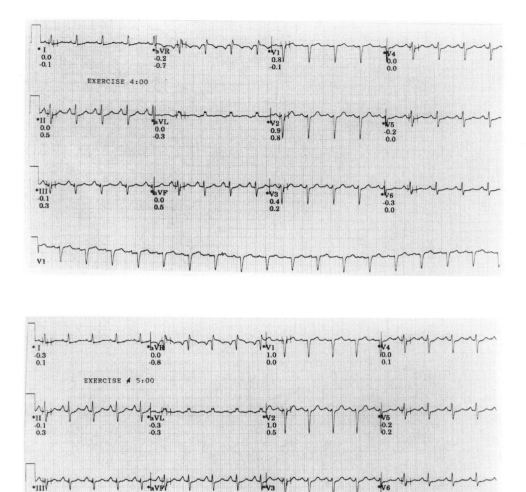

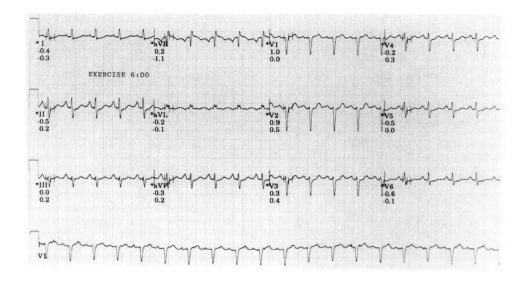

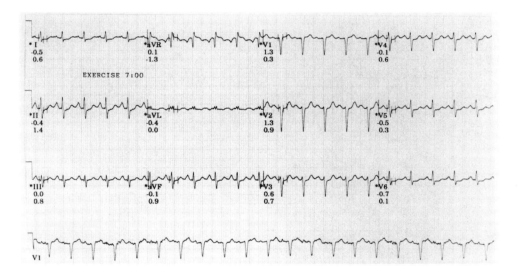

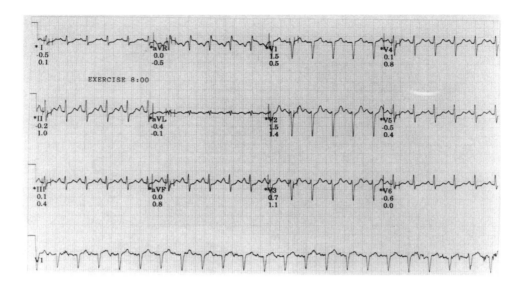

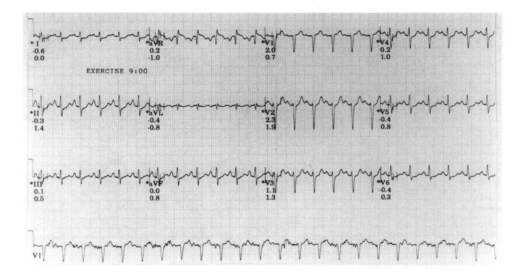

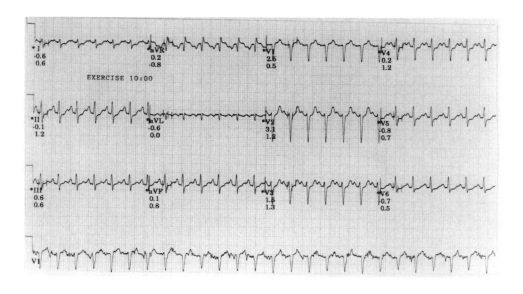

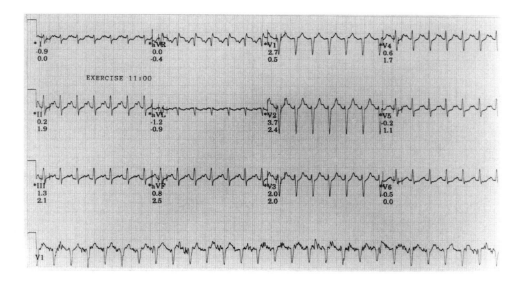

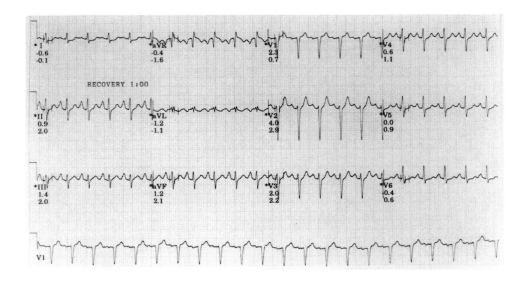

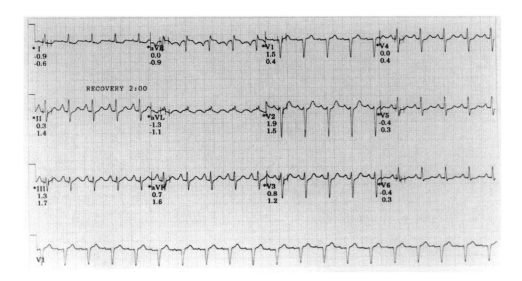

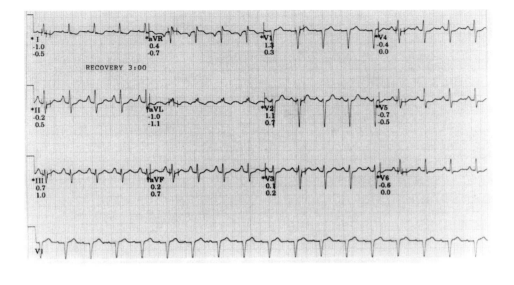

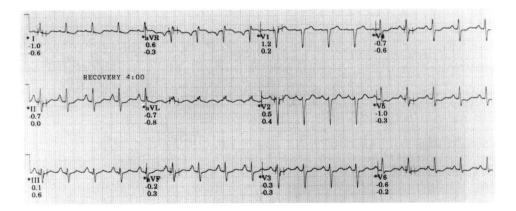

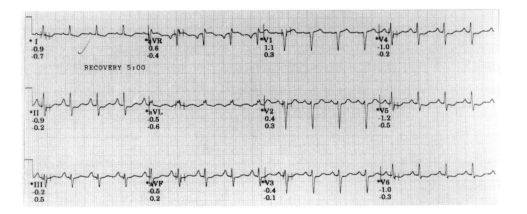

REFERENCES

1. Bruce, R.A. and P.F. Cohn. Exercise testing. In Cohn, P.F. (Ed.). *Diagnosis and Therapy of Coronary Artery Disease.* Boston, MA: Martinus Nijhoff, pp. 135–167, 1985.
2. Bruce, R.A. Clinical exercise testing. A review of personal and community practice experience. In Evans, C.H. (Ed.). *Exercise Testing. Primary Care Clinics in Office Practice.* Philadelphia, PA: W.B. Saunders, p. 405, 1994.
3. Master, R., et al. The EKG and step exercise. *Am. J. Med. Sci.* 207:435–450, 1944.
4. Chung, E.K. *Principles of Cardiac Arrythmias.* Baltimore, MD: Williams and Wilkins, 1989.
5. Mason, R.E. and I. Likar. A new system of multiple-lead exercise electrocardiography. *Am. Heart J.* 71:196–205, 1966.
6. Miranda, C.P., Liu, J., Kadar, A., et al. Usefulness of exercise-induced ST segment depression in the inferior leads during exercise testing as a marker for coronary artery disease. *Am. J. Cardiol.* 69:303–307, 1992.
7. Koppes, G., Mckierman, T., Bassan, M. and V.F. Froelicher. Treadmill exercise testing. *Curr. Probl. Cardiol.* 7:1–44, 1977.
8. Froelicher, V.F., Myers, J., Follansbee, W.P. and A.J. Labovitz. *Exercise and the Heart,* 3rd Edition. St. Louis, MO: Mosby-Yearbook, 1993.
9. Fletcher, G.F., Froelicher, V.F., Hartley, L.H., Haskell, W.L. and M.L. Pollock. Exercise Standards: American Heart Association Exercise Scientific Statement. *Circulation.* 82:6, 2286–2322, 1990.
10. Schlant, R.C., Blomqvist, C.G., Brandenburg, R.O., et al. Guidelines for exercise testing: A report of the joint ACC and AHA Task Force on Assessment of Cardiovascular Procedures. *Circulation.* 74:3, 653-A, 1986.
11. Ellested, M.H. *Stress-Testing, Principles and Practice*, 3rd Edition. Philadelphia, PA: F.A. Davis Company, 1986.
12. McHenry, P.L., Morris, S.N. and M. Kavalier. Exercise-induced arrhythmias — recognition, classification and clinical significance. *Cardiovasc. Clin.* 6:245, 1974.
13. Braunwald, E. *Heart Disease: A Textbook of Cardiovascular Medicine*, 4th Edition. Philadelphia, PA: W.B. Saunders, 1992.
14. Lachterman, B., Lehmann, K.G., Abrahamson, D., and V.F. Froelicher. "Recovery only" ST-segment depression and predictive accuracy of the exercise test. *Ann. Intern. Med.* 112:11, 1990.
15. Mark, D.B., Hlatky, M.A., Lee, K.L., et al. Localizing coronary artery obstructions with the exercise treadmill test. *Ann. Intern. Med.* 106:53, 1987.
16. Dunn, R.F., Freedman, B., Bailey, I.K., et al. Localization of coronary artery disease with exercise electrocardiography: correlation with thallium-201 myocardial perfusion scanning. *Am. J. Cardiol.* 48:837–843, 1981.
17. Sriwattanakomen, S., Ticzon, A.R., Zubritzky, S.A., et al. ST segment elevation during exercise: electrocardiographic and artiographic correlation in 38 patients. *Am. J. Cardiol.* 45:762–768, 1980.
18. Arora, R., Ioachim, L, Matza, D. and S.F. Horowitz. The role of ischemia and ventricular asynergy in the genesis of exercise-induced ST elevation. *Clin. Cardiol.* 11:127–131, 1988.
19. Diamond, G.A. Bayes' theorem: a practical aid to clinical judgement for diagnosis of coronary artery disease. *Prac. Cardiol.* 10(6):47–77, 1984.
20. Detrano, R. and V.F. Froelicher. Exercise testing: uses and limitations considering recent studies. *Prog. Cardiovasc. Dis.* 31:173–204, 1988.

Chapter 9

Radionuclide Exercise Testing

Miqdad Khan and Steven C. Port

CONTENTS

I. INTRODUCTION

The application of radionuclides to the study of the cardiovascular system began more than 50 years ago but widespread clinical applications did not begin until approximately 1975. At that time, advances in the technology of gamma cameras and, most especially, the progress in computer hardware and software led to a rapid expansion of the research and clinical applications of nuclear cardiology procedures. The next 10 years saw the refinement of clinical protocols and definition of the roles of myocardial perfusion and ventricular function imaging in diagnosis and prognosis of individuals with heart disease. From the mid-1980s to the present, another surge of technological breakthroughs in gamma camera technology, computer hardware and software, and most recently radiopharmaceuticals has left the field of nuclear cardiology with many more options for answering a host of clinical and research questions related to those suspected of or afflicted with heart disease, especially coronary artery disease.

Current clinical applications of nuclear cardiology can be divided into two broad categories, myocardial perfusion imaging and ventricular function imaging. There are applications that do not fit into those categories but they play a relatively minor role in the average clinical laboratory. In this chapter, we will define and characterize the types of perfusion and function imaging techniques and specifically address their individual strengths and weaknesses and how they relate to clinical exercise testing.

II. CORONARY FLOW RESERVE AND EXERCISE TESTING

The remarkable ability of the coronary circulation to autoregulate maintains coronary blood flow at normal resting levels despite marked reductions in the caliber of the epicardial coronary arteries. Resting flow may be normal even when there is an 80 to 90% luminal diameter stenosis of a major coronary artery. However, peak flow begins to decrease with stenoses in the 50% range and may be markedly reduced when stenoses reach the 75 to 90% range.[1] Consequently, in order to detect most coronary stenoses, it is necessary to evaluate flow reserve, i.e., the magnitude of the increase in flow when a maximum or near maximum stimulus to flow is applied. Clinically, the classic approach to evaluating flow reserve is to perform maximum symptom-limited aerobic exercise which typically results in flow increases of three- to fivefold over resting flow.[2] At peak demand, stenotic arteries deliver less blood than do normal or less severely involved arteries. Such regional heterogeneity of coronary flow is the hallmark of coronary artery disease and can be detected by injection of tracers that localize in the myocardium or by visualization of the effect of subnormal flow on regional ventricular function. Imaging heterogeneous coronary flow and/or regional variations in ventricular function form the basis of all radionuclide exercise testing.

III. MYOCARDIAL PERFUSION IMAGING

The discovery of radiopharmaceuticals that were extracted by the myocardium after intravenous injection and which had appropriate gamma photon energies for detection with commercially available gamma cameras enabled physicians to visualize myocardial blood flow. Various radionuclides were used early on, but the agent that became adopted as the universal standard for imaging myocardial perfusion was thallous chloride or thallium-201. Thallium, a cyclotron by-product, is a potassium analogue and is distributed in the potassium space of the body. It is taken up by cardiac muscle in direct proportion to tissue blood flow across a wide physiological range of flows.[3] When first introduced into clinical practice, the most common acquisition protocol involved separate-day exercise and resting injections and imaging. Typically thallium is injected at peak exercise and the subject continues to exercise for at least 1 min thereafter. Thallium has a high first-pass extraction by the myocardium and its concentration in the myocardium peaks at about 10 min after the injection.[4] For that reason, imaging is usually performed at that point in time. Regional differences in thallium concentration will be apparent on images obtained immediately after exercise if a significant coronary stenosis is present. Postexercise images can then be compared with images acquired after thallium is injected at rest when myocardial blood flow is more hemogeneous. Not long after its introduction into clinical use, the pharmacokinetics of thallium were described in patients and it became apparent that the regional distribution of thallium began changing soon after its concentration in myocardial tissue peaked. In fact, thallium showed a fairly linear clearance from normal myocardium with the average time to reach 50% of peak concentration being approximately 4 h.[5] In contrast, myocardium rendered ischemic by exercise showed slower tracer clearance or occasionally a net increase in tracer concentration during the same time period.[6] Consequently, regional differences in thallium uptake due to ischemia that were detected on immediate postexercise images became less apparent or disappeared altogether when imaging was repeated 4 h later. That phenomenon was named thallium redistribution. Subsequently, it has been shown that the redistribution process may take considerably longer than 4 h and seems to be prolonged in proportion to the severity of stenosis and, by inference, the severity of the flow reduction.[7] Current protocols frequently use 24-h delayed imaging to enhance the detection of reversible ischemia. Alternatively, there are protocols that use reinjection of a small amount of thallium 4 h after the postexercise imaging.[8,9] That strategy has been shown to increase the detection of reversible ischemia and, in many cases, obviate the need for additional delayed imaging such as the 24-h image.

Within the past few years, new radiopharmaceuticals have been developed for myocardial perfusion imaging. Several technetium-99m–based agents have been tested and two have reached clinical use. To date, the most accepted is technetium-99m sestamibi. Its pharmacokinetics are very different from those of thallium and, as a result, the imaging protocols are quite different. Technetium-99m sestamibi is taken up by the myocardium proportional to blood flow over a wide range of flows much like thallium. However, unlike thallium, the sestamibi molecule is very slow to clear from the myocardium. In fact, there is little redistribution over a period of many hours.[10] Since there is minimal redistribution, a second injection of sestamibi must be made under resting conditions to determine whether an abnormality is reversible or not. Either the resting or the exercise imaging can be performed first although there is a theoretical advantage to performing the resting study first if the studies are performed on the same day. The rest and exercise sessions can take place on different days. In contrast to thallium, where imaging must be performed within 10 min of the injection, imaging may be delayed for hours following injection of sestamibi. An interval of 10 to 15 min is recommended after exercise since the hepatobiliary clearance of the radionuclide results in increasing accumulation in the bowel over time and bowel loops can be situated close enough to the heart to create problems in interpretation. A major advantage of sestamibi is the higher photon energy of technetium (twice that of thallium), which yields images with much better spatial resolution. As will be discussed later, use of a technetium agent allows coupling of ventricular function imaging to the perfusion imaging. The other clinically available technetium agent is technetium-99m teboroxime. Its pharmacokinetics differ from both thallium and sestamibi. It is more rapidly extracted by the myocardium than is sestamibi, but it is also much more rapidly cleared. In fact, its clearance is measured in minutes. Imaging must start immediately after injection and must be completed in a few minutes.[10] The major advantage to its use is the fact that rest and exercise imaging can be completed in a very short time.

There are other radionuclides that can be used to image myocardial blood flow such as the positron agents N-13 ammonia and O-15 water. Those radionuclides are accelerator produced, have short half-lives, and must be imaged with a positron emission tomograph (PET) scanner. Rubidium-82 is a positron agent with a longer half-life and which can be produced with an on-site generator. None of the positron emitters has achieved any significant application in exercise imaging although use with pharmacological testing has been reported.[11]

A. PLANAR VS. TOMOGRAPHIC IMAGING

Myocardial perfusion imaging can be performed using either planar or tomographic methods. Historically, planar imaging was the first method available, but over the past several years the trend has been to a steady transition to tomographic imaging. As the name implies, the planar method involves imaging the heart from various predefined angles or planes and reproducing those angles for the exercise and subsequent delayed or resting images. Traditionally, three views were obtained for every study, an anterior, a shallow left anterior oblique or "best septal" view, and a steep oblique or left lateral view (Figure 1). Those three views typically revealed enough of the left ventricle to be able to interrogate all three major coronary vascular distributions. Planar imaging is two dimensional and, as such, is not ideally suited to representing a complex three-dimensional object with activity surrounding it, hence, the appeal of tomographic imaging or single photon emission computed tomography (SPECT). During tomographic imaging, a large number of static images, usually 30 to 60, are acquired by a gamma camera that rotates around the subject or rotating the subject in front of the gamma camera. The set of images is then subjected to filtered back-projection to arrive at the three-dimensional object of interest. Once the object of interest is reconstructed from its individual projections, it can then be "sliced" and displayed from any angle (Figure 2). SPECT imaging offers the ability to examine the ventricle throughout its depth and relatively free of surrounding activity.

Both planar and tomographic techniques lend themselves to quantitative analysis, and it has been shown that quantitation improves interpretive accuracy for both methods.[12-15] Typically, quantitative data are generated for each view of a planar study or for each slice of a tomographic study and the data are then compared with normal reference files. A variety of formats can then be used to display the severity and extent of image abnormalities (Figure 3). Quantitative analysis cannot replace visual interpretation

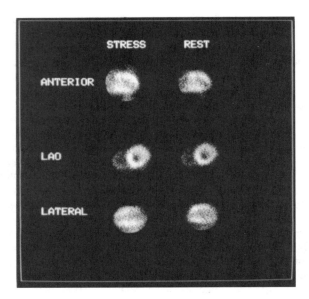

Figure 1   Planar perfusion imaging is typically performed in three or four views, here displayed as anterior, left anterior oblique (LAO) or best septal, and lateral views. The resting images must be acquired using the same patient positioning and camera angles as those of the stress study in order to be able to directly compare the two sets of images.

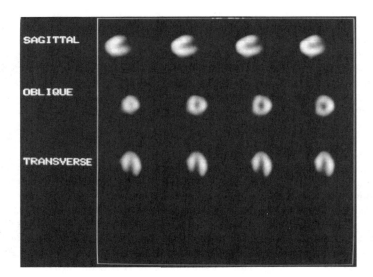

Figure 2   With a tomographic approach, the heart is reconstructed in three dimensions which allows display of the ventricle in any projection and visualization of multiple "slices" in each projection. One is able to interrogate the entire chamber from septal side to free wall (top row, left to right), apex to base (middle row, left to right), and inferior to anterior (bottom row, left to right).

of images but, in effect, adds another "expert" opinion to which the interpreting physician can look for assistance. It is particularly useful as a research tool.

B. SENSITIVITY AND SPECIFICITY: COMPARISON WITH ELECTROCARDIOGRAPHY

In every study published on the subject, the addition of myocardial perfusion imaging to a diagnostic exercise rest significantly increased the sensitivity for the detection of coronary artery disease compared with exercise electrocardiography (ECG).[16] It should be noted that the sensitivity and specificity of the

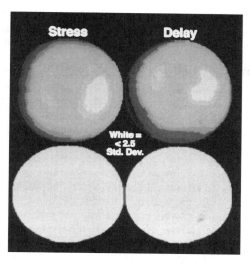

Figure 3 For quantitative analysis and comparison with normal reference standards, the tomographic images may be displayed in a bull's-eye format (upper images). The bull's-eye, itself, is a display of the peak count at 6° intervals around each short axis slice (middle row, Figure 2) with the apical data in the center of the bull's-eye and the data from the base of the chamber at the perimeter of the image. This two-dimensional polar map display conveniently shows the entire three-dimensional peak count data for the ventricle. The lateral wall (right side of bull's-eye) tends to be hotter (white pixels) than the septum (left), anterior wall (top), or inferior wall (bottom). If a normal reference data base is available, the composite bull's-eye of the normals may be compared with the bull's-eye of any individual to detect and quantify any pixels whose values exceed the normal limits by any desired number of standard deviations, in this case 2.5. All pixels that do not exceed the normal limits are coded white.

exercise ECG will depend upon the inclusion or exclusion of subjects with baseline abnormalities of the ECG, such as left ventricular hypertrophy, conduction abnormalities, and so-called nonspecific ST segment abnormalities. A distinct advantage of exercise myocardial perfusion imaging is the fact that, aside from left bundle branch block, resting abnormalities of the ECG do not affect the accuracy of the method. Left bundle branch block completely precludes exercise ECG analysis and can cause both reversible and fixed abnormalities on exercise myocardial perfusion scans in the anteroseptal and septal walls of the left ventricle in the absence of coronary artery disease.[17,18] Perfusion imaging after administration of a coronary vasodilator appears to have better specificity in the presence of left bundle branch block.[19] Myocardial perfusion imaging is subject to artifacts induced by tissue attenuation which can be particularly troublesome in very large individuals or in large-breasted women. The exercise ECG is largely immune to such difficulties.

C. SENSITIVITY AND SPECIFICITY: COMPARISON OF AVAILABLE RADIONUCLIDES

As indicated above there are three single-photon radionuclides currently approved for myocardial perfusion imaging, thallium-201, technetium-99m sestamibi, and technetium-99m teboroxime. The sensitivity and specificity of thallium-201 has been compared with that of technetium-99m sestamibi in multicenter trials using both planar and SPECT imaging. For the diagnosis of coronary artery disease, there were no significant differences between the sensitivity or specificity of the two agents. Sestamibi was noted to be more sensitive for detection of disease in individual coronary arteries.[20] Imaging with technetium-99m teboroxime has also been compared with imaging with thallium-201, and again the sensitivities and specificities for the diagnosis of coronary artery disease were found to be similar.[21] More ischemic segments were, however, detected with the teboroxime than with thallium. In one study, planar thallium, sestamibi, and teboroxime imaging were all performed in the same patients. In general, there was good agreement among the three agents with a slightly but not significantly better correlation between thallium and sestamibi.[22] It should be noted that teboroxime, because of an extremely rapid myocardial clearance, has largely been used with planar imaging. SPECT imaging with teboroxime can be performed using a very rapid acquisition protocol and a multiheaded detector, but image quality is frequently suboptimal.

D. PHARMACOLOGICAL ASSESSMENT OF CORONARY FLOW RESERVE

There are many patients who are unable to exercise at all or who are unable to achieve an adequate heart rate because of coexisting medical illness, physical constraints, or medications or in whom exercise carries too great a risk. Fortunately, there are pharmacological methods for challenging the coronary circulation. The most widely used are the coronary vasodilators, dipyridamole[23] and adenosine.[24] Dobutamine is also being used, but its sensitivity has not, as yet, been as rigorously studied as that of the vasodilators.[25] Dipyridamole and adenosine are potent coronary vasodilators. They act directly on the arterioles to decrease coronary vascular resistance, thereby increasing flow.

When adenosine is given as a continuous intravenous infusion of 0.14 mg/kg/min for 4 to 6 min, coronary blood flow increases three- to fivefold over resting flow. It has a very short half-life, measured in seconds, so any unwanted or untoward side effects disappear rapidly after reducing or discontinuing the infusion. One particularly important side effect is the appearance of varying degrees of heart block due to its depressant effect on AV conduction. It must, therefore, be administered with very careful ECG monitoring. Dipyridamole is typically given as an intravenous infusion of 0.15 mg/kg/min for 4 min. It acts by inhibition of the metabolism of endogenous adenosine and has a much longer half-life than intravenous adenosine itself. Coronary flow may remain elevated for more than an hour. Both agents cause systemic vasodilation as well, and blood pressure typically drops modestly while the heart rate increases by 10 to 20 beats/min on average. Myocardial oxygen demand is minimally, if at all, increased since the double product usually increases only slightly. As such, it is important to recognize that administration of these agents is not a surrogate stress test. The often used terms *dipyridamole* and *adenosine stress testing* are misnomers to be avoided. Common side effects of both agents include headache, nausea, flushing, and dizziness, as well as nonanginal chest discomfort. They are rarely severe and always reversible by either discontinuing the infusion in the case of adenosine or by administration of the adenosine receptor antagonist, aminophylline, in the case of dipyridamole. Unlike adenosine, dipyridamole does not cause heart block. Either agent can be coupled with imaging by injection of a myocardial perfusion imaging agent. Ample data exist to substantiate the diagnostic accuracy of myocardial perfusion imaging with either dipyridamole or adenosine.[26,27] The sensitivity and specificity appear to be comparable with exercise testing.

There is one group of patients that cannot be studied with dipyridamole or adenosine, and that is the group with reactive airways disease. Both agents can cause severe bronchospasm in susceptible individuals. The drugs are absolutely contraindicated in patients with a history of asthma. For those patients, intravenous infusion of dobutamine has been safely used for perfusion imaging. The drug is started at 5 μm/kg/min and increased gradually up to a peak dose of 50 μg/kg/min or until side effects preclude additional increments. In contrast to the coronary vasodilators, dobutamine infusion is a form of stress test since its effect on coronary flow is related to a substantial increase in myocardial oxygen demand by virtue of the increases in heart rate and contractility. Blood pressure may also increase, but not to the levels typically achieved during exercise.[28]

IV. VENTRICULAR FUNCTION IMAGING

By temporarily labeling the circulating blood pool with a radionuclide, it is possible to image the changes in size and shape of the ventricular chambers during the cardiac cycle. There are two approaches to so-called blood pool imaging, the first-pass[29] and the gated equilibrium methods.[30] In the first-pass technique, a bolus of a radionuclide, typically technetium-99m in one form or another, is rapidly injected into a peripheral vein and a gamma camera records the passage of the radionuclide through the chambers of the central circulation. Once the bolus clears the left ventricle on its first pass through the heart, the acquisition is over. Only the relatively few beats that occurred during the initial transit of the radionuclide through the heart can be used for image analysis. In the gated equilibrium technique, a stable red blood cell tag is created such that the entire blood pool is simultaneously visualized. Separation of the cardiac chambers relies on the imaging angles. In contrast, in the first-pass technique, there is a temporal separation of chambers as the radionuclide bolus makes its way from one cardiac chamber to the next. Both techniques lend themselves to quantitation since the concentration of the radionuclide in any chamber is directly proportional to the volume of the chamber. Changes in recorded radioactive counts within a chamber can be used as a surrogate for changes in volume. Consequently, ejection fraction and chamber volumes can be measured with count-based techniques that are largely free of geometric assumptions about ventricular shape. The ejection fraction of either ventricle is calculated as ED-ES* counts/ED counts with a correction for background activity.[29] Several methods for volume calculation are available, some requiring reference blood sampling and others that do not require blood sampling.[31] In addition to the volume and ejection fraction measurements, the images can be displayed in a cinematic format such that regional wall motion can also be evaluated. With either radionuclide technique, the measurements of ejection fraction and chamber volumes have been shown to closely correlate with those made by contrast ventriculography. In fact, the radionuclide approaches may actually be more accurate since they are free of the geometric assumptions about ventricular shape inherent in the contrast angiographic approach to such measurements. Several other quantitative variables can be calculated from radionuclide ventriculograms, such as ejection rates[32] and the many parameters used to describe diastolic function: rapid filling rate, time to peak filling rate, atrial filling rate, and filling fractions.[33,34] Diastolic function has received increasing clinical attention recently, but radionuclide descriptors of diastolic function are only accurate at relatively low heart rates, that is, less than 100 beats/min. Consequently, there is very little literature on diastolic function during exercise.

A. FIRST-PASS IMAGING

For first-pass imaging of ventricular function, it is necessary to use a gamma camera with high count rate capability since only a few cardiac cycles are available for data analysis. The primary advantage of the first-pass technique for the evaluation of ventricular function during exercise is its short acquisition time. As indicated above, the study takes as long as the transit time of the radionuclide bolus through the central circulation, which at peak exercise may be less than 10 s. Such a short acquisition time is ideally suited to the evaluation of peak exercise in a patient population whose exercise tolerance is often quite limited because of age, deconditioning, or ischemia. The major disadvantage of the technique is that each measurement of ventricular function requires a separate injection of the radionuclide, and therefore the number of measurements during an exercise session is limited to at most three, including a resting study. Study quality is very dependent upon the integrity of the injected bolus, and therefore the site and method of injection are important variables that do not have to be considered in other types of imaging. Large bore veins as close to the central veins as possible are the routes of choice, and either the medial antecubital or the external jugular vein is the most commonly used injection site. One advantage of the technique is that it can theoretically be performed in many views. Practically, the most commonly used views are the straight anterior (Figure 4) and the shallow right anterior oblique views. Since there are just a few beats available during injection at peak exercise, it is important to keep the subject's chest as immobilized as possible during the 10 to 20 s of acquisition. Because of the potential confounding influence of chest motion on the quality of the first-pass study, it has traditionally been performed during upright bicycle exercise where the chest, especially in the anterior view, can be easily stabilized against the gamma camera during exercise. More recently, a technique for tracking chest wall motion and then correcting the image data for such motion has allowed application of first-pass imaging to treadmill exercise.[35] Preliminary results suggest that by using a motion correction scheme, exercise ejection fraction and wall motion can be accurately assessed at peak exercise on a treadmill.

B. GATED BLOOD POOL IMAGING

Gated equilibrium blood pool imaging is known by several other names including the most often used name, MUGA, which was an abbreviation for multigated acquisition. It is also frequently called radionuclide ventriculography (RNV). As indicated above, it differs from the first-pass technique by virtue of the fact that the entire blood pool is simultaneously labeled by creating a stable red blood cell tag, a process that takes about 20 to 30 min. The count flux in such a study is considerably lower than that seen in first-pass imaging, and the study can be performed with most conventional gamma cameras. Because of the low count rate, information form hundreds of cardiac cycles must be stored for adequate image construction and quantitation. By using an ECG signal as trigger or "gate," the data from all cardiac cycles are stored as a single representative beat. Alternatively, one can acquire equilibrium data in a "list mode" fashion, where scintigraphic events, time markers, and the ECG signal are recorded continuously. Following acquisition, the data are reformatted into a single cardiac cycle using any number of cycles and cycle lengths desired. Since the blood pool tag is stable for hours, the gated blood pool

---

* ED = End-diastolic; ES = End-systolic

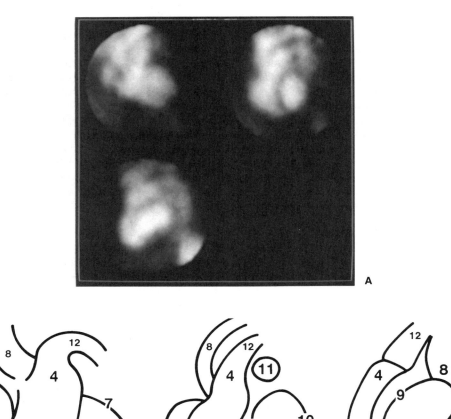

Figure 4   A, The typical resting gated equilibrium radionuclide angiogram (MUGA) is acquired in three views, anterior (top left), a left anterior oblique view that best separates the right and left ventricles (top right), and a steep left anterior oblique or lateral view (bottom). B, The relevant chambers in the gated equilibrium study are shown diagrammatically for the anterior (left), best septal (middle), and lateral (right) views. 1 = Right atrium; 2 = RV inflow; 3 = RV apex; 4 = RV outflow tract; 5 = inferior wall of LV; 6 = apex of LV; 7 = anterior wall of LV; 8 = ascending aorta; 9 = septal wall of LV; 10 = posterior wall of LV; 11 = left atrium; 12 = pulmonary artery.

technique has the distinct advantage of allowing multiple acquisitions over time including the imaging of as many stages of a graded exercise test as desired. The major disadvantages of the technique are the length of time necessary for acquiring an adequate image, 2 min at a minimum, and the need to perform imaging in a view that separates the ventricular chambers, typically a 30 to 60° left anterior oblique projection (Figure 5). In addition, because of the need to electrocardiographically gate the acquisition, variability of the heart rate is problematic. As a result, 3-min exercise stages are recommended in order to provide 1 min for the heart rate to stabilize and 2 min for acquisition. Because of the requisite imaging angle and the time necessary for acquisition, gated equilibrium blood pool imaging cannot be performed during treadmill exercise.

C. VENTRICULAR FUNCTION DURING EXERCISE

Radionuclide ventriculography has given us information about the response of the ventricle that was not available with any other technique. An extensive literature has evolved which describes the changes in left ventricular and right ventricular ejection fractions, as well as end-diastolic and end-systolic volumes during and following graded exercise. Changes in ventricular function have been studied during aerobic[36]

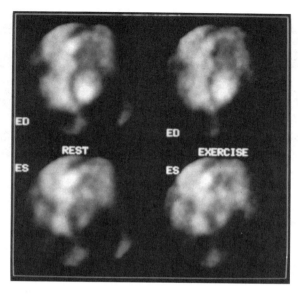

Figure 5 Gated equilibrium imaging may be performed during exercise. The left anterior oblique view must be acquired during exercise so that the LVEF may be calculated. The end-diastolic images (top) and end-systolic images (bottom) at rest and at peak exercise are shown in this figure for a normal subject.

and isometric exercise,[37] during sudden strenuous exercise,[38] and immediately after exercise,[39,40] as well as during supine[41] and upright exercise.[42-44]

During upright exercise in normal volunteers, one can expect to see a decrease in end-systolic volume and either a mild increase or no change in end-diastolic volume. Consequently, left ventricular ejection fraction typically increases. That idealized response may vary with age or gender. Women appear to rely more heavily on an increase in end-diastolic volume with a smaller change in ejection fraction, while men tend to rely more on a decrease in end-systolic volume and an increase in ejection fraction.[45] Older volunteers show a less predictable rise in ejection fraction during exercise than do younger subjects, and, not infrequently, ejection fraction may actually fall with exercise.[44] The type of exercise protocol also influences the ejection fraction response[38] and, in particular, pure isometric exercise such as handgrip may cause a drop in ejection fraction.[37]

When exercise is stopped, rapid changes in ventricular volume and ejection fraction occur. After cessation of upright exercise, end-diastolic volume decreases and ejection fraction increases. That is true in normal individuals as well as in patients with exercise-induced ischemia. By simply lowering the work load as exercise is continued, ejection fraction increases and ischemic wall motion abnormalities improve,[40] which suggests that, for diagnostic and especially for prognostic information, imaging should be performed during peak exercise, not after exercise, and work loads should not be reduced in an effort to prolong the exercise for the sake of the imaging.

The typical response of the left ventricle to exercise in patients with ischemic heart disease includes a regional wall motion abnormality, an increase in end-systolic volume, a variable increase in end-diastolic volume, a decrease in left ventricular ejection fraction, and a subnormal increase or no change in stroke volume. Cardiac output invariably increases as a result of the increased heart rate (Figure 6). The magnitude of those changes will vary with the severity of the ischemia and the extent of coronary disease.[46]

V. CLINICAL APPLICATIONS OF RADIONUCLIDE EXERCISE TESTING

A. SCREENING FOR CORONARY ARTERY DISEASE

When a diagnostic test is applied to screening for a disease, its value depends not only upon the sensitivity and specificity of the test, but also upon the prevalence of the disease in the population to be screened. For example, exercise myocardial perfusion imaging can be performed with a sensitivity of 90% and specificity of 90% for the detection of ≥70% diameter occlusions of a coronary artery. If such a test were applied to an average asymptomatic, adult population in whom the prevalence of significant

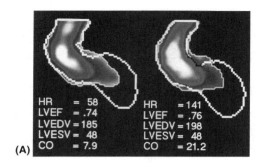
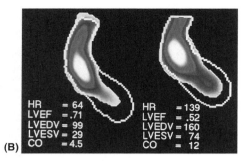

Figure 6 The first-pass radionuclide angiogram allows display of one ventricle at a time, in this case the left ventricle along with the ascending aorta. The end-diastolic perimeter and the end-systolic volume are displayed at rest and during exercise in a normal subject (A) and in a subject with coronary artery disease (B). Note the much larger increase in end-diastolic volume (EDV), the increase in end-systolic volume (ESV), the drop in ejection fraction (LVEF), and the smaller increase in cardiac output (CO) in the subject with the ischemic response.

coronary disease is approximately 5%, then the number of false positive results would exceed the number of true positives by over a 2:1 margin. If, on the other hand, the test were applied to a population of middle-aged male smokers with hypertension, diabetes, and hyperlipidemia where the prevalence of coronary disease was 25%, then the number of true positives would exceed the number of false positives by a similar margin.

The ultimate value of a screening test also depends upon the risk of an adverse outcome in the group with the disease, the adverse outcomes of all the testing and treatment applied to the group with the disease, and the long-term benefit of the treatment when successfully applied. In general, radionuclide exercise testing has too low a specificity to be applied in a cost-effective, safe manner to the screening of populations with a low prevalence of disease and could only be justified for populations with very high pretest likelihoods of coronary artery disease.

B. DIAGNOSIS OF CORONARY ARTERY DISEASE

Radionuclide exercise testing is most frequently applied to the diagnosis of coronary artery disease in symptomatic individuals. As indicated above, radionuclide imaging increases the sensitivity of stress testing for the detection of coronary disease. However, the exercise ECG may still be the test of choice for subjects at the low and high extremes of probability of disease. Someone with a very high pretest likelihood of coronary artery disease (for example, a hypertensive, hyperlipidemic, middle-aged male with typical angina pectoris) needs a cost-effective confirmatory diagnostic test. That individual's posttest likelihood of coronary disease will not change substantially by either a negative or a positive exercise test; therefore, it is not a cost-effective strategy to perform a much more expensive study simply for the sake of diagnosis. Similarly, an individual with a very low pretest likelihood of coronary artery disease (for example, a young woman with no risk factors but with atypical chest pain) will not have a much higher posttest likelihood of the disease even if the test is positive. In that case, the false positives outnumber the true positives and so the strategy cannot be cost effective. Ideally, then, exercise radionuclide imaging should be applied to the diagnosis of coronary artery disease in individuals with an intermediate pretest likelihood of the disease. It should also be used for individuals at the extremes of probability when the exercise ECG gives unexpected results, i.e., the low probability subject with a positive exercise ECG and the high probability subject with a negative exercise ECG. Obviously, the latter two strategies result in two exercise tests for many people, but for the majority the single, less expensive test would suffice.

Of the two types of exercise radionuclide imaging, perfusion and function imaging, which is best suited for the diagnosis of coronary disease? That is a controversial issue and depends on the criteria being used to consider a test positive. For the perfusion scan, all investigators agree that the finding of a reversible perfusion defect during exercise or pharmacological manipulation is the *sine qua non* for the diagnosis of coronary disease. The sensitivity and specificity of that finding are approximately 87% and 87%, respectively.[17] For ventricular function imaging, some authors have used a failure to increase the ejection fraction by at least 0.05 as a criterion for stress-induced ischemia,[47] while others have used a new or worsened regional wall motion abnormality during exercise as the criterion for ischemia.[48] Ejection fraction criteria have higher sensitivity but lower specificity, while regional wall motion criteria have lower sensitivity and higher specificity. There are many possible explanations for a decrease or a failure to increase the ejection fraction during exercise other than coronary artery disease, whereas there are few causes of a regional perfusion abnormality or wall motion abnormality other than coronary artery disease. In direct comparisons between perfusion and function imaging, perfusion imaging usually is more sensitive for detecting coronary disease.[49] That should not be surprising since the first event in the so-called ischemic cascade is a reduction in regional blood flow which is directly imaged on a perfusion scan. The ventricular function scan images the mechanical consequences of the reduction in blood flow and may fail to detect mild functional abnormalities when the surrounding myocardium is contracting vigorously. Furthermore, exercise ventricular function imaging is typically performed in one view only which limits the amount of the ventricle in direct view. A logical approach to the application of radionuclide testing would be to use exercise perfusion imaging as the primary diagnostic test. If the exercise ECG and perfusion scan are equivocal or contradictory, then an exercise function study can be of particular benefit. In some situations exercise function imaging may be more sensitive than perfusion imaging. For example, patients with multivessel coronary disease in whom there are comparable flow reductions throughout the entire myocardium can have a perfusion scan with homogeneous tracer uptake. There is no way to know that the uptake, although homogeneous, is reduced. However, a ventricular function study in such a situation would be very abnormal since there is global ischemia. Similarly, there are cases in which function imaging will have better specificity. Subjects likely to have perfusion scan artifacts, such as obese individuals or large-breasted women, may be more appropriately studied with ventricular function imaging.

C. COMBINED FUNCTION–PERFUSION IMAGING

The availability of technetium-based myocardial perfusion agents makes it possible to perform both ventricular function and myocardial perfusion imaging with a single injection. At peak exercise, a first-pass study can be acquired, and some minutes later, the perfusion scan is acquired. No other imaging modality can, as yet, deliver such a comprehensive simultaneous assessment of ventricular function and myocardial perfusion. Clinical experience with combined function–perfusion imaging is limited at the present time. There are no published trials to indicate how and when the combination of the two types of data is potentially helpful, but preliminary experience suggests that while the diagnostic power of the perfusion study exceeds that of the simultaneously acquired function study, the function data do have independent diagnostic power and the combination of the two provides maximum diagnostic power.[49,50] The function data may be particularly helpful in clarifying equivocal perfusion scans and frequently eliminates the need for another diagnostic test. Addition of first-pass data to the perfusion data may detect noncoronary causes of symptoms, such as diastolic dysfunction or valvular insufficiency, conditions that are not detectable on perfusion imaging alone. Perhaps most important will be the added prognostic information from the exercise ventricular function study as discussed below.

In addition to the ability to perform first-pass ventricular function studies, the technetium perfusion agents also permit high-resolution gated perfusion imaging. In such a study, the perfusion data, which are normally collected without any ECG signal, are acquired using an ECG gate. That allows creation of the perfusion images at different times during the cardiac cycle. By viewing the end-diastolic to end-systolic perfusion images in a cinematic display, one can visualize wall motion and wall thickening, quite analogous to two-dimensional echocardiography. In a recent comparison, wall motion and wall thickening were evaluated using both gated tomographic perfusion imaging and echocardiography.[51] However, it should be emphasized that the wall motion and thickening images represent resting ventricular function at the time of imaging, which is typically 15 min to 1 h after exercise. Gated perfusion scans do not provide information about ventricular function during exercise as does the first-pass study.

D. PROGNOSIS IN STABLE CORONARY ARTERY DISEASE

Both myocardial perfusion imaging and ventricular function imaging play important prognostic roles in patients with coronary artery disease. The significance of resting ventricular function in the prognosis of patients with stable coronary disease was recognized over 20 years ago using data from contrast ventriculography.[52] Subsequently, similar results were obtained using the noninvasively obtained radionuclide left ventricular ejection fractions both at rest and during exercise. Radionuclide ventriculography remains the only practical method to measure the exercise ejection fraction. In the largest trial ever published on the subject, a multivariate analysis showed that the exercise left ventricular ejection fraction was the most powerful noninvasive variable for predicting subsequent mortality in patients treated medically.[53] Data from perfusion imaging were not, however, included in that analysis. In other studies, the change in ejection fraction from rest to exercise was as important or more so than the absolute exercise or resting ejection fraction.[54] It appears that when the population being studied has normal or only mildly reduced ejection fractions at rest, then the change in ejection fraction during exercise is prognostically significant, but when the population has a broad range of resting ejection fractions, then the absolute exercise ejection fraction may be the most important prognostic variable.

There are also several prognostic indexes available from myocardial perfusion images. Both the extent and the severity of perfusion abnormalities appear to have prognostic power which appear to be additive.[55] Dilatation of the left ventricle on an exercise perfusion study carries an increased risk of a subsequent adverse outcome.[56] Perhaps most significant prognostically is the finding of increased uptake of thallium in the lungs during exercise or pharmacological testing.[57] Unfortunately, to date, no large scale trials are available that compare the prognostic information contained in perfusion images with that available from ventricular function imaging.

E. PROGNOSIS FOLLOWING MYOCARDIAL INFARCTION

Many studies in the prethrombolytic era have addressed the issue of post-myocardial infarction (post-MI) risk stratification. Significant univariate predictive power has been demonstrated for clinical variables such as early congestive heart failure,[58] post-MI angina, high-grade or frequent ventricular ectopy at rest,[59] and coexisting right ventricular infarction.[60] For patients without any manifest predictors of an adverse post-MI course, exercise testing has been widely applied for risk stratification. Exercise test variables associated with a recurrent infarction or death post-MI include exercise-induced angina and ST segment depression. In a fairly large consecutive series of patients studied in the prethrombolytic, preangioplasty era, exercise ECG, cardiac catheterization, and exercise thallium imaging variables were all compared for their relative prognostic power. The data that best discriminated between patients at high and low risk for subsequent adverse outcomes were the exercise/redistribution thallium results.[61] Other investigators have shown that the exercise left ventricular ejection fraction was also predictive of subsequent outcome.[62]

At this point in time, the prognostic value of routine post-MI stress testing is not as clear as it appeared to be 10 years ago. With the widespread application of thrombolytic therapy and early angioplasty in acute MI, the coronary anatomy and ventricular function of the predischarge, post-MI patient is changing. However, radionuclide exercise or pharmacological testing may be of particular value in the early postthrombolytic patient for deciding whether or not early catheterization and angioplasty are necessary. The radionuclide study adds critical information about the location, extent, and severity of any ischemia and helps in the evaluation of myocardial viability. The assessment of myocardial viability becomes especially relevant in that clinical situation (see below).

F. DETECTION OF RESTENOSIS FOLLOWING PERCUTANEOUS TRANSLUMINAC CORONARY ANGIOPLASTY (PTCA)

The application of radionuclide exercise testing following coronary angioplasty remains controversial. For patients who become symptomatic following PTCA, radionuclide exercise testing, in particular, myocardial perfusion imaging may be especially useful in confirming recurrent ischemia and in localizing the ischemia to either the vessel previously dilated or to myocardium remote from the previous PTCA site. However, for asymptomatic patients post-PTCA, radionuclide exercise testing may be abnormal even though the dilated vessel has not restenosed. We have noted a 25% prevalence of abnormal exercise thallium scans obtained within 1 week of successful PTCA, and others have shown that this phenomenon can extend out to 6 months post-PTCA.

If radionuclide exercise testing is to be used in asymptomatic patients post-PTCA, it should probably be delayed for at least 3 and possibly 6 months after the procedure. The test of choice is most likely an exercise SPECT myocardial perfusion scan, since it is more sensitive than exercise radionuclide ventriculography[48,49] and better at localizing ischemia to individual vessels.

G. NONCORONARY HEART DISEASE

Radionuclide exercise testing plays a small, if any, role in the assessment of patients with noncoronary heart disease. The radionuclide evaluation of right and left ventricular function at rest is of major clinical

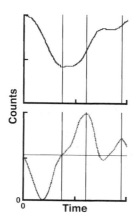
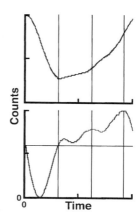

Figure 7 A normal left ventricular volume curve (upper left) and its first derivative (lower left) are compared with those of a subject with abnormal left ventricular diastolic function (right). The vertical lines indicate end-systole, the peak of rapid filling, and the peak rate of atrial filling. Notice the markedly delayed and decreased early diastolic filling in the abnormal case and the concomitant increase in the relative contribution of the atrium to ventricular filling.

significance in the management of patients with valvular disease, congenital heart disease, and the various cardiomyopathies. However, similar measurements during exercise have little diagnostic or known prognostic value. One exception is the use of combined radionuclide and gas exchange measurements to distinguish cardiac from pulmonary causes of dyspnea on exertion or effort intolerance.

H. LEFT VENTRICULAR DIASTOLIC FUNCTION

Although radionuclide testing is most frequently thought of as a method to evaluate myocardial perfusion or systolic ventricular function, radionuclide ventriculography can be used to qualitatively and quantitatively evaluate diastolic function of the left ventricle. In fact, this application is clinically quite important in evaluating patients with unexplained heart failure or dyspnea on exertion.[63] Typically, diastolic dysfunction is detected on resting studies. The most common presentations include a delayed and decreased rapid filling phase, an exaggerated atrial contribution to filling, and occasionally a prolongation of the isovolumic relaxation period. Such findings may also be present during exercise (Figure 7). All of those parameters can be measured using the radionuclide ventriculogram.[33] Subjects with normal diastolic function at rest may have diastolic dysfunction during exercise-induced ischemia, but it is more difficult to quantify since the normal pattern of diastolic filling at high heart rates cannot be adequately assessed with the typical sampling time of radionuclide studies.

VI. ASSESSMENT OF EXERCISE TRAINING

Radionuclide imaging may be of value in assessing the effects of training on myocardial perfusion and ventricular function. There is some animal data to suggest that exercise may stimulate the development of coronary collateral circulation.[64] Todd et al.[65] studied a group of 40 patients with chronic stable angina that was radomized to either an exercise program or to a sedentary life-style for 1 year.[65] Using planar thallium imaging, the group that exercised was shown to have a 35% reduction in the level of ischemia after 1 year. In a similar study that added dietary modification to the exercise training, myocardial perfusion improved at 1 year in the treatment group.[66] The perfusion scans improved in subjects who had both exercised for more than 3 h/week and followed a low-fat diet. Regression of coronary artery disease was noted in 7 of 18 subjects while no change occurred in the remaining 11 subjects in the treatment group. Except for one individual, control subjects who received "usual care" were noted to have progression of their coronary disease.

The effects of vigorous exercise training on left ventricular function have been evaluated in a group of competitive swimmers. Rest and exercise radionuclide angiography was performed before and after 6 months of intensive physical training.[67] The results showed that there was no change in peak exercise left ventricular ejection fraction but end-diastolic volume did increase which resulted in a higher peak cardiac output.

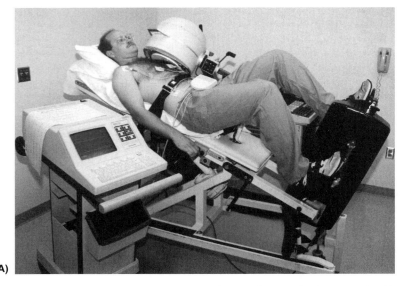

(A)

Figure 8   Several models of ergometer tables are available that allow semisupine or supine bicycle ergometry (A). The tables are narrow enough to allow close approximation of the gamma camera to the chest. Some tables may be placed in the fully upright position (B) although some gamma camera configurations will not allow the detector to reach the necessary height to perform this type of stress imaging.

VII. ORGANIZATION OF THE NUCLEAR CARDIOLOGY LABORATORY

Historically, nuclear imaging and diagnostic stress testing were the provinces of different laboratories, in fact, different clinical departments. That precedent has deep roots and remains a controversial issue to this day. There is certainly no good reason to keep the functions apart if there are personnel on site who are trained in both exercise testing and imaging.

A. EXERCISE VENTRICULAR FUNCTION IMAGING

Exercise testing has usually been performed in an imaging laboratory when a stress ventricular function study is performed, since the stress test must be performed in front of the gamma camera. Occasionally, a portable gamma camera may be brought to the stress laboratory to accomplish the same task. Various pieces of exercise equipment have been used during exercise ventricular function imaging. For gated equilibrium imaging during exercise, tables with attached exercise ergometers have been popular because it is easy to stabilize the patients chest during image acquisition. The simplest of those tables allows supine and semisupine bicycle ergometer exercise and is narrow enough to facilitate close approximation of the gamma camera to the patient's chest (Figure 8A). More-sophisticated tables can be elevated to put the patient in an upright position, which is a much better tolerated exercise position for the typical clinical subject (Figure 8B). However, most gamma cameras cannot reach high enough to image a patient when the imaging table is elevated to 90° because at that angle the length of the table and the necessary clearance for the ergometer bring the patient's chest more than 6 ft above the floor. If the exercise table is abandoned and a simple upright bicycle ergometer is used, imaging is much more easily accomplished, but it is more difficult to stabilize the chest for the relatively long time necessary for gated equilibrium acquisition. First-pass imaging is easily performed during exercise without the need for exercise tables since the chest can be satisfactorily stabilized against the gamma camera detector for the brief acquisition period (Figure 9).

B. EXERCISE MYOCARDIAL PERFUSION IMAGING

In the case of exercise myocardial perfusion imaging, it is typical to have the exercise test performed in a standard cardiac stress laboratory and then have the subject moved to a nuclear medicine laboratory which may be quite remote from the stress laboratory. With thallium imaging, there is a premium on the time from injection to the time of imaging since peak myocardial thallium concentration occurs about 10 min following injection during exercise, after which it begins washing out of the heart.

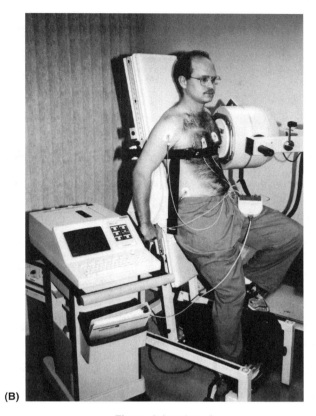

(B)

Figure 8 (continued)

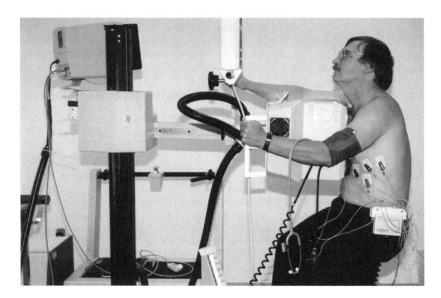

Figure 9 Gamma cameras designed specifically for first-pass radionuclide imaging have been configured for bicycle exercise. In the example shown, the detector is small enough to be easily stabilized against the chest during the imaging which only lasts for 15 to 30 s.

Therefore, patients have to be promptly dispatched to the imaging laboratory which occasionally prematurely terminates the recovery phase of the stress test. That problem has been overcome with the newer agent technetium sestamibi since imaging can be delayed for a long time after injection. In contrast, the problem has been seriously aggravated by the use of technetium teboroxime because the ultrafast myocardial washout of that agent forces the exercise and imaging equipment to be virtually right next to each other.

In the traditional two laboratory setup, a nuclear medicine technologist has to be present in the stress laboratory in order to inject the radionuclide, which removes that technologist from performing any other specialized tasks related to imaging other patients. Because of the somewhat unnatural and time-wasting shuffling of personnel and patients between stress and imaging laboratories, many high-volume laboratories have merged the two functions such that stress testing, pharmacological testing, and all imaging are performed in a single facility, the nuclear cardiology laboratory. The personnel in such a laboratory may still have specialized tasks such as radionuclide injection and gamma camera operations, but a considerable amount of cross training facilitates patient flow and prevents laboratory slowdowns. For example, nuclear technologists can be trained to place ECG monitoring equipment, record ECGs during testing, take and record blood pressures, and administer pharmacological agents such as dipyridamole, adenosine, and dobutamine. Similarly, traditional stress laboratory personnel can be trained to start intravenous lines and administer pharmacological agents, as well as assist nuclear technologists wherever possible. All personnel working in the laboratory should be BCLS and, if possible, ACLS trained. The single nuclear cardiology laboratory also benefits the entire staff since personnel are exposed to all aspects of the stress test, from obtaining a history to imaging the patient. All personnel thus become better educated and sophisticated in the care and testing of cardiac patients.

Combining the stress and imaging laboratories obviously increases the space requirements for the single facility compared with each separate laboratory. The imaging equipment tends to be bulky and requires more clearance than most stress laboratory equipment. For a single gamma camera, treadmill, bicycle ergometer, ECG recorder, computer, patient setup table, emergency equipment, and hot laboratory (for radionuclide preparation and storage), a minimum of 345 f^2 is necessary. For every additional gamma camera, an average of 112 f^2 is necessary as is an extra 82 f^2 for additional treadmills or bicycle ergometers.

VIII. SUMMARY

Radionuclide exercise testing provides qualitative and quantitative information about myocardial perfusion and ventricular function that cannot be generated with any other imaging modality. Widespread application of radionuclide imaging during exercise has expanded our knowledge of cardiac physiology and pathophysiology. The addition of radionuclide imaging to the exercise test has significantly improved diagnostic sensitivity and specificity for the detection of coronary artery disease. Although, historically, radionuclide exercise testing has been a combined effort of a stress laboratory team and a nuclear medicine group, the field is evolving toward a single nuclear cardiology laboratory that combines both the exercise and imaging capabilities.

REFERENCES

1. Klocke FJ. Measurements of coronary blood flow and degree of stenosis: current clinical implications and continuing uncertainties. *J. Am. Coll. Cardiol.* 1:31–41, 1983.
2. Nabel EG, Selwyn AP, Ganz P. Paradoxical narrowing of atherosclerotic coronary arteries induced by increases in heart rate. *Circulation* 81:850, 1990.
3. Nielsen AP, Morris KG, Murdock BS, Bruno EP, Cobb MD. Linear relationship between the distribution of thallium-201 and blood flow in ischemic and nonischemic myocardium during exercise. *Circulation* 61:797–801, 1980.
4. Weich HF, Strauss W, Pitt B. The extraction of thallium-201 by the myocardium. *Circulation* 56:188–191, 1977.
5. Beller GA, Watson DD, Pohost GM. Kinetics of thallium distribution and redistribution. Clinical applications in sequential myocardial imaging. In Strauss HW, Pitt B (eds): *Cardiovascular Nuclear Medicine,* 2nd ed. St. Louis, CV Mosby, 1979.
6. Wackers FJT. Myocardial perfusion imaging. In Gottschalk A, Hoffer PB, Potchen EJ (eds): *Diagnostic Nuclear Medicine,* 2nd ed. Baltimore, Williams and Wilkins, 1988, p. 291.
7. Kiat H, Berman DS, Maddahi J, et al. Late reversibility of tomographic myocardial thallium-201 defects: an accurate marker of myocardial viability. *J. Am. Coll. Cardiol.* 12:1456–63, 1988.

8. Dilsizian V, Rocco TP, Freedman NMT, et al. Enhanced detection of ischemic but viable myocardium by the reinjection of thallium after stress-redistribution imaging. *N. Engl. J. Med.* 323:141, 1990.
9. Rocco TP, Dilsizian V, McKusick KA, et al. Comparison of thallium redistribution with rest "reinjection" imaging for the detection of viable myocardium. *Am. J. Cardiol.* 66:158, 1990.
10. Seldin DW, Johnson LL, Blood D, et al. Myocardial perfusion imaging with technetium-99m SQ30217: comparison with thallium-201 and coronary anatomy. *J. Nucl. Med.* 30:312, 1989.
11. Go RT, Marwick TH, MacIntyre WJ, et al. A prospective comparison of rubidium-82 PET and thallium-201 SPECT myocardial perfusion imaging utilizing a single dipyridamole stress in the diagnosis of coronary artery disease. *J. Nucl. Med.* 31:1899, 1990.
12. Tamaki N, Yonejura Y, Mukai T, et al. Stress thallium-201 transaxial emission-computed tomography: quantitative versus qualitative analysis for evaluation of coronary artery disease. *J. Am. Coll. Cardiol.* 4:1213, 1984.
13. DePasquale EE, Nody AC, DePuey EG, et al. Quantitative rotational thallium-201 tomography for identifying and localizing coronary artery disease. *Circulation* 77:316, 1988.
14. Maddahi J, Van Train K, Prigent F, et al. Quantitative single photon emission-computed thallium-201 tomography for detection and localization of coronary artery disease: optimization and prospective validation of a new technique. *J. Am. Coll. Cardiol.* 14:1689, 1989.
15. Mahmarian JJ, Boyce TM, Goldberg RK, Cocanougher MK, et al. Quantitative exercise thallium-201 single photon emission computed tomography for the enhanced diagnosis of ischemic heart disease. *J. Am. Coll. Cardiol.* 15:318–329, 1990.
16. Gregoire J, Theroux P. Detection and assessment of unstable angina using myocardial perfusion imaging: comparison between technetium-99m Sesta-MIBI: SPECT and 12-lead electrocardiogram. *Am. J. Cardiol.* 66:42E, 1990.
17. DePuey EG, Guertler-Krawczynska E, Robbins WL. Thallium-201 SPECT in coronary artery disease patients with left bundle branch block. *J. Nucl. Med.* 29:1479, 1988.
18. Hirzel HO, Senn M, Neusch K, Buettner C, et al. Thallium-201 scintigraphy in complete left bundle branch block. *Am. J. Cardiol.* 53:764, 1984.
19. Burns RJ, Galligan L, Wright LM, Lawand S, et al. Improved specificity of myocardial thallium-201 single-photon emission computed tomography in patients with left bundle branch block by dipyridamole. *Am. J. Cardiol.* 68:504–508, 1991.
20. Kahn JK, McGhie I, Akers MS, Sills MN. Quantitative rotational tomography with 201-TI and 99-m-Tc 2-methoxy-isonitrile. *Circulation* 79:1282–1293, 1989.
21. Iskandrian AS, Heo J, Nguyen T, Beer S, et al. Tomographic myocardial perfusion imaging with technetium-99m teboroxime during adenosine-induced coronary hyperemia: correlation with thallium-201 imaging. *J. Am. Coll. Cardiol.* 19:307–312, 1992.
22. Taillefer R, Lambert R, Essiambre R, Phaneuf DC, et al. Comparison between thallium-201, technetium-99m-sestamibi and technetium-99m-teboroxime planar myocardial perfusion imaging in detection of coronary artery disease. *J. Nucl. Med.* 33:1091–1098, 1992.
23. Zhu YY, Chung WS, Botvinick EH, et al. Dipyridamole perfusion scintigraphy: the experience with its application in one hundred seventy patients with known or suspected unstable angina. *Am. Heart J.* 121:133, 1991.
24. Verani MS, Mahmarian JJ, Hixson JB, et al. Diagnosis of coronary artery disease by controlled coronary vasodilation with adenosine and thallium-201 scintigraphy in patients unable to exercise. *Circulation* 82:80–87, 1990.
25. Mason JR, Palac RT, Freeman ML, Virupannavar S. Thallium scintigraphy during dobutamine infusion: nonexercise-dependent screening test for coronary disease. *Am. Heart J.* 107:481, 1984.
26. Francisco DA, Collins SM, Go RT, Ehrhardt JC, et al. Tomographic thallium-201 myocardial perfusion scintigrams after maximal coronary artery vasodilation with intravenous dipyridamole. *Circulation* 66:370–379, 1982.
27. Nishimura S, Mahmarian JJ, Boyce TM, Verani MS. Equivalence between adenosine and exercise thallium-201 myocardial tomography: a multicenter, prospective, crossover trial. *J. Am. Coll. Cardiol.* 20:265–275, 1990.
28. Hays JT, Mahmarian JJ, Cochran AJ, et al. Dobutamine thallium-201 tomography for evaluating patients with suspected coronary artery disease unable to undergo exercise or vasodilatory pharmacologic testing. *J. Am. Coll. Cardiol.* 21:1583–1590, 1993.
29. Gal R, Grenier RP, Carpenter J, Schmidt DH, et al. High count rate first-pass radionuclide angiography using a digital gamma camera. *J. Nucl. Med.* 27:198–206, 1986.
30. Zaret BL, Strauss HW, Hurley PJ, Natarajan TK, et al. A noninvasive scintiphotographic method for detecting regional ventricular dysfunction in man. *N. Engl. J. Med.* 284:1165–1170, 1971.
31. Callahan RJ, Froelich JW, McKusick KA, et al. A modified method for the in vivo labeling of red blood cells with Tc-99m: concise communication. *J. Nucl. Med.* 23:315, 1982.
32. Bonow RO, Bacharach SL, Green MV, Kent KM, et al. Impaired left ventricular diastolic filling in patients with coronary artery disease: assessment with radionuclide angiography. *Circulation* 64:315–323, 1981.
33. Magorien DJ, Shaffer P, Bush C, Magorien RD, et al. Hemodynamic correlates for timing intervals, ejection rate and filling rate derived from the radionuclide angiographic volume curve. *Am. J. Cardiol.* 53:567–571, 1984.
34. Magorien DJ, Shaffer P, Bush CA, Majorien RD, et al. Assessment of left ventricular pressure-volume relations using gated radionuclide angiography, echocardiography, and micromanometer pressure recordings. *Circulation* 67:844:853, 1983.

35. Port S, Gal R, Grenier R, Acharya K, et al. First-pass radionuclide angiography during treadmill exercise: evaluation of patient motion and a method for motion correction. *J. Nucl. Med.* 30:770, 1989.
36. Gibbons RJ, Lee KL, Cobb FR, Coleman BE, et al. Ejection fraction response to exercise in patients with chest pain, coronary artery disease and normal resting ejection fraction. *Circulation* 66:643–648, 1982.
37. Peter CA, Jones RH. Effects of isometric handgrip and dynamic exercise on left ventricular function. *J. Nucl. Med.* 21:1131, 1980.
38. Foster C, Dymond DS, Anholm JD, et al. Effect of exercise protocol on the left ventricular response to exercise. *Am. J. Cardiol.* 51:859, 1983.
39. Rozanski A, Elkayam U, Berman DS, et al. Improvement of resting myocardial asynergy with cessation of upright bicycle exercise. *Circulation* 67:529, 1983.
40. Seaworth JF, Higginbotham MN, Coleman RE, Cobb FR. Effect of partial decreases in exercise workload on radionuclide indexes of ischemia. *J. Am. Coll. Cardiol.* 2:522, 1983.
41. Borer JS, Kent KM, Bacharach SL, et al. Sensitivity, specificity and predictive accuracy of radionuclide cineangiography during exercise in patients with coronary artery disease. *Circulation* 60:572, 1979.
42. Berger H, Reduto J, Johnstone D, et al. Global and regional left ventricular response to bicycle exercise in coronary artery disease assessment by quantitative radionuclide angiography. *Am. J. Med.* 66:13, 1979.
43. Jengo JA, Oren V, Conant R, et al. Effects of maximal exercise stress on left ventricular function in patients with coronary artery disease using first-pass radionuclide angiocardiography. A rapid, noninvasive technique for determining ejection fraction and segmental wall motion. *Circulation* 59:60, 1979.
44. Port SC, Cobb, FR, Coleman RE, Jones RH. The effect of age on left ventricular function at rest and during exercise. *N. Engl. J. Med.* 303:1131, 1980.
45. Higginbotham MB, Morris KG, Coleman RE, Cobb FR. Sex-related differences in the normal cardiac response to upright exercise. *Circulation* 70:357, 1984.
46. Morris KG, Palmeri ST, Califf RM, et al. Value of radionuclide angiography in predicting specific cardiac events after acute myocardial infarction. *Am. J. Cardiol.* 55:318–324, 1985.
47. Dymond DS, Foster C, Grenier RP, Carpenter J, et al. Peak exercise and immediate postexercise imaging for the detection of left ventricular functional abnormalities in coronary artery disease. *Am. J. Cardiol.* 53:1532–1437, 1984.
48. Herman MV, Heinle RA, Klein MD, Gorlin R. Localized disorders in myocardial contraction. *N. Engl. J. Med.* 277:222–232, 1967.
49. Borges-Neto S, Coleman RE, Potts JM, Jones RH. Combined exercise radionuclide angiocardiography and single photon emission computed tomography perfusion studies for assessment of coronary artery disease. *Sem. Nucl. Med.* 21:223–229, 1991.
50. Larock MP, Cantineau R, Legrand V, Kulbertus, et al. 99m-Tc-MIBI (RP-30) to define the extent of myocardial ischemia and evaluate ventricular function. *Eur. J. Nucl. Med.* 16:223–230, 1990.
51. Albin G, Rahko PS. Comparison of echocardiographic quantitation of left ventricular ejection fraction to radionuclide angiography in patients with regional wall motion abnormalities. *Am. J. Cardiol.* 65:1031–1032, 1990.
52. Mock MB, Ringqvist I, Fisher LD, Davis KB. Survival of medically treated patients in the coronary artery surgery study (CASS) registry. *Circulation* 66:562–568, 1982.
53. Pryor DB, Harrell FE, Lee KL, Rosati RA, et al. Prognostic indicators from radionuclide angiography in medically treated patients with coronary artery disease. *Am. J. Cardiol.* 53:18–22, 1984.
54. Bonow RO, Kent KM, Rosing DR, et al. Exercise-induced ischemia in mildly symptomatic patients with coronary artery disease and preserved left ventricular function: identification of subgroups at risk of death during medical therapy. *N. Engl. J. Med.* 311:1339, 1984.
55. Iskandrian AS, Hakki AH, Kane-Marsch S. Prognostic implications of exercise thallium-201 scintigraphy in patients with suspected or known coronary artery disease. *Am. Heart J.* 110:135–143, 1985.
56. Weiss AT, Berman DS, Lew AS, et al. Transient ischemic dilation of the left ventricle on stress thallium-201 scintigraphy: a marker of severe and extensive coronary artery disease. *J. Am. Coll. Cardiol.* 9:752, 1987.
57. Boucher CA, Zir LM, Beller GA, et al. Increased lung uptake of thallium-201 during exercise myocardial imaging: clinical, hemodynamic and angiographic implications in patients with coronary artery disease. *Am. J. Cardiol.* 46:189, 1980.
58. Forrester J, Diamond G, Swan HJC. Correlative classification of clinical and hemodynamic function after myocardial infarction. *Am. J. Cardiol.* 39:137:145, 1977.
59. Moss MD, Bigger JT, Case RB, Gillespie JA, et al. Risk stratification and survival after myocardial infarction. *N. Engl. J. Med.* 309:331–336, 1983.
60. Zehender M, Kasper W, Kauder E, Schonthaller M, et al. Right ventricular infarction as an independent predictor of prognosis after acute inferior myocardial infarction. *N. Engl. J. Med.* 328:981–988, 1993.
61. Gibson RS, Watson DD, Craddock GB, et al. Prediction of cardiac events after uncomplicated myocardial infarction: a prospective study comparing predischarge exercise thallium-201 scintigraphy and coronary angiography. *Circulation* 68:321–328, 1983.
62. Hung J, Goris ML, Nash E, Kraemer HC, et al. Comparative value of maximal treadmill testing, exercise thallium myocardial perfusion scintigraphy and exercise radionuclide ventriculography for distinguishing high- and low-risk patients soon after acute myocardial infarction. *Am. J. Cardiol.* 53:1221–1227, 1984.

63. Cohn JN, Johnson G and the Veterans Administration Cooperative Study Group. Heart failure with normal ejection fraction. *Circulation* 81(Suppl. III)4A, 1990.
64. Eckstein RW. Effect of exercise and coronary artery narrowing on coronary collateral circulation. *Circ. Res.* 5:230–235, 1957.
65. Todd IC, Bradnam MS, Cooke MBD, Ballantyne D. Effects of daily high-intensity exercise on myocardial perfusion in angina pectoris. *Am. J. Cardiol.* 68:1593–1599, 1991.
66. Schuler G, Hambrecht R, Schlierf G, Grunze M, et al. Myocardial perfusion and regression of coronary artery disease in patients on a regimen of intensive physical exercise and low fat diet. *J. Am. Coll. Cardiol.* 19:34–42, 1992.
67. Rerych SK, Scholz PM, Sabiston DC, Jones RH. Effects of exercise training on left ventricular function in normal subjects: a longitudinal study by radionuclide angiography.

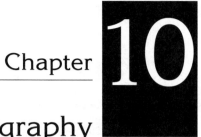

Chapter 10

Stress Echocardiography

Larry C. Kuo

CONTENTS

0-8493-4593-6/97/$0.00+$.50

I. INTRODUCTION

While exercise electrocardiography remains a basic tool in the diagnosis of coronary artery disease (CAD), it has substantial limitations in certain patient groups, yields a limited amount of pathophysiological information, and has many associated causes of false positive and false negative results. Subsequently, many refinements have been described. The primary enhancement to electrocardiogram (ECG) stress testing couples it with an imaging modality. Iodine contrast ventriculography, thallium or technetium isonitrile imaging, radionuclide ventriculography, two-dimensional echocardiography (2-D echo), positron emission tomography (PET), ultrafast cine computed tomography, and magnetic resonance imaging have all been utilized with ECG stress testing.

Since the earlier descriptions of echocardiography-assisted stress testing[68] more than a decade ago, this examination has gained wide clinical acceptance. Stress echocardiography (stress echo) and radionuclide myocardial perfusion stress imaging are now both frequently utilized and are generally regarded as the most accurate noninvasive diagnostic tests for detection of clinically significant coronary artery disease. (Some modalities, such as PET scanning may have higher accuracy, but are available only at a few medical centers).

Echocardiography provides ECG-independent information, such as myocardial contractility, change in ejection fraction, valvular function, and hemodynamic measurements, as well occasionally detecting alternative etiologies of chest pain. Stress echo is an alternative to ECG treadmill testing in nearly all patient populations and, for some, is now the procedure of choice. This chapter will review the fundamental principles underlying stress echo and clinical aspects of selecting and utilizing this examination.

II. ECHOCARDIOGRAPHY

Echocardiography is ultrasound imaging of the heart, and thus it involves no ionizing radiation exposure to the patient or the operator. There are three major components to echo: M-mode, 2-D, and Doppler.

A. M-MODE ECHOCARDIOGRAPHY

M-mode provides an "ice-pick" view of the cardiac structures, plotting lines that represent each echogenic structure intersected by the ultrasound beam on a y-axis, with time along the x-axis. M-mode permits excellent temporal resolution and allows easy caliper measurement of cardiac structures. Except for certain narrowly focused applications, however, these advantages are outweighed by many disadvantages. M-mode is technically difficult, being very sensitive to small changes in transducer angulation, shows very limited portions of the heart at any one time, and is not diagnostically useful when performed from the important apical location or window, leaving many "blind spots" in the assessment of regional wall motion.

B. 2-D ECHOCARDIOGRAPHY

By far, 2-D echo is the most important diagnostic component for stress testing. Real-time, tomographic planes of moving cardiac structures are depicted on a television or monitor. Detection of CAD is based primarily on identifying abnormally contracting myocardial segments during rest and physiological stress. The 2-D examination can be expected to identify all the important segments of myocardium in approximately 95% of patients at rest, with only slightly decreased success rates during various stresses. Ejection fraction, the fraction of blood volume that is ejected from the ventricle during each cardiac cycle (systole), is the next most valuable indicator of CAD. Ejection fraction may be determined subjectively by viewing the beating heart from several angles or may be mathematically derived from any of several geometrically based formulas.[67] In technically difficult studies, indirect estimates of ventricular function may be obtained;[1] this type of patient is, however, not an ideal candidate for echocardiographic stress testing.

In addition, 2-D echo routinely visualizes valvular morphological abnormalities, cardiac chamber enlargement, ventricular hypertrophy, pericardial disease or effusions, and most intracardiac masses or congenital anomalies. Not rarely, the baseline 2-D echo will yield diagnoses which either explain the patient's referred symptoms or may contraindicate the planned exercise portion of the test.

C. DOPPLER ECHOCARDIOGRAPHY

Doppler echo permits an audio and visual representation of any intracardiac blood which has detectable motion; no Doppler signal is generated from static structures. Using the "Doppler equation" and variations of Bernoulli's formulas, any detectable velocity of blood flow generates a predictable shift in the frequency property of the ultrasound beam. To the echocardiographer, this may be displayed directly as a velocity of blood flow or as a calculated pressure gradient between two adjacent intracardiac locations. There are three formats of Doppler in frequent clinical use. Gated spectral Doppler is obtained as the operator limits the time during which the echo machine can process returning ultrasound information from the heart. Specifying electronic time "gates" effectively localizes the Doppler information to a specific depth or location within the heart. Gated Doppler allows the operator to interrogate flow velocity or pressure information from a selected point of interest. However, the spatial localization advantage is at a cost of maximal velocity range available. The Nyquist limit is the maximal velocity that can be detected by gated Doppler, varying inversely with the depth of the desired location, the transducer frequency, and the rate at which the ultrasound beam sweeps the heart. This Nyquist limit is frequently exceeded in clinical settings, more so when interrogating a structure far from the transducer and when using a higher-frequency transducer or color Doppler mapping (see below). When this limit is exceeded, not only can the true blood flow velocity usually not be measured, but the direction of blood flow (toward or away from the transducer) may be ambiguous or nondeterminable. Interested readers are referred to Hatle and Angelsen.[19]

Color Doppler mapping is a computer-enabled enhancement of gated Doppler. In essence, numerous electronic gates are placed within a user-selected imaging wedge or sector; the ultrasound beam rapidly and repetitively sweeps this sector and assigns a color (usually red or blue) to represent direction of blood flow within each of the hundreds of gates. The resulting television image superimposes the color Doppler data on 2-D pictures of the cardiac structures, thus showing red or blue "blood" moving to and fro within cardiac chambers and great vessels. Although differing in several respects from contrast ventriculography obtained at cardiac catheterization, color Doppler may be viewed as an easily repeatable noninvasive equivalent of a right and left ventriculogram and aortogram — without the iodine contrast material or ionizing radiation exposure. In the baseline prestress study, color Doppler allows a rapid and accurate detection of valvular or subvalvular stenosis or regurgitation. In the setting of routine stress testing, the practical value of color or standard gated Doppler is limited to the detection of exercise- or ischemia-induced valvular regurgitation, as from ischemic papillary muscle dysfunction.

Continuous wave Doppler, the third Doppler modality, consists of non-gated ultrasound velocity information. All flow data along a line (or ultrasound beam) of interrogation are displayed together. After mathematical transformation of the Doppler signals — such as by Fourier transform — the displayed data show velocities of blood flow as amplitude, while the density of blood cells at each velocity–time coordinate correlates with the intensity of the Doppler signal. At any given time, the velocity data represent numerous depths or locations within the heart. In return for the inability to localize the origin of a Doppler signal, however, the echocardiographer can detect essentially all velocities of flow. Higher velocities, associated with stenotic valves, can be measured, permitting quantification of the severity of valvular stenosis; the Nyquist limit is no longer a constraint, as with the other two Doppler modalities.

Hemodynamic data obtained from Doppler echocardiography have been the focus of much clinical research recently. Among the relevant applications are the quantification of valvular stenosis, valvular regurgitation,[55] intraventricular obstruction, stoke volume or cardiac output,[27] diastolic ventricular and left atrial[24,54] parameters, estimation of left atrial or pulmonary capillary wedge, and pulmonary artery pressures. That these calculations or estimations can be obtained noninvasively is a major clinical breakthrough, as all of these data previously required cardiac catheterization.

All of these Doppler-derived data have considerable clinical importance and can potentially be assessed with exercise. However, most stress echo laboratories currently find a limited role for Doppler echo. Adequate increase in stroke volume[29] or in systolic flow acceleration[14] parameters may be used to indicate normality of ventricular contractile response to stress. Continuous wave Doppler from the suprasternal notch is the method of choice, due to good access even with simultaneous treadmill walking and relative freedom from respiratory and chest motion artifact at this location. However, an abnormal systolic Doppler response is nonspecific and may be due to any number of cardiac disorders or to changes in afterload, myocardial contractility, and ventricular filling characteristics. Conversely, ischemia involving a small segment of myocardium may not alter the (global) Doppler parameters at all.

III. MYOCARDIAL STRESSORS

Except for the diagnosis of myocardial infarction, most noninvasive techniques require a myocardial stressor in order to elicit and then detect clinically significant CAD. The type of stress may be classified as either increasing myocardial oxygen demand or creating maldistribution of coronary arterial flow (without increasing myocardial work). We will discuss only the more commonly utilized clinical stressors.

A. INCREASED MYOCARDIAL DEMAND
1. Exercise

There are practical advantages and disadvantages of each exercise modality, which will determine the appropriate choice for a laboratory or for an individual patient. Treadmill or bicycle (supine or upright) exercise are the earliest and most widely studied of all the myocardial stressors used with echocardiography. Exercise is well known to induce ischemia by causing the myocardium to work at a level which exceeds the perfusion or flow capacity of a stenotic coronary artery. Major advantages include the "physiologic" nature of exercise, availability of exercise equipment, patient familiarity with exercise, clinical applicability to daily activities which induce ischemia, and the extensive literature on pathophysiological and prognostic information derived from exercise ECG testing (independent of imaging). Aerobic functional capacity and the "double product" of systolic blood pressure and heart rate are frequently useful clinical data.

Treadmill exercise is the most commonly used modality in this country, both for its physiological advantages and patient familiarity. Generally, higher levels of myocardial oxygen consumption are achieved with treadmill than with bicycle stress, although this is patient dependent. Unlike bicycle ergometry, during treadmill walking, there is less reliance on the patient to maintain a constant work load for any given stage. Submaximal peak heart rates are more common with bicycling. Commonly, leg fatigue during supine bicycling results in lower peak levels of myocardial stress; typically, lower peak heart rates but somewhat higher blood pressures are achieved. Upright bicycling seems intermediate in its physiological and hemodynamic consequences, between (upright) treadmill and supine bicycling.

As it is not easy to image a walking individual, echo is performed with the patient lying in a partial left lateral decubitus position before and immediately after treadmill exercise. Generally, imaging is performed from two or more windows. With treadmill exercise, the patient tends to achieve a higher level of exertion and exceed his/her ischemic threshold more frequently than with alternative exercise modalities; the ischemia tends to persist longer into the recovery phase, allowing imaging from several views before evidence of ischemia disappears. Nevertheless, the diagnostic yield will diminish progressively as time passes after stopping exercise.

Conversely, bicycle exercise, particularly supine or semierect, permits imaging during actual exercise. Among the attendant advantages are the ability to detect the onset of ischemia and the lack of concern about quick resolution of ischemia findings when exercise terminates. Such brief-lived ischemia (which could be missed by posttreadmill imaging) is expected to be of less clinical severity, however. Although customized equipment has helped, imaging during exercise is technically challenging, which may result in a lower-quality examination than with postexercise imaging. Furthermore, because of these technical considerations, many operators will obtain 2-D images from only one window (often apical or subcostal) during bicycling. Imaging immediately *after* bicycle exercise is reported[5] occasionally to yield more informative and a greater selection of images than during peak exercise; ischemia, however, will often be undetectable if not imaged within 90 to 120 s after termination of exercise.[51]

Respiratory and other chest wall motion may degrade the echocardiographic image quality for both treadmill and bicycle studies. Arm ergometry and isometric (such as handgrip) exercise do not achieve high enough levels of myocardial stress in most individuals and are usually inadequate as isolated stressors. As addressed in more detail elsewhere in this book, patient characteristics and physical limitations may be the overriding factors in choosing the stressor modality or agent.

Many patients, however, cannot achieve an adequate diagnostic exercise level because of pulmonary or peripheral vascular disease or musculoskeletal limitations. Zoghbi et al.[70] reported that one third (34%) of 4700 patients referred in 1 year for exercise testing could not achieve a diagnostic maximal exercise test. Furthermore, exercise is often curtailed in certain clinical situations, including the critical early period after a myocardial infarction. Thus, nonexercise stress has a major role in modern stress testing; several nonexercise stressors are described in the following discussion.

2. Atrial Pacing

An alternative method of increasing the myocardial work load is to electronically control the heart rate. In some respects, pacing is ideal for echocardiographic imaging, as the patient may be positioned optimally, does not have to move and is not tachypneic, and the level of stress (i.e., heart rate) can be controlled with precision. Furthermore, an unusual potential advantage exists — imaging the heart at nearly identical pre- and poststress heart rates, which is optimal for subjective wall motion analysis. After increasing the heart rate to desired peak levels for the desired duration, the pacemaker can be shut off, with the patient's heart rate usually abruptly returning to its baseline, while ischemic changes can be expected to persist for a short time.

However, pacing has several notable logistic and theoretical disadvantages. The transvenous technique is invasive and requires more-specialized physician skills, with infrequent but potentially serious complications. The transesophageal technique[36] is semi-invasive, unfamiliar to most patients, and not uncommonly causes patient esophageal discomfort from the small electronic pacing discharges. The major theoretical drawback to pacing is its "non-physiologic" nature. Artificially increasing the heart rate does not produce the same increase in myocardial contractility seen with exercise or with adrenergic stressors, for example.

A percutaneous, transvenous pacemaker catheter can be positioned within the right atrium or right ventricle. Ventricular pacing has the major disadvantage that the myocardial activation sequence is altered, leading to wall motion abnormalities, particularly of the interventricular septum. This has obvious adverse impact on any echocardiographic attempt to detect new ischemic wall motion abnormalities. Atrial pacing is more "physiologic," resulting in no intrinsic myocardial contractile abnormalities, but often may fail to achieve a high enough ventricular rate as a result of development of atrioventricular nodal block as atrial rates increase.

3. Pharmacological Stressors

Drugs that have been used for stress testing include dipyridamole, dobutamine, adenosine, atropine, dopamine, arbutamine, and isoproterenol. By far, dipyridamole and dobutamine have the greatest acceptance; several recent studies utilized adenosine instead of dipyridamole. The majority of dipyridamole publications originated in Europe, more specifically, Italy. More recently, dobutamine has also gained acceptance and is now the dominant pharmacological stressor used in the United States.

Catecholamine administration may be used to increase the myocardial oxygen demand. Catecholamines may increase heart rate, myocardial contractility or blood pressure in variable proportions, depending on the specific agent. In this category, there is now common use of only dobutamine, a predominant beta$_1$ receptor agonist, with lesser beta$_2$ and alpha$_1$ cardiovascular activity.[65] Dobutamine exerts both a positive chronotropic (heart rate) and inotropic (contractility) effect on the myocardium. Clinically, dobutamine increases heart rate to a lesser degree than dopamine, isoproterenol, or norepinephrine. Experimental investigations suggest that dobutamine is superior to dopamine in increasing myocardial oxygen demand, with a corresponding increase in sensitivity for detecting significant coronary stenoses.[39] Interestingly, dobutamine influences coronary artery perfusion and hemodynamics differently in patients with and without coronary disease.[42] In addition to the expected increase in myocardial work load and demand, dobutamine seems to cause inhomogeneous coronary perfusion patterns in the presence of significant coronary stenosis. Ischemia may be induced by any or all of these effects. Although less arrhythmogenic than dopamine and isoproterenol (which have also been used as physiological stressors), dobutamine may induce or exacerbate supraventricular or ventricular ectopy.

B. CORONARY FLOW MALDISTRIBUTION
1. Pharmacological Stressors

The primary physiological principle for dipyridamole testing is the concept of coronary artery vasodilation leading to flow maldistribution. A potent coronary vasodilator, intravenous dipyridamole inhibits adenosine cellular uptake, resulting in adenosine accumulation. In the presence of a flow-restricting stenosis in an epicardial coronary artery, maximal pharmacological vasodilation produces a vascular "steal" phenomenon. Nonstenotic arteries dilate and "steal" flow from the stenotic artery which cannot dilate normally because of the atherosclerotic changes in the vessel wall. This inappropriate diversion of coronary flow may be "horizontal," to another epicardial artery through collateral vessels, or "vertical," from subendocardium to subepicardium. Although heart rate–blood pressure double product does not increase substantially, transient regional contractile dysfunction is induced by this maldistribution of coronary flow.[47]

Adenosine itself has more recently been utilized by some centers in place of intravenous dipyridamole. Adenosine theoretically produces coronary vasodilation more directly, has quicker onset of action and a shorter half-life (less than 10 s); thus, side effects are transient and less consequential.

More recently, improved sensitivity has been reported with a dual-drug protocol which starts with a typical dipyridamole infusion protocol, followed immediately by dobutamine infusion in those patients with nondiagnostic dipyridamole examinations.[43]

2. Cold Pressor

Pheripheral exposure to intense cold results in a systemic alpha-adrenergic discharge, resulting in an abrupt increase in vascular resistance and systemic blood pressure. While the normal heart responds successfully to the increased myocardial oxygen demand, a severely diseased coronary artery may not be able to overcome the alpha-adrenergic vasoconstriction, resulting in reduced coronary perfusion to the affected myocardial segments. Coronary vasospasm may also occasionally be provoked by cold stress.

The patient's hand is immersed completely in an ice-water bath for as long as tolerated, preferably for longer than 1 full minute, but rarely greater than 5 min. ECG and blood pressure monitoring is performed routinely. Echocardiographic images are obtained before, during, and for a few minutes after ice-water immersion.

IV. LABORATORY FACILITY

A. EQUIPMENT

A standard echocardiography imaging unit is, of course, the central piece of equipment. As expected, the higher-priced machines have more features and often produce sharper images in a greater percentage of patients. The most important characteristic for stress echocardiography is image quality, with specific attention paid to the ability to display endocardial movement. Perceived image quality will be affected by many factors, including transducer frequency, image frame rate, depth of tissue being scanned, number of phased array elements, sonographic power output, image conversion computer algorithms, monitor resolution, and individual patient physical characteristics. While generally not necessary for routine stress echocardiography, it is prudent to possess Doppler capability, including continuous wave and color Doppler. Colorization of myocardial tissue or automatic and real-time edge detection capabilities are more recent developments which may be of value, but have not been well validated in this setting, and are not used by most stress laboratories.

The other crucial unit is a digitizer. Such a module should be able to "grab" images from the echocardiography machine and transform (if necessary) the image to digitized, computer-compatible images. Once digitized, computer software will generally be able to display a single, user-selected cardiac cycle from desired imaging projections for both stress and baseline studies. The representative heart cycles are shown as a repeating "cine-loop," with resting and the stress images adjacent to each other for easier interpretative comparisons. The different images can also be synchronized to start at the same point of the cardiac cycle. We typically capture and display parasternal long and short axis as well as apical two-chamber and four-chamber views. The digitizer unit may be a component of the echo machine or may be separately purchased.

For exercise studies, the exercise equipment is no different than for nonechocardiographic examinations, being generally a motorized treadmill or a bicycle ergometer. Pharmacological stress tests require intravenous solutions, tubing, and accurate infusion devices, but have the advantage of not requiring exercise equipment. All forms of cardiac stress testing must include real-time ECG monitoring capability and intermittent blood pressure monitoring.

B. PERSONNEL

Adequately trained personnel are vital for both patient safety as well as to assure quality of diagnostic data. The roles needed follow logically from the previous discussions.

First, patient safety mandates attendance of one person experienced in clinical cardiology assessment — to obtain a screening medical history; to reject inappropriate candidates for cardiac stress; to assess symptoms, physiological and ECG changes during stress; and to determine an appropriate stopping point. We feel a cardiologist should be in attendance or immediately available.

An experienced echocardiographer is vital to the acquisition of quality, interpretable images. Especially for exercise testing, the technologist must be able to find the best windows (usually determined on the resting study) quickly and skillfully in the immediate postexercise period or during peak bicycle exercise. This is a challenge in a tachypneic and hyperpneic (and sometimes moving) patient. In most laboratories, the technologist must be experienced enough to select the best few cardiac cycles for digitizing. In some laboratories, this may be the only image data the interpreting physician will see.

The interpreting physician must be experienced in adult echocardiography. Training for stress image interpretation should probably include an additional 100 supervised stress imaging cases, before a reliable and high level of interpretative accuracy can be expected.[46] Experienced echocardiographers who were relative beginners at stress echocardiography showed a predictive accuracy of 62%, compared with 85% for more seasoned (>100 stress studies) echocardiographers. Correlation with other clinical diagnostic procedures is also important. This may be in the form of hard clinical events, cardiac catheterization, surgical outcome, or nuclear cardiology studies (if these have had independent successful correlation) at the same institution.

V. STRESS PROTOCOLS

A. EXERCISE

Physical exercise protocols are not substantially different than for nonimaging tests, with selection based on the individual patient's clinical circumstances, as discussed in other chapters of this book. Most commonly, we use a symptom-limited, maximal Bruce treadmill protocol. For treadmill testing, the recovery phase is modified to permit the patient to move as quickly as possible to a partial left lateral decubitus position, immediately after conclusion of walking. ECG and blood pressure monitoring proceed at usual intervals, all while the echocardiographer is scanning. The echocardiographer is asked to scan first from the best sonographic window, as determined on the preexercise study. The first images can usually be obtained within 15 or 20 s after exercise. Preferably one full set of images (such as parasternal short and long axis and apical four- and two-chamber views) will be completed within 1 min. Imaging continues until the 2-min recovery mark; after that, ischemic changes will often have resolved. If the patient has symptoms later in the recovery phase, it is valuable to obtain simultaneous echocardiographic data.

With bicycle exercise, imaging is performed during actual supine or upright exercise, as well as during the recovery phase. Blomstrand et al.[5] and Presti et al.[51] found better diagnostic sensitivity at peak exercise, compared with postexercise imaging alone. Applegate et al.[3] and Sawada et al.[60] found no difference in clinical information obtained after (bicycle) exercise or during peak exercise. Contraindications to exercise are well described elsewhere in this book and are unchanged by the addition of echocardiographic imaging.

B. DIPYRIDAMOLE AND ADENOSINE

Intravenous dipyridamole protocols have been studied extensively, particularly in Europe and South America.[45] Picano and associates[48] reported only 56% sensitivity when using 0.56 mg/kg, compared with 74% sensitivity when using a "high dose" protocol of 0.84 mg/kg.[48] In the multicenter Echo-Persantine International Cooperative Study (EPIC), over 10,000 tests were performed. After a 3-h fast, with specific attention to avoidance of xanthine products, resting ECG and echocardiographic information are obtained. ECG and blood pressure monitoring were then performed every 1 to 4 min. Continuous ultrasound scanning and intermittent recording are performed as 0.56 mg/kg of dipyridamole is infused over 4 min, followed by 4 min of no drug, and then 0.28 mg/kg over 2 more minutes — for a total dose of 0.84 mg/kg. By comparison, the standard dose used with thallium scintigraphy is 0.56 mg/kg over 4 min.[20]

Adenosine has also been utilized, with several different dosing protocols reported. Zoghbi et al.[70] used progressive 1-min dosing of 50, 75, 100, and 140 mcg/kg; the highest tolerated dose was maintained

Table 1 Stress Echocardiography: End Points to Testing

Symptomatic limits (exhaustion, bronchospasm, nausea, chest pain, etc.)
Hypotension (>20 mmHg drop)
Severe hypertension
Reached 85% of predicted maximal heart rate for age
Achieved maximal dose of pharmacological stressor
Echocardiographic findings of significant myocardial ischemia
Significant, new ECG abnormalities: severe ischemia, arrythmias, heart block

for a total of 4 min. Martin infused 140 mcg/kg/min for 6 min.[31] Marwick et al.[33] used 100, 140, and 180 mcg/kg/min.

Contraindications in our laboratory to dipyridamole and adenosine administration include bronchospastic disease, severe obstructive lung disease requiring methylxanthine (theophylline) therapy, severe hypotension, second- or third-degree heart block unprotected by a pacemaker, and ongoing unstable (resting) angina pectoris. In patients referred with persistent but atypical chest pain, the attending clinician may choose to proceed with stress testing if the prestress echo shows normal myocardial contractility.

C. DOBUTAMINE

Baseline ECG, blood pressure, and echocardiographic data are obtained. Dobutamine is infused with a perfusion pump, according to one of several protocols. A typical initial dose is 5 or 10 mcg/kg/min. Subsequent doses are 20, 30, and 40 mcg/kg/min; some laboratories stop at 30 or 50 mcg/kg/min. Each dosage stage may last 3 to 8 min. Some investigators have added atropine (such as increments of 0.25 mg every minute up to 1.0 mg) to increase heart rate in patients who do not reach 85% predicted maximal exercise heart rate. In our laboratory, we use 3-min stages for 5, 10, 20, 30, 40, and 50 mcg/kg/min of dobutamine; if an endpoint is not attained, the attending clinician may administer atropine (0.5 mg initially, then 0.25 mg increments up to 1.0 mg total).

Contraindications in our laboratory to dobutamine testing include history of clinically significant tachyarrhythmia, severe hypertension or hypotension, and ongoing unstable (resting) angina pectoris.

VI. END POINTS AND ADVERSE EFFECTS

Many of the end points listed in Table 1 are common to any myocardial stress test, with some variability due to the specific stressor and the testing environment. For example, an experienced cardiologist in a hospital laboratory may well exercise a patient to moderate angina, while a noncardiologist in a free-standing office may choose to terminate the test with onset of only mild angina pectoris. Pragmatically, when real-time imaging (such as echocardiography) is available, there may be upward or downward modification of the threshold for terminating the test compared with standard exercise ECG testing or myocardial scintigraphic stress testing. This results from the ability of the echocardiographer to instantaneously detect normal or deteriorating ventricular contractile response during stress.

A. EXERCISE

In Chapter 8 there is a more detailed discussion of the reasons to terminate an exercise test. As in many laboratories, we often use symptom limitation as an end point, rather than a percentage of the maximum predicted heart rate. Side effects of exercise echocardiography are those of any similar exercise test. Leg fatigue and hypertensive exercise response appear to be more frequent end points with bicycle than with treadmill exercise.

B. DIPYRIDAMOLE

End points to dipyridamole testing are listed in Table 1. Compared with adenosine and dobutamine, intravenous dipyridamole has a relatively long half-life (of approximately 30 to 60 min), requiring longer observation for ischemic or adverse effects. Fortunately, aminophylline directly and promptly counteracts the pharmacological effects of dipyridamole. In the multicenter EPIC study, aminophylline (80 to 240 mg i.v. infusion over 1 to 3 min) was available, in case prompt reversal of dipyridamole was needed;[45] lesser doses (40 to 70 mg over 1 min) of aminophylline were routinely administered even with negative examinations, usually at the 15th or 17th minute.

With the routine use of aminophylline by the EPIC investigators, significant side effects (including major adverse reactions and minor but limiting side effects) occurred in only 113 patients (1.2%). Of the seven major reactions, six were felt to be related to echocardiographically detected ischemia. They included one prolonged, drug-resistant asystole (fatality), two other myocardial infarctions, one pulmonary edema, one short-lived asystole, and one sustained ventricular tachycardia. The one nonischemic major event was cardiac asystole, which responded to aminophylline and atropine. An additional 89 patients had significant dipyridamole-related events, 21 with apparent ischemia and 68 with no echocardiographic evidence of associated ischemia. Cardioinhibitory reactions were the most frequent side effects, consisting of hypotension and/or bradycardia, often accompanied by pallor, nausea, and sweating. Acute heart failure, supraventricular tachyarrhythmias, ventricular tachycardia, bronchospasm, and ischemic chest pain were among the other side effects.

Aminophylline was usually successful in reversing the adverse effects. Sometimes atropine or antianginals (usually nitrates) were required; thrombolysis may be advisable if myocardial infarction occurs. The remaining 17 (of 113) significant side effects occurred after aminophylline administration. Interestingly, 13 of these patients (7 with an otherwise negative test) developed transient ST segment elevation with echocardiographic regional dyssynergy. These patients had variant angina; 5 had not been previously diagnosed.

In contrast to the infrequent "significant" side effects, milder side effects are relatively frequent; palpitations, headache, nausea, flushing, and mild chest pain are often experienced. Typical reported rates are in the 40 to 70% range, with 46% having previously been reported by the Intravenous Dipyridamole Thallium Imaging Study Group.[53]

Clinical, hemodynamic, and ECG end points are similar to standard treadmill ECG stress tests, as described elsewhere in this book. The test should also be stopped if the echo shows obvious worsening of or development of new segmental dyssynergy involving a substantial amount of myocardium; the drug infusion should be discontinued. Intolerable pharmacological side effects may also force termination of the test.

C. DOBUTAMINE

Test end points are listed in Table 1. We consider a heart rate greater than 85% of predicted maximum to be a reason to stop the drug infusion. In a series of 1118 patients (420 of whom also received atropine), the major reasons for test termination were achievement of target heart rate (52.1%), maximum dose of drug (22.8%), and angina pectoris (13%).[41]

Several side effects reported with dobutamine are similar to those experienced with dipyridamole. There is no large multicenter dobutamine study of quite the magnitude of the EPIC study. However, most investigators report (in highly variable proportions) chest pain (often nonanginal), headache, diaphoresis, vomiting, palpitations, symptomatic hypotension, and dyspnea. The Echo Dobutamine International Cooperative Study Group reported the largest prospective, multicenter study of dobutamine-atropine stress echocardiography; 2949 tests were reported, involving 2799 patients and 24 experienced laboratories.[49] The maximal dobutamine infusion rate was 50 mcg/kg/min, with the optional addition of up to 1.0 mg of atropine, in 1-min increments of 0.25 mg; unfortunately, the proportion of patients receiving atropine was not reported. "Dangerous events" (life-threatening, or requiring hospital admission, or lasting more than 3 h and requiring treatment) occurred in only 14 tests (0.47%). Of these, 9 were cardiac (3 ventricular tachycardia, 2 ventricular fibrillation, 2 myocardial infarctions, 1 resistant ischemia, 1 severe, resistant hypotension), and 5 were extracardiac (hours-duration hallucinations from atropine, requiring hospital admission, and without apparent ischemia or hypotension). Of interest, the 2 infarctions and 1 ventricular fibrillation occurred 11 to 20 min after the dobutamine infusion was terminated. All 5 of the atropine toxic reactions occurred in patients older than 56 years, which was coincidentally the mean overall patient age for this study.

In this multicenter study, an additional 341 tests (12% of all tests) were terminated because of less-dangerous side effects. These events include complex ventricular tachyarrhythmias in 134 (4.5%), nausea and/or headache in 71 (2.4%), hypotension and/or bradycardia in 62 (2.1%), supraventricular tachyarrhythmias in 44 (1.5%), hypertension in 24 (0.81%), and other events in 20 (0.68%).

Most side effects (except significant ischemic episodes) resolve within 2 or 3 min after discontinuing intravenous dobutamine. However, in addition to the standard "crash cart" medications, it is prudent to have an intravenous beta blocker immediately available, such a inderal or the shorter-acting esmolol. Chest pain is typically treated with prompt termination of infusion, sublingual nitroglycerine and intravenous beta blocker, in that order. Interestingly, hypotension during dobutamine stress appears commonly (20 to 40%) and, unlike with exercise testing, often does not indicate significant ischemic disease, unless wall motion abnormalities are also present.[56]

D. ADENOSINE

Theoretically, adenosine has the same side effects as dipyridamole; the latter drug prevents cellular reuptake of adenosine, which then produces coronary and systemic vasodilation. Most investigators report some side effects in the vast majority of patients during adenosine administration. However, the need to reverse effects with aminophylline or cardiac medications is very uncommon, due the rapid disappearance of adenosine after termination of infusion. Adverse responses will sometimes subside if the infusion rate is decreased, allowing continuation of the test.

VII. ECHOCARDIOGRAPHY INTERPRETATION

A new or deteriorating regional wall motion abnormality is considered an abnormal response with any stressor modality. Among several reported and validated methods, we use a 16-segment anatomical scheme[67] to describe location of regional wall motion. In addition to the left ventricular apex, the basal, mid, and apical segments are identified for the anterior, septal, lateral, inferior, and posterior walls. Each segment may be described as hyperkinetic (=4), normal (=3), mildly hypokinetic (=2), hypokinetic (=1), akinetic (=0), or dyskinetic (=−1). Wall motion scores may be assigned to each segment and/or summed for the entire left ventricle at rest and after exercise. The American Society of Echocardiography proposes a slightly different 16-segment scheme[62] with a wall motion scoring system which does not differentiate hyperkinetic from normal contractility, nor mild from more-severe hypokinesis. New mitral regurgitation occurred in 4 of 50 patients studied by Mazeika[58] with dobutamine stress echocardiography, presumably due to papillary muscle ischemia; incorporating this color Doppler finding increased sensitivity slightly (78 to 81%) without diminishing specificity.[38]

With exercise and dobutamine (but not with pacing or dipyridamole), a normal echocardiographic response to stress also should include a substantial increase in myocardial contractility, including all segments, and often to the point near obliteration of the left ventricle. By using the more traditional exercise radionuclide criteria, a normal response is an absolute increase in global ejection fraction of at least 5%. The arbitrary increment should probably be adjusted for individual circumstances, such as amount of exercise performed,[25] and may not be valid for women.[23] With graded dobutamine stress echo, patients with abnormalities seen at heart rates less than 126 beats/min had a higher incidence of multivessel disease, confirmed by quantitative angiography.[63]

Compared with exercise, whether bicycle or posttreadmill, imaging performed during pharmacological stress is easier for the technologist and often of better visual quality. In the latter situation, the patient is generally quiet, not physically moving, not tachypneic, and can be positioned optimally on the bed. Furthermore, for any given dosage (or stage), the technologist usually has several minutes to obtain images.

Blomstrand et al.[5] found that 96% of myocardial segments (out of 594 total segments in 66 patients) were adequately visualized when the patients were recumbent at rest, the position used preexercise and with pharmacological stress. As expected, lower success rates were noted recumbent immediately after exercise (92%), seated before exercise (80%), and seated during peak bicycle exercise (72%). These rates may be expected to differ with experience of the technologist, supine instead of upright bicycling,[5] and with the positional and imaging flexibility of the exercise equipment or bed.

It has been suggested that an appropriate learning curve for clinically accurate interpretation of stress echocardiographic studies involves approximately 100 examinations. Personal observations suggest that undertrained interpreters tend toward a low sensitivity (or a high false negative rate), while with radionuclide scintigraphic perfusion studies, the novice will tend to have an unacceptably high false positive rate.

VIII. CLINICAL VALIDATION AND APPLICATIONS

For all practical purposes, ischemic CAD is the major clinical arena for stress echocardiography, as summarized in Table 2. Less frequently, congestive heart failure (including diastolic dysfunction) or valvular heart disease may be investigated with this tool; these and other less common clinical applications are not discussed any further.

A. DETECTION OF ISCHEMIC HEART DISEASE

Treadmill ECG, radionuclide techniques, and stress echocardiography each have a wide range of reported predictive accuracy, sensitivity, or specificity. Treadmill ECG testing has an overall sensitivity of approx-

Table 2 Stress Echocardiography: Clinical Applications

Baseline, prestress ECG is significantly abnormal (left bundle branch block, etc.)
Pharmacological stress in patients who cannot exercise
Stratify risk in patients with known CAD
Substitute for stress thallium or radionuclide study (bedside, etc.)
Preoperative risk stratification in moderate- or high-risk patients
Prognosticate and stratify risk post-MI in moderate-risk patients
Detect viability in potentially "stunned" or "hibernating" myocardium

imately 60 to 65% with a specificity of approximately 80%. Thallium tomographic imaging (SPECT) has sensitivity and specificity generally reported in the 85% range. Tremendous variability in reported values relates to many factors, including the exercise or imaging protocol used, the experience of the laboratory, the prevalence of actual disease in the patient population tested, pre- or posttest referral bias, the "gold standard" chosen, and the choice of arbitrary, subjective, or quantitative criteria for designating a test as normal or abnormal.

In 228 patients undergoing both exercise echocardiography and coronary arteriography, Crouse et al.[13] reported much higher sensitivity (97 vs. 51%) for stress echocardiography vs. stress ECG, but similar specificity (64 vs. 62%). Salustri et al.[59] summarized published exercise echo studies with coronary angiogram confirmation. Exercise echocardiography had sensitivity and specificity ranging from 70 to 100%. The median (among the reviewed studies) sensitivity was 71% with median specificity of 92%. Corresponding values were 54 and 91% for exercise ECG. Subsequently, in one of the larger series to date, involving 309 patients who underwent upright bicycle exercise echocardiography and coronary angiography (within an average of 9 days between tests), Ryan et al.[58] reported sensitivity and specificity of bicycle echo as 91 and 78%. Exercise ECG alone yielded 40% sensitivity and 89% specificity. Of 104 patients with nondiagnostic exercise ECGs, stress echo correctly identified 95% of those with coronary disease and 75% of those with no disease. Of those without resting or baseline wall motion abnormalities (n = 183), stress echo had a sensitivity and specificity of 83 and 84%. As is typical with other studies of nearly all stress testing, sensitivity for multivessel disease was higher (95%) than for single-vessel disease (86%). There was a high (75%) prevalence of significant coronary disease in this patient group.

Various factors may reduce the predictive accuracy of exercise echo. Marwick et al.[32] reported posttreadmill echo with cardiac catheterization in 150 patients, with a demonstrated 76% prevalence of significant coronary disease. Overall sensitivity and specificity of exercise echo was 84 and 86%. Age, gender, body weight, and image quality did not seem to significantly influence the test accuracy. However, submaximal exercise performance, single-vessel disease, and moderate (50 to 70%) stenoses did lead to more false negative results — i.e., a lower sensitivity. Sensitivity rose to 90% after excluding patients with submaximal exercise performance. Among 54 patients without previous infarctions and with adequate exercise, sensitivity for detection of multivessel disease was 96%, compared with 79% for single-vessel disease.

Segar et al.[63] reported on 85 patients who underwent both dobutamine stress echocardiography (to physiological end point or to a maximum of 30 mcg/kg/min) and quantitative coronary angiography. Of this group, 66 had significant (diameter stenosis ≥50%) coronary disease. The overall sensitivity for detection of CAD was 95% with specificity of 82% and accuracy of 92%. Sensitivity for detection of disease was similar in all three artery distributions — 79% for anterior descending, 70% for circumflex, and 77% for right coronary arteries. Multivessel disease was found in 11 of 16 patients who had abnormal echocardiographic findings at heart rates below 126 beats/min.

Because of its nondependence on adrenergic stress, sensitivity of dipyridamole or adenosine testing is not significantly affected by heart rate response. A more recent technique, adenosine echocardiography, has been reported to have a lower diagnostic sensitivity. Martin et al.[31] found its sensitivity inadequate (40%), when compared with dobutamine and dipyridamole; however, Zoghbi et al.[70] reported 85% sensitivity and 92% specificity. In comparing adenosine and dobutamine echocardiography and scintigraphy, Marwick et al.[33] found adenosine echocardiography to have the lowest sensitivity (58%) and accuracy (69%) among these four modalities. Acceptable sensitivity of dobutamine stress has been reported by some investigators to depend on adequate heart rate response.[12,40] Conversely, others find that continued therapy with beta-blocker medications did not adversely affect sensitivity of dobutamine testing.[2,61]

Table 3 Sensitivity and Specificity for Various Stress Tests

Stress Test	Approximate Sensitivity (%)	Approximate Specificity (%)
Exercise ECG[a]	40–80	60–90
Exercise SPECT	85–90	85
Dipyridamole SPECT	80	85
Exercise Echo[a]	85	85–90
Dipyridamole Echo	80	90
Dobutamine Echo	85	85
Adenosine Echo	65	85–90

Note: Echo = echocardiography, ECG = electrocardiogram, SPECT = single photon emission computed tomography (thallium or sestamibi).

[a] Accuracy for exercise tests assumes adequate peak exercise.

In summary, one may reasonably consider competently performed stress echocardiography (with the possible exception of adenosine echocardiography) to have similar clinical accuracy to competently performed stress nuclear scintigraphy. This has been demonstrated by numerous investigators, comparing exercise or pharmacological echocardiography against radionuclide ventriculography, thallium-201, or technetium-99m sestamibi stress scintigraphy.[18,22,28,37,50,52] Table 3 summarizes approximate sensitivity and specificity for various stress tests. Although all of these noninvasive modalities can provide important physiological information not available with coronary arteriography, arteriography remains the clinical gold standard for detection of CAD.

B. POST-MYOCARDIAL INFARCTION STRATIFICATION

Among the CAD population, those who have already suffered a myocardial infarction (MI) are at risk for future fatal and nonfatal cardiac events. Thus, a major clinical benefit of diagnostic modalities is the ability to distinguish those at high risk for cardiac events. Health care resources and intensity of follow-up care can then be more effectively allocated. Resting echocardiography has long established its ability to stratify risk by accurate determination of global ventricular contractile function, usually expressed as an ejection fraction.[67] After MI, stress testing is frequently performed (1) to estimate the amount of still-viable tissue in the infarct zone, especially with nontransmural MI or after thrombolytic therapy and (2) to identify significant stenoses in the remaining noninfarcted zones.

Stress echocardiography has the ability to provide postinfarction clinical data with an accuracy comparable with the more traditional nuclear cardiology techniques. As may be expected, both of these imaging modalities can provide substantially more information than standard ECG exercise testing alone. Berthe et al.[4] showed that dobutamine echocardiogrphy can be performed safely early (5 to 10 days) after MI, with 85% sensitivity for detection of multivessel disease. Jaarsma et al.[21] showed that transient asynergy in noninfarct myocardium seen in early (within 3 weeks of MI) exercise echocardiogrphy could identify patients with a higher likelihood of multivessel disease and future ischemic events. Similarly, Applegate et al.[3] and Ryan et al.[57] found that inducible ischemia on postinfarction exercise echo predicted a higher risk for further cardiac events. High-dose dipyridamole stress echocardiography has more recently been shown to have similar efficacy in this clinical population, when correlated with coronary angiography.[6]

In addition, dipyridamole and low-dose dobutamine testing may be able to identify myocardium within the infarct region which is perfused but "stunned"[7,64] or chronically ischemic, "hibernating" myocardium in patients without clinical infarction.[11] Such muscle is characterized by resting hypokinesis which may show improved contractility with mild stress (such as at 5 or 10 mcg/kg/min dobutamine dosages) or reversible deterioration with moderate or higher stress (such as standard dobutamine and dipyridamole dosages).

The ability to identify viable myocardium is particularly important after a subendocardial MI or after acute thrombolytic treatment of MI; such patients frequently have residual ischemic myocardium, subjecting them to future cardiac events.[69] Patients without inducible ischemia or evidence of viable, ischemic myocardium can be stratified as having a low risk of cardiac events in the next year. Alternatively, in the absence of MI, hibernating myocardium may present as a clinical cardiomyopathy and will show substantial or complete recovery if identified and surgically revascularized.[9] Unfortunately, the detection of myocardial viability is still subject to a considerable false negative rate, whether by myocardial radionuclide scintigraphy or by these echocardiographic techniques.

C. PREOPERATIVE ASSESSMENT OF CARDIAC RISK

Preoperative stratification of perioperative complication risk is clinically desirable. In particular, risk of serious cardiovascular mortality and morbidity can be predicted by preoperative evaluation. Patients who undergo vascular surgery are at particularly high risk for serious perioperative cardiac events and thus have significant potential benefit from risk assessment. Dipyridamole thallium scintigraphy has been extensively reported to successfully identify vascular patients at highest risk for surgery.

Dipyridamole echocardiography has comparable accuracy. In a study of 109 patients undergoing major vascular surgery, 8 had abnormal preoperative dipyridamole ECGs, of whom 7 experienced perioperative ischemic events, compared with only 1 patient with a negative preoperative dipyridamole study.[66] Preoperative dobutamine echocardiography has also been studied in undergoing vascular surgery; perioperative cardiac events occurred in 20 and 0% of patients with positive and negative dobutamine studies, respectively.[15]

Massie and Mangano[35] make the sobering observation that our knowledge in this area is still incomplete, however. Current diagnostic tests can stratify perioperative risk, but there is still meager proof that the additional procedural risk of coronary revascularization favorably alters eventual clinical outcome.

D. FOLLOW-UP OF CORONARY ARTERY REVASCULARIZATION

As might be expected, stress echocardiography may also aid in evaluation of revascularization procedures. Improved exercise echocardiographic wall motion score (in 81% of patients[10]) or improved ejection fraction was noted after successful coronary angioplasty.[26] Using dobutamine and atropine echocardiography, McNeill et al.[40] found inducible ischemia in 71% of preangioplasty patients. Although McNeill reported a need for atropine in 50% of their positive examinations, Akosah et al.[2] reported good (88%) sensitivity of dobutamine stress alone in their 35 preangioplasty patients. Wall motion score at peak dobutamine (maximum of 40 mcg/kg/min) infusion rate improved in 90% of patients after angioplasty.[2] Of interest, Akosah's study population showed the improved contractile function early (24 to 48 h) after angioplasty. This contrasts with reports of persistent thallium perfusion defects seen in nearly one third of patients 4 to 18 days after angioplasty.[30] Thus, dobutamine echocardiography may be a better method to assess early success after angioplasty. Bongo et al.[8] showed good predictive accuracy with high-dose dipyridamole echocardiography performed in the first postoperative month.

IX. HOW TO USE STRESS ECHOCARDIOGRAPHY

A. PATIENT POPULATION: EFFECT ON TESTING ACCURACY

The proper selection of any testing modality requires that the clinician incorporate data from the medical history, physical examination, and composite clinical presentation, in addition to knowledge of the advantages and disadvantages of a particular test. The true prevalence (or pretest probability) of disease in the tested population can dramatically affect the predictive accuracy of the subsequent test results, an expression of Bayes's theorem of conditional probability.[16]

For illustration, let us assume optimistically that stress echocardiography has a 90% sensitivity and 90% specificity and that the pretest clinical probability of coronary disease is only 5%, which is the approximate disease prevalence for an asymptomatic 50-year-old male without other CAD risk factors. Then, of all positive stress echo examinations, less than one third (32%) will prove (by coronary angiography) to actually have significant CAD. This is the positive predictive value. In this low-prevalence population, a negative test increases the likelihood of not having CAD from 95% (pretest prediction) to 99%.

Conversely, if a patient presenting for stress echocardiography clinically has a 50/50 chance of actually having CAD (such as a 55-year-old male with atypical chest pain), either a positive or negative stress ECG (again assuming 90% sensitivity and specificity) will yield a predictive accuracy of 90%.

Thus, one could argue that even a very accurate stress echo test would not have much clinical utility in the first example, since two thirds of patients with an abnormal test will not actually have CAD, while a negative test will only slightly improve the 95% pretest predictive accuracy for having no CAD. However, in the second example, much clinical benefit is derived from this single test which increased

Table 4   Choosing the Most Appropriate Stress Test

Characteristic	Exercise ECG	Exercise SPECT	Dipyridamole SPECT	Rest-redist SPECT	Exercise Echo	Dipyridamole Echo	Dobutamine Echo
Clinical accuracy[a]	−	++	+	0	++	+	+
Abnormal ECG, LBBB	−	+	++	0	+	+	+
Bronchospasm	0	0	− −	0	0	− −	+
Tachyarrhythmia	0	0	+	0	0	+	− −
Unstable angina	− −	− −	− −	++	− −	− −	− −
Heart block, no pacemaker	0	0	− −	0	0	− −	+
Can't exercise	− −	− −	++	0	− −	++	++
Large breasts	0	−	−	−	0	0	0
Emphysema, pectus deformity	0	+	+	0	−	−	−
Unable to lie still	0	−	−	−	0	0	0
LV contractility	−	−	−	−	++	++	++
Valvular disorder	−	−	−	−	++	+	++
Operator dependent "subjective"	+	0	0	0	− −	−	−
Myocardial "viability"	−	0	0	+	0	0	+
On beta blocker: detect any CAD	− −	−	++	−	−	++	0
On beta blocker: still ischemic?	+	++	+	0	++	+	+
Avoid radiation	++	−	−	−	0	0	0
Quantitate myocardial areas	−	++	++	++	+	+	+
Abnormal resting wall motion	0	+	+	0	−	−	−
Predict functional capacity	++	++	−	−	++	−	0
ICU/CCU or immobile patient	− −	− −	− −	− −	− −	+	+
Cost: equipment, supplies	++	−	− −	−	0	0	0
Test time: beginning to end	++	− −	− −	−	0	0	0

Note: Advantage or disadvantage: ++ is most favorable, 0 is neutral, − − is least favorable.

Abbreviations: SPECT = single photon emission computed tomography (could use thallium or sestamibi isotope), redist = redistribution, Echo = echocardiography, ECG = electrocardiogram, LBBB = left bundle branch block, LV = left ventricular, CAD = coronary artery disease, ICU = intensive care unit, CCU = coronary care unit.

[a]   Accuracy for exercise tests assumes adequate peak exercise.

the diagnostic accuracy from 50 to 90%. It is beyond the scope of this chapter to further discuss the statistical principles alluded to above, or to expound on the cost-effectiveness of various clinical testing strategies. It is generally true, however, that patients with an intermediate probability for disease will benefit the most from a diagnostic test. Testing should be used more discriminately for patients in whom good clinical judgment predicts a very low or very high clinical probability for CAD.[44]

B. ADVANTAGES AND DISADVANTAGES OF THE COMMON STRESS TESTS

It is clear from the preceding discussion that stress echocardiography or stress scintigraphy are relatively equivalent in predictive accuracy (and that both are more accurate than ECG stress testing without imaging). The choice of nuclear or ultrasound imaging should rest with the experience and track records of available laboratories or departments. For individual patients, however, there may be advantages to selecting the specific type of stress test, as outlined Table 4. Gender does not appear to play a significant role in diagnostic accuracy of exercise or dipyridamole echocardiography.[34,60] Although debatable, I prefer an exercise test to a pharmacological test, if the patient can exercise, as there is significant functional and prognostic information related to exercise performance.

Echocardiography may be preferable to scintigraphy in women with large amounts of breast tissue or implants, which result in artifactual defects that cannot usually be distinguished with certainty from a myocardial scar. Recently described techniques may be able to correct for scintigraphic attenuation defects, reducing this relative disadvantage of scintigraphy. Echocardiography is also preferable when valvular disease is expected to worsen with exercise; for example, optionally requested Doppler echocardiography permits assessment of exertional increase in pulmonary pressures in mitral stenosis or ischemia-induced mitral regurgitation. Less frequently, ultrasound may be selected to avoid even low doses of radiation (as in a pregnant or pediatric patient) or when a patient can lie still for only brief periods — too brief for most nuclear imaging protocols. Echocardiography equipment is much more portable than nuclear cameras, an advantage for the former in the more disabled or ill population. The equipment and supplies for stress echocardiography are generally less expensive than their nuclear counterpart.

Conversely, nuclear scintigraphy is preferred in patients known to have poor echocardiographic windows. The assessment of stress-induced wall motion defects often is more difficult when baseline hypokinesis is present; thus, stress echocardiography may be less desirable in patients with previous MIs. With tomographic (SPECT) nuclear perfusion imaging, the protocol has less time-urgency demands for the technologist after completion of strenuous treadmill exercise. Recently described equipment and processing modifications may substantially diminish the frequently encountered attenuation perfusion defects.[17] When quantification of abnormal myocardial territories is desirable, nuclear computer software algorithms hold a distinct advantage over currently available echocardiographic analysis tools.

X. CONCLUDING COMMENTS

Stress echocardiography has assumed a prominent position among physiological examinations of the heart. In some clinical laboratories, stress echocardiography may be used more frequently than radio-nuclide scintigraphy — with equivalent overall predictive accuracy. In other laboratories, the ultrasound and nuclear examinations complement each other, providing accurate, noninvasive stress testing capability for nearly all patients with CAD.

REFERENCES

1. Abinader EG, Kuo LC, Rokey R, Quinones MA: Mitral-septal angle: a new two-dimensional echocardiographic index of left ventricular performance. *Am. Heart J.* 110:381–385, 1985.
2. Akosah KO, Porter TR, Simon R, Funai JT, Minisi AJ, Mohanty PK: Ischemia-induced regional wall motion abnormality is improved after coronary angioplasty: demonstration by dobutamine stress echocardiography. *J. Am. Coll. Cardiol.* 21:584–589, 1993.
3. Applegate RJ, Dell'Italia LJ, Crawford MH: Usefulness of two-dimensional echocardiography during low-level exercise testing early after uncomplicated myocardial infarction. *Am. J. Cardiol.* 60:10–16, 1987.
4. Berthe C, Pierard LA, Hiemaux M, Trotteur G, Lempereur P, Carlier J, Kulbertus HE: Predicting the extent and location of coronary artery disease in acute myocardial infarction by echocardiography during dobutamine infusion. *Am. J. Cardiol.* 58:1167–1172, 1986.
5. Blomstrand P, Engvall J, Karlsson JE, Bjorkholm A, Wallentin L, Wranne B: Exercise echocardiography: a methodological study comparing peak-exercise and post-exercise image information. *Clin. Physiol.* 12:553–565, 1992.
6. Bolognese L, Sarasso G, Aralda D, Bongo AS, Rossi L, Rossi P: High dose dipyridamole echocardiography early after uncomplicated acute myocardial infarction: correlation with exercise testing and coronary angiography. *J. Am. Coll. Cardiol.* 14:357–363, 1989.
7. Bolognese L, Sarasso G, Bongo AS, Rossi L, Aralda D, Piccinino C, Rossi P: Dipyridamole echocardiography test: a new tool for detecting jeopardized myocardium after thrombolytic therapy. *Circulation* 84:1100–1106, 1991.
8. Bongo AS, Bolognese L, Sarasso G, Cernigliaro C, Aralda D, Carfora A, Piccinino C, Campi A, Rossi L, Rossi P: Early assessment of coronary artery by pass graft patency by high dose dipyridamole echocardiography. *Am. J. Cardiol.* 67:133–136, 1991.
9. Braunwald E, Rutherford JD: Reversible ischemic left ventricular dysfunction: evidence for the "hibernating myocardium. "*J. Am. Coll. Cardiol.* 8:1467–1470, 1986.
10. Broderick TS, Sawada S, Armstrong WF, Ryan T, Dillon JC, Bourdillon PD, Feigenbaum H: Improvement in rest and exercise-induced wall motion abnormalities after coronary angioplasty: an exercise echocardiographic study. *J. Am. Coll. Cardiol.* 15:591–599, 1990.
11. Cigarroa CG, deFilippi CR, Brickner E, Alvarez LG, Wait MA, Grayburn PA: Dobutamine stress echocardiography identifies hibernating myocardium and predicts recovery of left ventricular function after coronary revascularization. *Circulation* 88:430–436, 1993.

12. Cohen JL, Green TO, Ottenweller J, Bineenbaum SZ, Wilchfort SD, Kim CS, Alston JR: Dobutamine digital echocardiography for detecting coronary artery disease. *Am. J. Cardiol.* 67:1311–1318, 1991.

13. Crouse LJ, Harbrecht JJ, Vacek JL, Rosamond TL, Kramer PH: Exercise echocardiography as a screening test for coronary artery disease and correlation with coronary arteriography. *Am. J. Cardiol.* 67:1213–1218, 1991.

14. Daley PJ, Sagar KB, Wann LS: Doppler echocardiographic measurement of flow velocity in the ascending aorta during supine and upright exercise. *Br. Heart J.* 54:562, 1985.

15. Davila-Roman V, Waggoner AD, Sicard GA, Geltman EM, Schechtman KB, Perez JE: Dobutamine stress echocardiography predicts surgical outcome in patients with an aortic aneurysm and peripheral vascular disease. *J. Am. Coll. Cardiol.* 21:957–963, 1993.

16. Diamond GA, Forrester JS: Analysis of probability as an aid in the clinical diagnosis of coronary-artery disease. *N. Engl. J. Med.* 300:1350–1358, 1979.

17. Frey EC, Tsui MBW, Perry JR: Simultaneous acquisition of emission and transmission data for improved thallium-201 cardiac SPECT imaging using a technetium-99m transmission source. *J. Nucl. Med.* 33:2238–2245, 1992.

18. Grayburn PA, Popma JJ, Pryor SL, Walker BS, Simon TR, Smitherman TC: Comparison of dipyridamole-Doppler echocardiography to thallium-201 imaging and quantitative coronary arteriography in the assessment of coronary artery disease. *Am. J. Cardiol.* 63:1315–1320, 1989.

19. Hatle L, Angelsen B (editors): Doppler ultrasound in cardiology: physical principles and clinical applications. 2nd edition. Lea & Febiger, Philadelphia, 1982.

20. Haynie MP, Gould KL, Gerson MC: Methods alternative to dynamic leg exercise for detecting chronic coronary artery disease. In Gerson MC (ed.): Cardiac Nuclear Medicine. 2nd ed. McGraw-Hill, New York, 1991, pp. 273–298.

21. Jaarsma W, Visser CA, Kupper AJF, Res JCJ, van Eenige MJ, Ross JP: Usefulness of two-dimensional exercise echocardiography shortly after myocardial infarction. *Am. J. Cardiol.* 57:86–92, 1986.

22. Jain A, Suarez J, Mahmarian JJ, Zoghbi WA, Quinones M, Verani MS: Functional significance of myocardial perfusion defects induced by dipyridamole using thallium-201 single photon emission computed tomography and two-dimensional echocardiography. *Am. J. Cardiol.* 66:802–806, 1990.

23. Jones RH, McEwan P, Newman GE, Port S, Rerych SK, Scholz PM, Upton MT, Peter CA, Austin EH, Leong KH, Gibbons RJ, Cobb FR, Coleman RE, Sabiston DC Jr: Accuracy of diagnosis of coronary artery disease by radionuclide measurement of left ventricular function during rest and exercise. *Circulation* 64:586–601, 1981.

24. Kuo LC, Quinones MA, Rokey R, Sartori M, Abinader EG, Zoghbi WA: Quantification of atrial contribution to left ventricular filling by pulsed Doppler echocardiography and the effect of age in normal and diseased hearts. *Am. J. Cardiol.* 59:1179–1182, 1987.

25. Kuo LC, Bolli R, Thornby J, Roberts R, Verani MS: Effects of exercise tolerance, age and gender on the specificity of radionuclide angiography: sequential ejection fraction analysis during multistage exercise. *Am. Heart J.* 113:1180–1189, 1987.

26. Labovitz AJ, Lewen M, Kern MJ, Vandormael M, Mrosek DG, Byers SI, Pearson AC, Chaitman BR: The effects of successful PTCA on left ventricular function: assessment by exercise echocardiography. *Am. Heart J.* 117:1003–1008, 1989.

27. Lewis JF, Kuo LC, Nelson JG, Limacher MC, Quinones MA: Pulsed Doppler echocardiographic determination of stroke volume and cardiac output: clinical validation of two new methods utilizing the apical window. *Circulation* 70:425–431, 1984.

28. Limacher MC, Quinones MA, Poliner LR, Nelson JG, Winters WL Jr, Waggoner AD: Detection of coronary artery disease with exercise two-dimensional echocardiography. Description of a clinically applicable method and comparison with radionuclide ventriculography. *Circulation* 67:1211–1218, 1983.

29. Loeppky JA, Green ER, Hoekenga DE, Caprihan A, Luft UC: Beat-by-beat stroke volume assessment by pulsed Doppler in upright and supine exercise. *J. Appl. Physiol.* 50:1173, 1981.

30. Manyari DE, Knudtson M, Kloiber R, Rogh D: Sequential thallium-201 myocardial perfusion studies after successful percutaneous transluminal coronary angioplasty: delayed resolution of exercise induced scintigraphic abnormalities. *Circulation* 77:86–95, 1988.

31. Martin TW, Seaworth JF, Johns JP, Pupa LE, Condos WR: Comparison of adenosine, dipyridamole, and dobutamine in stress echocardiography. *Ann. Intern. Med.* 116:190–196, 1992.

32. Marwick TH, Nemec JJ, Pashkow FJ, Stewart WJ, Salcedo EE: Accuracy and limitations of exercise echocardiography in a routine clinical setting. *J. Am. Coll. Cardiol.* 19:74–81, 1992.

33. Marwick T, Willemart B, D'Hondt AM, Baudhuin T, Wijns W, Detry JM, Melin J: Selection of the optimal nonexercise stress for the evaluation of ischemic regional myocardial dysfunction and malperfusion. Comparison of dobutamine and adenosine using echocardiography and 99mTc-MIBI single photon emission computed tomography. *Circulation* 87:345–354, 1993.

34. Masini M, Picano E, Lattanzi F, Distante A, L'Abbate A: High dose dipyridamole echocardiography test in women: correlation with exercise-electrocardiography test and coronary arteriography. *J. Am. Coll. Cardiol.* 12:682–685, 1988.

35. Massie BM, Mangano DT: Risk stratification for noncardiac surgery. How (and why)? [editorial; comment] *Circulation* 89:913–914, 1994.

36. Matthews RV, Haskell RJ, Ginzton LE, Laks MM: Usefulness of esophageal pill electrode atrial pacing with quantitative two-dimensional echocardiography for diagnosing coronary artery disease. *Am. J. Cardiol.* 64:730–735, 1989.

37. Maurer G, Nanda NC: Two-dimensional echocardiographic evaluation of exercise-induced left and right ventricular asynergy: correlation with thallium scanning. *Am. J. Cardiol.* 48:720–727, 1981.
38. Mazeika PK, Nadazdin A, Oakley CM: Dobutamine stress echocardiography for detection and assessment of coronary artery disease. *J. Am. Coll. Cardiol.* 19:1203–1211, 1992.
39. McGillem MJ, DeBoe SF, Friedman HZ, Mancini GBJ: The effects of dopamine and dobutamine on regional function in the presence of rigid coronary stenoses and subcritical impairments of reactive hyperemia. *Am. Heart J.* 115:970, 1988.
40. McNeill AJ, Fioretti PM, El-Said ME, Salustri A, Forster T, Roelandt J: Enhanced sensitivity for detection of coronary artery disease by addition of atropine to dobutamine stress echocardiography. *Am. J. Cardiol.* 70:41–46, 1992.
41. Mertes H, Sawada SG, Ryan T, Segar DS, Kovacs R, Foltz J, Feigenbaum H: Symptoms, adverse effects, and complications associated with dobutamine stress echocardiography. *Circulation* 88:15–19, 1993.
42. Meyer SL, Curry GC, Donsky MS, Twieg DB, Parkey RW, Willerson JT: Influence of dobutamine on hemodynamics and coronary blood flow in patients with and without coronary artery disease. *Am. J. Cardiol.* 38:103–108, 1975.
43. Ostojic M, Picano E, Beleslin B, Dordjevic-Dikic A, Distante A, Stepanovic J, Reisenhofer B, Babic R, Stojkovic S, Nedeljkovic M, Stankovic G, Simeunovic S, Kanjuh V: Dipyridamole-dobutamine echocardiography: a novel test for the detection of milder forms of coronary artery disease. *J. Am. Coll. Cardiol.* 23:1115–1122, 1994.
44. Patterson RE, Horowitz SF: Importance of epidemiology and biostatistics in deciding clinical strategies for using diagnostic tests: a simplified approach using examples from coronary disease. *J. Am. Coll. Cardiol.* 13:1653–1665, 1989.
45. Picano E and others on behalf of the Echo-Persantine International Cooperative Study Group: Safety of intravenous high-dose dipyridamole echocardiography. *Am. J. Cardiol.* 70:252–258, 1992.
46. Picano E, Lattanzi F, Orlandini A, Marini C, L'Abbate A: Stress echocardiography and the human factor: the importance of being expert. *J. Am. Coll. Cardiol.* 17:666–669, 1991.
47. Picano E: Dipyridamole echocardiography test: the historical background and physiologic basis. *Eur. Heart J.* 10:365–376, 1989.
48. Picano E, Lattanzi F, Masini M, Distante A, L'Abbate A: High dose dipyridamole echocardiographic test in effort angina pectoris. *J. Am. Coll. Cardiol.* 8:848:854, 1986.
49. Picano E, Mathias W Jr, Pingitore A, Gigi R, Previtali M, on behalf of the Echo Dobutamine International Cooperative Study Group: Safety and tolerability of dobutamine-atropine stress echocardiography: a prospective, multicentre study. *Lancet* 344:1190–1192, 1994.
50. Pozzoli MMA, Fioretti PM, Salustri A, Reijis AEM, Roelandt JRTC: Exercise echocardiography and technetium-99m MIBI single-photon emission computed tomography in the detection of coronary artery disease. *Am. J. Cardiol.* 67:350–355, 1991.
51. Presti C, Feigenbaum H, Armstrong WF: Comparison of echo at peak exercise and after bicycle exercise in evaluation of patients with known or suspected CAD. *J. Am. Soc. Echocardiogr.* 1:119–126, 1988.
52. Quinones MA, Verani MS, Haichin RN, Mahmarian JJ, Suarez JM, Zoghbi WA: Exercise echocardiography versus thallium-201 single photon emission computed tomography in the evaluation of coronary disease: analysis of 292 patients. *Circulation* 85:1026–1031, 1992.
53. Ranhosky A, Kempthorn-Rawson J: The safety of intravenous dipyridamole thallium myocardial perfusion imaging. Intravenous Dipyridamole Thallium Imaging Study Group. *Circulation* 81:1205–1209, 1990.
54. Rokey R, Kuo LC, Zoghbi WA, Limacher MC, Quinones MA: Determination of left ventricular diastolic filling parameters with pulsed Doppler echocardiography: comparison with cineangiography. *Circulation* 71:543–550, 1985.
55. Rokey R, Sterling LL, Zoghbi WA, Sartori MP, Limacher MC, Kuo LC, Quinones MA: Determination of regurgitant fraction in isolated mitral or aortic regurgitation by pulsed Doppler two-dimensional echocardiography. *J. Am. Coll. Cardiol.* 7:1273–1278, 1986.
56. Rosamond TL, Vacek JL, Hurwitz A, Rowland AJ, Beauchamp GD, Crouse LJ: Hypotension during dobutamine stress echocardiography: initial description and clinical relevance. *Am. Heart J.* 123:403–407, 1992.
57. Ryan T, Armstrong WF, O'Donnell J, Feigenbaum H: Risk stratification following myocardial infarction using exercise echocardiography. *Am. Heart J.* 114:1305–1315, 1987.
58. Ryan T, Segar DS, Sawada SG, Berkovitz KE, Whang D, Dohan AM, Duchak J, White TE, Foltz J, O'Donnell JA: Detection of coronary artery disease with upright bicycle exercise echocardiography. *J. Am. Soc. Echocardiogr.* 6:186–197, 1993.
59. Salustri A, Pozzoli MMA, Reijs AEM, Fioretti PM, Roelandt JRTC: Comparison of exercise echocardiography with myocardial perfusion scintigraphy for the diagnosis of coronary artery disease. *Herz.* 16:388–394, 1991.
60. Sawada SG, Ryan T, Fineberg NS, Armstrong WF, Judson WE, McHenry PL, Feigenbaum H: Exercise echocardiographic detection of coronary artery disease in women. *J. Am. Coll. Cardiol.* 14:1440–1447, 1989.
61. Sawada SG, Segar DS, Ryan T, Fineberg NS, Armstrong WF, Judson WE, McHenry PL, Feigenbaum H: Echocardiographic detection of coronary artery disease during dobutamine infusion. *Circulation* 83:1603–1614, 1991.
62. Schiller NB, Shah PM, Crawford M, DeMaria A, Devereaux R, Feigenbaum H, Gutgesell H, Reichek N, Sahn D, Schnittger I, Silverman HN, Tajik AJ: Recommendations for quantitation of the left ventricle by two-dimensional echocardiography. *J. Am. Soc. Echocardiogr.* 2:358–367, 1989.
63. Segar DS, Brown SE, Sawada SG, Ryan T, Feigenbaum H: Dobutamine stress echocardiography: correlation with coronary lesion severity as determined by quantitative angiography. *J. Am. Coll. Cardiol.* 19:1197–1202, 1992.

64. Smart SC, Sawada S, Ryan T, Segar D, Atherton L, Berkovitz K, Bourdillon PDV, Feigenbaum H: Low-dose dobutamine echocardiography detects reversible dysfunction after thrombolytic therapy of acute myocardial infarction. *Circulation* 88:405–415, 1993.
65. Sonnenblick EH, Frishman WH, Lejemtel TH: Dobutamine: a new synthetic cardioactive sympathetic amine. *N. Engl. J. Med.* 300:17–22, 1979.
66. Tischler MD, Lee TH, Hirsch AT, Lord CP, Goldman L, Creager MA, Lee RT: Prediction of major cardiac events after peripheral vascular surgery using dipyridamole echocardiography. *Am. J. Cardiol.* 68:593–597, 1991.
67. Van Reet RE, Quinones MA, Poliner LR, Nelson JG, Waggoner AD, Kanon D, Lubetkin SJ, Pratt CM, Winters WL: Comparison of two-dimensional echocardiography with gated radionuclide ventriculography in the evaluation of global and regional left ventricular function in acute myocardial infarction. *J. Am. Coll. Cardiol.* 3:243–252, 1984.
68. Wann LS, Faris JV, Childress RH, Dillon JC, Weyman AE, Feigenbaum H: Exercise cross-sectional echocardiography in ischemic heart disease. *Circulation* 60:1300–1308, 1979.
69. White CW: Recurrent ischemic events after successful thrombolysis in acute myocardial infarction: the Achilles' heel of thrombolytic therapy. *Circulation* 80:1482–1485, 1989.
70. Zoghbi WA, Cheirif J, Kleiman NS, Verani MS, Trakhtenbroit A: Diagnosis of ischemic heart disease with adenosine echocardiography. *J. Am. Coll. Cardiol.* 18:1271–1279, 1991.

Chapter 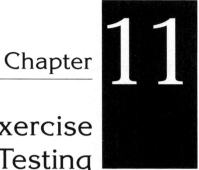 11

Cardiopulmonary Exercise Testing

Thomas Chick

CONTENTS

I. PURPOSES OF EXERCISE TESTING

Evaluation of exercise capacity in the clinical or physiology laboratory addresses the following three key questions:

What is the maximal oxygen uptake (V_{O_2max})? V_{O_2max}, which is the standard measurement of work capacity, is defined as the highest oxygen uptake (V_{O_2}) which can be attained during graded exercise testing. The importance of determining V_{O_2max} lies in the principle that the cardiopulmonary demands of a particular exercise of constant intensity depend on the relative power requirement (fraction of maximal exercise, E_{max}, capacity) of the exercise.

What is the power output the subject or patient can perform for a prolonged period? In order to sustain a given exercise intensity, the cardiopulmonary system must be able to maintain an adequate nutrient supply, to prevent accumulation of metabolites within working muscle, and to dissipate heat generated during muscle contraction. Failure of any of these functions results in muscle fatigue or excessive hyperthermia. The exercise evaluation can determine the absolute and relative exercise intensity at which fatigue will occur if exercise is carried on for a prolonged period. Alternatively, exercise testing allows prediction of the likelihood a given work requirement can be tolerated without excess strain or fatigue and also permits diagnostic and prognostic evaluation of disease conditions.

What is the mechanism of exercise impairment in patients with cardiovascular and pulmonary diseases? Using exercise testing, clinicians can determine the contribution of disorders of the heart and lungs to dyspnea and fatigue. Evaluation of changes in disease status or activity and assessment of therapy can be enhanced by determination of exercise capacity and the pattern of cardiopulmonary response to submaximal exercise.

The objectives of this chapter will be to (1) describe the physiological limits of the oxygen transport system, (2) describe the equipment required to determine the physiological responses of the oxygen transport system during exercise, (3) describe methods used in testing, (4) describe the handling of the data obtained during submaximal exercise and at E_{max}, and (5) discuss changes in exercise performance attributable to gender, age, and cardiopulmonary disease.

II. PHYSIOLOGICAL LIMITS OF THE COMPONENTS OF THE OXYGEN TRANSPORT SYSTEM

An individual's capacity to perform work can be measured in the physiology laboratory by determination of V_{O_2max}. In practice, the subject performs graded exercise (the work load is increased at regular intervals) and the test proceeds until the subject is exhausted and unable to continue. Testing is usually performed using a motor-driven treadmill or a cycle ergometer. Sophisticated measurement devices such as gas analyzers and pneumotachygraphs interfaced with computers enable the physiologist or clinician to fully characterize the response of the components of the oxygen transport system at rest and during each stage of the exercise test.[1]

In normal individuals, V_{O_2max} represents an approximately tenfold increase in V_{O_2} over resting values. This high level of oxygen transport is achieved by activating all components in the oxygen transport system: ventilation, diffusion, pulmonary gas exchange, and cardiac output and its distribution. In this section, the capacities of each of these components will be described. It will be seen that the bottleneck to maximal oxygen transport is at the level of the cardiac output and its distribution.[2]

For purposes of illustration, we will consider the exercise response of a normal male subject who is 35 years old, 182 cm in height, and 70 kg in weight. Pulmonary function testing results are as follows:

	Observed	(% predicted)
FVC, l	5.60	(101)
FEV$_1$, l	4.70	(102)
MVV, l/min	195	(108)
DLCO, ml/min/mmHg	35	(100)

where FVC is forced vital capacity, FEV_1 is forced expiratory volume in 1 s, MVV is maximal voluntary ventilation, and DLCO is lung diffusing capacity.

During performance of a graded cycle exercise test the work load is increased 20 W/min. Measurements of gas exchange variables and heart rate (HR) are recorded at 15-s intervals. Values obtained at rest and at E_{max}:

	Rest	E_{max}
V_E, l/min	8	135
V_{O_2}, l/min	0.30	2.71
HR, beats/min	72	182

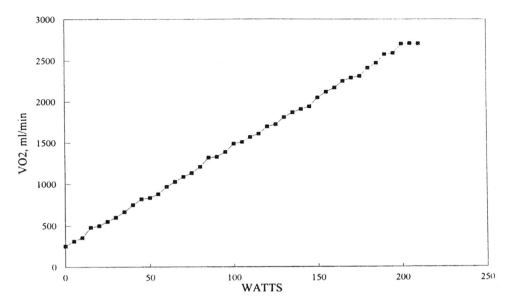

Figure 1 Graph of V_{O_2} vs. watts. V_{O_2} increases linearly with respect to work load. At E_{max} there is a plateau of V_{O_2}.

Predicted V_{O_2max} is 2.99 l/min.[3] Figure 1, a graph of V_{O_2} vs. work rate on the cycle ergometer, shows a linear increase in V_{O_2} until a work load of 200 W is reached, and then a plateau occurs for three consecutive intervals, corresponding to a V_{O_2} of 2.71 l/min.

A. VENTILATION (V_E)

During exercise the increase in V_E is accomplished by increases in both tidal volume and repiratory frequency. Each tidal breath comprises two portions: dead space ventilation and alveolar ventilation. Dead space ventilation is the portion of the ventilation which subtends the conducting airways and unventilated alveoli and does not undergo gas exchange; it can be thought of as wasted ventilation. Alveolar, or effective, ventilation is the portion of ventilation which reaches perfused alveoli and undergoes gas exchange (O_2 and CO_2 transfer between air and blood). With increasing exercise intensity the dead space volume increases because of distension of the conducting airways in response to increased transpulmonary pressures brought about by exercise hyperpnea. Because of the increase in cardiac output and pulmonary blood flow, alveoli which are unperfused at rest, become perfused during low levels of exercise and then participate in gas exchange, augmenting alveolar ventilation. As a result of these changes during exercise, the increase in alveolar ventilation far exceeds the increase in dead space ventilation. The ratio of dead space to tidal volume decreases from 0.3 at rest to approximately 0.12 to 0.15 at V_{O_2} 1.0 l/min and greater. The changes in the breathing pattern from rest to E_{max} are as follows: increased $\dot{V}_E$ from rest to approximately 40% of E_{max} is achieved primarily by an increased tidal volume; maximal tidal volume corresponds to about 50% of vital capacity.[4] At low exercise intensity, the increase in tidal volume is accomplished by increasing end-inspiratory lung volume. At moderate and high exercise intensities, further increase in tidal volume is achieved by reduction of end-expiratory lung volume, an adaptation which requires active expiration. The reduction of end-expiratory lung volume results in generation of an inspiratory recoil pressure which augments diaphragm force generation. The increase in V_E above 40% E_{max} is achieved primarily by an increase in breathing frequency; at E_{max} breathing frequency reaches 35 to 45 breaths/min from a normal value of 10 to 15 breaths/min at rest. The diaphragm force requirement for V_{Emax} does not exceed the threshold for fatigue in short-term exercise, so that respiratory muscle exhaustion does not contribute to limitation of E_{max} in normal individuals.[5] The ventilatory capacity can be measured directly by determination of MVV. During this maneuver, the subject is instructed to breathe as hard and fast as possible for 15 s into a spirometer, and the V_E achieved during this 15-s maneuver is then expressed as liters per minute. The normal value for MVV corresponds to $FEV_1 \times 40$ l/min. In order to detect ventilatory limitation, ventilatory reserve (VR) is calculated as follows:

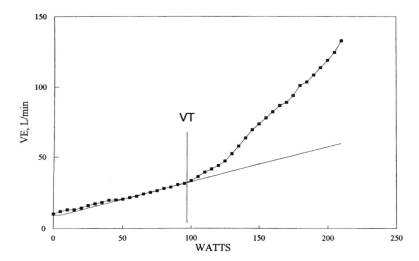

Figure 2 V_E plotted vs. watts. At low-to-moderate work loads V_E increases in proportion to watts; VT is identified by inflection of V_E followed by disproportionate increase in V_E.

$$VR = (1 - [V_{Emax}/MVV]) \times 100\%$$

In normal individuals and patients with cardiovascular limitation, the expected value is >30.[6]

Figure 2 displays V_E plotted vs. work load in watts. It can be seen that the ventilatory response is curvilinear, with an inflection at 100 W followed by a disproportionate increase in V_E; this pattern will be discussed in detail below. V_{Emax} was 135 l/min and VR was 31%. This finding indicates that exercise was not limited by ventilatory capacity.

B. DIFFUSION

The next component of the oxygen transport system is the passive transfer of oxygen from alveolar air into pulmonary capillary blood along a concentration gradient. During exercise, the partial pressure of oxygen in alveolar air is 100 to 120 mmHg whereas, in the pulmonary capillaries, oxygen tension is below 25 mmHg as blood enters the pulmonary circulation. As blood traverses the pulmonary capillaries, oxygen diffuses from the high-concentration region (alveolar air) to the low-concentration region (capillary blood) until complete equilibration is reached, at the end-capillary region. In this transfer, oxygen molecules encounter the resistances of the alveolar–capillary membrane (composed of the alveolar epithelial cell, the capillary endothelial cell, and the blood plasma). The completion of the transfer of oxygen into the blood requires the combination of oxygen with hemoglobin molecules within the erythrocyte. In each step of the diffusion process during exercise, complex adaptations must take place. In order to facilitate O_2 diffusion, the alveolar–capillary membrane surface area increases primarily on the basis of an increase in end-inspiratory lung volume. The diffusing capacity of the alveolar capillary membrane increases from 90 ml/min/mmHg at rest to 115 ml/min/mmHg at E_{max}. The volume of the pulmonary capillaries increases approximately three–fold, from 70 ml at rest to greater than 200 ml at E_{max}. The diffusing capacity of the lung increases from 45 ml/min/mmHg at rest to 80 ml/min/mmHg at E_{max}.[7] These functional changes serve to enhance the diffusion of O_2. However, erythrocyte transit time through the pulmonary capillary decreases from 1 s at rest to 0.4 s at E_{max}, due to the increased velocity of pulmonary blood flow.[7] This shortened erythrocyte transit time partially counteracts the diffusion-enhancing effects of the increase in membrane diffusing capacity and capillary blood volume. Calculation of the diffusion limitation of O_2 transport using E_{max} DLCO of 80 ml/min/mmHg (which corresponds to a diffusing capacity for O_2 of 98 ml/min/mmHg) and assuming a mean alveolar–capillary O_2 tension gradient of 65 mmHg shows that diffusion can accommodate a V_{O_2max} of 6370 ml/min (DLCO $\times$ 1.23 $\times$ [mean alveolar–capillary O_2 tension gradient] = 80 $\times$ 1.23 $\times$ 65 = 6370), which is considerably greater than the measured value of 2710 ml/min in the subject. Therefore, diffusion is not the limiting factor in V_{O_2max}.

C. PULMONARY GAS EXCHANGE

Arterial blood gas changes during graded exercise: In normals, alveolar–arterial O_2 tension difference ($AaPO_2$) progressively widens as V_{O_2} exceeds 50% V_{O_2max}. The mechanism of the increase in $AaPO_2$ is unclear, but probably involves increased dispersion of ventilation/perfusion ratios and incomplete O_2 equilibration across the alveolar–capillary membrane.[8] Arterial P_{CO_2} decreases moderately and pH increases (repiratory alkalosis) at low and moderate exercise intensities; above anaerobic threshold (AT), metabolic acidosis due primarily to accumulation of lactic acid in blood develops.[8]

D. CARDIAC OUTPUT AND ITS DISTRIBUTION

This next step in O_2 transport to working muscle consists of the cardiovascular system, composed of a central, or cardiac, component and a peripheral component, the vasodilator reserve of the muscular arterioles and the microanatomy of the skeletal muscle systemic capillaries and the skeletal muscle fibers. With regard to the central component, cardiac output is determined by the product of HR and stroke volume. During graded exercise, HR increases continuously or linearly with work load or V_{O_2}; however, stroke volume and left ventricular ejection fraction increase from rest to approximately 50% E_{max} and then reach a plateau.[9] The increase in HR reflects combined effects of decreased parasympathetic activation and restrained activation of the sympathetic nervous system. The maximal HR (HR_{max}) corresponds to a value equal to 220 minus the age of the subject in years. It is this age-related decline in HR_{max} (due mainly to decreased response to sympathetic stimulation[10]) which contributes to the decline in V_{O_2max} with advancing years. The increase in stroke volume is due to two factors: (1) the Starling mechanism, whereby augmented venous return from the exercising muscles gives rise to increases in left ventricular filling, end-diastolic volume, and myocardial stroke work and (2) enhanced myocardial contractility and decreased end-systolic volume in response to sympathetic nervous system activation.[9] The peripheral component of the cardiovascular system, the vasodilator reserve, and the microcirculatory anatomy are to be considered next. During exercise blood must be redistributed from nonworking organs and tissues to exercising muscle. In addition, because exercising muscle generates heat, skin perfusion must be commensurate with the requirements for thermoregulation, mainly sweating and convective heat loss. Based on these considerations, it is obvious that arterioles in working muscles and exposed skin must dilate in order to achieve the functions of enhanced O_2 transport and heat dissipation, respectively. Blood flow to working muscles increases in proportion to the work performed, mediated by release of metabolites from working muscle and mechanoreceptor reflex activation of localized vasodilation.[11] Cardiac output increases from 4.5 to 6.5 l/min at rest to 15 to 25 l/min at E_{max}, a value which is consistent with observed values for V_{O_2max}.[9] To illustrate, assuming E_{max} arteriovenous O_2 content difference of 0.14 l/l and maximal cardiac output of 20 l/min, we calculate V_{O_2} according to the Fick principle:

$$\begin{aligned} V_{O_2} &= (\text{Cardiac output}) \times (\text{arteriovenous } O_2 \text{ content difference}) \\ &= 20 \text{ l/min} \times 0.14 \text{ l/l} \\ &= 2.8 \text{ l/min} \end{aligned}$$

which is very close to the observed value of 2.71 l/min and consistent with the observation that cardiac output and its distribution limit V_{O_2max} in normal individuals.

Because noninvasive measurements of cardiac output are not routinely available and it has been demonstrated that stroke volume reaches a maximal value at approximately 50% E_{max},[9] it is valid to use HR to determine the maximal cardiovascular response to exercise. HR response (HRR) and HR reserve are determined as follows:

$$HRR = (HR_{max} - HR_{rest})/(V_{O_2max} - V_{O_2rest})$$

$$HR \text{ reserve} = (1 - [HR_{max}/\text{predicted } HR_{max}]) \times 100\%$$

In normal individuals and in patients with cardiovascular disorders, HRR is <50 beats/min/l/min and HR reserve is <15%. In the subject under consideration, HRR is $(182 - 72)/(2.71 - 0.30) = 46$ beats/min/l/min and HR reserve is $(1 - 182/185) \times 100 = 2\%$. These values indicate that submaximal HR response is normal and that E_{max} resulted from attainment of predicted HR_{max}.

III. MANAGEMENT OF RESPIRATORY GAS EXCHANGE DATA

A. ANAEROBIC THRESHOLD

Up to this point we have discussed the cardiopulmonary variables at E_{max}. However, analysis of submaximal data allows the determination of AT, the exercise intensity at which O_2 demand begins to exceed O_2 supply;[12] this is a critical variable in exercise physiology because it is the exercise intensity which the subject can sustain for prolonged periods without development of muscle fatigue. When constant-intensity exercise exceeds AT, metabolites, such as lactic acid and diprotonated phosphate,[13] accumulate in exercising muscle and eventually cause muscle exhaustion by interfering with excitation–contraction coupling.

AT is defined as the V_{O_2} above which there is progressive accumulation of lactic acid in blood. It corresponds to the exercise intensity at which there is transition from aerobic to anaerobic metabolism. In order to understand the AT, one should consider the metabolic events in the exercising muscle during graded exercise. At low work loads energy demands are met by aerobic processes, and there is no significant accumulation of metabolites. However, as work intensity increases, O_2 supply becomes inadequate to completely meet the energy demands and a portion of energy must be derived from anaerobic sources, primarily anaerobic glycolysis. Lactic acid progressively accumulates in skeletal muscle cytoplasm and diffuses into systemic capillary blood as exercise intensity increases. In blood, the proton associated with lactic acid is buffered by plasma bicarbonate (HCO_3^-), yielding CO_2 by the following reaction:

$$H^+ + HCO_3^- \rightarrow H_2CO_3 \rightarrow H_2O + CO_2$$

This "nonmetabolic" source of CO_2 stimulates V_E above that required for the uptake of O_2 and accounts for the disproportionate increase in V_E at exercise intensities above AT. In Figure 2 the inflection of V_E is designated the ventilatory threshold (VT); this nomenclature is preferred because it is not possible to distinguish a true AT from the onset of hyperventilation when V_E alone is considered. A true AT is illustrated in Figure 3, where V_E/V_{O_2} increases at 100 W but V_E/V_{CO_2} does not increase until a higher exercise intensity is reached. (In the case of hyperventilation, both V_E/V_{O_2} and V_E/V_{CO_2} increase simultaneously.) Because adequate blood bicarbonate content exists to completely buffer the initial burden of protons, the early supra-AT inflection of V_E is associated with isocapnic hyperpnea and V_E/V_{O_2} rises but V_E/V_{CO_2} remains stable. As more lactic acid is liberated into blood with increasing exercise intensity blood bicarbonate is depleted and acidemia ensues, giving rise to further stimulation of V_E and an increase in V_E/V_{CO_2}. Above this point, the threshold of decompensated metabolic acidosis (TDMA), a disproportionate rise in V_E/V_{CO_2} is seen (Figure 3). TDMA is useful to verify that the subject's effort was maximal; that is, the absence of a TDMA indicates that the subject did not perform a maximal effort or that exercise is ventilatory limited. Because V_{CO_2} above AT increases out of proportion to V_{O_2}, the respiratory exchange ratio (RER) or (VCO_2/V_{CO_2}) increases to greater than 1.0 above AT. AT is also defined by an increase in exhaled O_2 concentration (F_{EO_2}) with no change in exhaled CO_2 concentration (F_{ECO_2}). To summarize, AT is determined by graphing V_{O_2} on the abscissa and V_E, V_E/V_{O_2}, V_E/V_{CO_2}, RER, F_{EO_2}, F_{ECO_2} on the ordinate; the following four inflection points are identified: (1) an inflection of V_E signaling the onset of a disproportionate increase in V_E, (2) the onset of increase V_E/V_{O_2} with no change in V_E/V_{CO_2}, (3) a systematic increase in RER, and (4) an increase in F_{EO_2} with no change in F_{ECO_2}. In most reports, AT is determined by methods 1 and 2. In the subject, Figure 2 shows that V_E increases linearly from rest to 100 W exercise and then begins an exponential increase. The AT is the V_{O2} corresponding to 100 W or 1450 ml/min V_{O_2}, as derived from Figure 1. Moreover, TDMA can be identified at 125 W and 1750 ml/min V_{O_2}, indicating that the subject's effort was maximal.

AT has proved to be a useful index of aerobic fitness and cardiopulmonary disease. Studies have shown that constant-intensity exercise performed just below AT can be carried out indefinitely, whereas the duration of constant-intensity exercise performed above AT is limited in proportion to the difference between the assigned work load and AT.[13] Of the variables derived from exercise physiology testing, AT is the strongest predictor of endurance exercise performance.[15]

B. DATA AT MAXIMAL EXERCISE

A common problem in interpretation of graded exercise studies is the subject who stops exercising for reasons other than physical exhaustion. This is especially problematical in disability evaluation. Data obtained from exercise physiology testing can determine whether a subject has achieved a true V_{O_2max} or has ceased exercising for nonphysiological reasons. The criteria for V_{O_2max} include a V_{O_2} plateau at

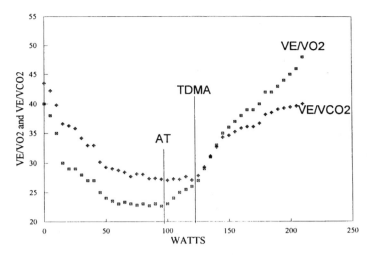

Figure 3 V_E/V_{O_2} and V_E/V_{CO_2} during exercise. AT is characterized by the onset of a systematic increase in V_E/V_{O_2} with no change in V_E/V_{CO_2}, occurring at 100 W. TDMA is seen at 125 W, signifying the onset of metabolic acidosis.

the highest exercise intensity achieved, RER greater than 1.1, evidence of metabolic acidosis (TDMA is detectable), and attainment of a physiological limit, such as HR_{max} greater than 85% of predicted HR_{max} in normal individuals and in patients with cardiac disease and V_{Emax} greater than 85% MVV in patients with pulmonary disease.[16]

IV. METHODS OF TESTING

Laboratory exercise testing is conventionally carried out with a motor-driven treadmill or a cycle ergometer. These are the most convenient forms of exercise for subjects who have the motor skills necessary to perform these modes of exercise. Normal standards have been established for both sexes, all ages, and varying fitness levels. However, in special circumstances, such as paraplegia and arthritis or deformity of the lower extremities, arm exercise is preferable. Because some rehabilitation programs use arm as well as leg training, testing of both these forms of exercise might be applicable.

A. CYCLE ERGOMETRY

Advantages of cycle ergometry are that virtually all subjects are able to perform this form of exercise, blood sampling during exercise can be accomplished more easily than during treadmill exercise, blood pressure measurements are less subject to movement artifact, and falls or other mishaps are less likely to occur. However, because cycle exercise does not involve weight bearing, V_{O_2max} is approximately 10% lower when compared with treadmill exercise in untrained subjects.[17] The cycle grade increments selected should result in an exercise test that is 7 to 17 min in duration; tests outside this range have been shown to underestimate V_{O_2max}.[18] In practice, the evaluator selects the work load increment based on the subject's age, size, and fitness. A small frail elderly woman would be most appropriately tested with 10-W/min stages. In contrast, a 30-year-old competitive cyclist would require stages of 30 to 50 W.

The duration of each stage in the exercise protocol is usually 1, 2, or 3 min. Because of the time requirements (see above), 1-min stages are preferred by some investigators. However, many laboratories use 3-min stages, in order to achieve stable cardiorespiratory variables at each stage and because, at low-to-moderate exercise intensities, blood lactate values reach a steady state in less than 3-min. Comparison of exercise protocols using 1-, 2-, and 3-min stages has shown no significant differences for AT and V_{O_2max} between the differing testing methods.[19]

B. TREADMILL EXERCISE

Treadmill testing offers the advantages of greater intensity of effort (due to weight bearing) and the assessment of a more commonly used activity (walking or running) than cycle ergometry. The Bruce protocol is the most commonly used testing procedure for evaluation of cardiac ischemia. The protocol consists of 3-min stages:

Stage	Speed, mph	Grade, %
1	1.7	0
2	1.7	5
3	1.7	10
4	2.5	12
5	3.4	14
6	4.2	16
7	5.0	18
8	5.5	20

Another commonly used protocol is the Balke protocol in which treadmill speed is kept constant and grade is increased in 1-min stages:

Stage	Speed, mph	Grade, %
1	3.3	1
2	3.3	2
3	3.3	3
4	3.3	4
5	3.3	5
6	3.3	6
7	3.3	7
8	3.3	8
9	3.3	9
10	3.3	10
11	3.3	11
12	3.3	12
13	3.3	13
14	3.3	14
15	3.3	15
16	3.3	16
17	3.3	17
18	3.3	18
19	3.3	19
20	3.3	20

V. VARIABLES MEASURED DURING EXERCISE TESTING

Metabolic carts measure the following variables: respiratory flow or volume, F_{EO_2}, F_{ECO_2}, and HR. Respired volume or V_E can be determined by pneumotachograph, the measurement of gas flow. V_E is calculated by differentiation of flow with respect to time. Alternatively, volume can be measured directly by a spirometer. Exhaled concentration of O_2 can be measured using mass spectrometry, paramagnetic, or fuel cell methodology. Exhaled CO_2 is usually measured with an infrared gas analyzer. Breath-by-breath techniques utilize rapid-responding gas analyzers which sample at the mouthpiece proximal to the pneumotachograph. The advantages of breath-by-breath analysis include collection of a large number of samples, which enhances the detection of trends and inflections. A typical exercise test would gather 300 to 500 data points. The alternative method for handling exercise data is the timed collection system; by this technique mixed exhaled gas is sampled at regular intervals of 5 to 60 s. Because fewer data points are obtained, results are more manageable if analyzed manually. However, in the era of inexpensive computerized data mamagement, breath-by-breath systems are preferred in order to more accurately detect trends and inflections.

VI. EFFECT OF AGING ON EXERCISE PERFORMANCE

V_{O_2max} decreases 0.02 to 0.03 l/min/year with age, beginning in the third decade of life.[3] Aging results in reduced capacity of all components of the oxygen transport system. Changes in pulmonary function include age-related declines in FVC, FEV_1, MVV, and respiratory muscle force and endurance; pulmonary gas exchange shows increased AaP_{O_2} with no change in P_{aCO_2}. During exercise, aged individuals show an excessive ventilatory response due to increased wasted ventilation.[20] Cardiovascular changes associated with aging consist of reduced maximal HR (probably related to reduced responsiveness to sympathetic stimulation), increased pulmonary and systemic vascular resistance, and greater dependence on the Starling mechanism for augmentation of left ventricular performance during exercise.[21] In addition, elderly individuals demonstrate reduced skeletal muscle mass.[22]

VII. EFFECT OF GENDER ON EXERCISE PERFORMANCE

Comparison of V_{O_2max} in normal men and women of equivalent fitness reveals values that are approximately 50% greater in men when expressed as liters per minute; when normalized to fat-free body weight (ml/min/kg) the difference in V_{O_2max} is reduced to approximately 15%.[23] When blood hemoglobin concentrations are equalized between men and women and V_{O_2max} is expressed as milliliters per minute per kilogram fat-free body weight, the gender difference disappears.[24]

VIII. EXERCISE TESTING IN CARDIOPULMONARY DISEASE

A. PULMONARY DISEASE

Pulmonary disease can be classified into two categories on the basis of spirometric abnormalities. Obstructive pulmonary disease, such as asthma, chronic obstructive pulmonary disease (COPD), and cyctic fibrosis, is defined as a reduction of expiratory flow due to increased resistance in the small intrapulmonary airways. The associated pulmonary mechanical and gas exchange abnormalities include lung hyperinflation, diaphragm muscle fiber shortening (due to the inspiratory position of the diaphragm), increased work of breathing, hypoxemia, and, in advanced disease, hypercapnia. Exercise limitation is most closely correlated with the severity of the obstructive ventilatory defect as measured by spirometry.[25] In moderate-to-severe obstructive pulmonary disease, exercise capacity is ventilatory limited; that is, E_{max} is reached when the patient's V_E corresponds to MVV. VR is low and arterial blood gases at E_{max} typically show increased arterial CO_2 tension (P_{aCO_2}).[26] Because many patients with COPD reach their ventilatory limit at low exercise intensities, AT may not be reached.[27] The cardiac output–V_{O_2} relationship is usually normal in patients with obstructive pulmonary disease uncomplicated by cardiovascular disorders. However, because increased pulmonary vascular pressure and right ventricular afterload impair right ventricular emptying, stroke volume is reduced and HR is increased at submaximal exercise intensities.[28] For example, a 60-year-old patient with COPD has the following spirometry and exercise findings:

Spirometry		
FEV$_1$ 1.0 l		
MVV 40 l/min		
Exercise study	**Rest**	**E_{max}**
V_{O_2}, l/min	0.35	0.95
V_E, l/min	12	40
HR, beats/min	95	120
pH$_a$, units	7.42	7.34
P_{aCO_2}, mmHg	42	48
P_{aO_2}, mmHg	75	62

Calculation of VR: $(1 - [V_{Emax}/MVV]) \times 100\% = (1 - 36/40) \times 100$ gives a value of 10%. In normal individuals and patients with cardiovascular limitation, the expected value is >30%. This finding indicates that exercise is limited by ventilatory impairment. Arterial blood gases indicate that CO_2 retention occurred at E_{max}, reflecting lack of adequate ventilatory reserve to eliminate metabolic CO_2 production.

To evaluate cardiovascular function during exercise, calculation of HRR:

$$(HR_{max} - HR_{rest})/(V_{O_2max} - V_{O_2rest}) = (120 - 95)/(0.95 - 0.35)$$

yields 42 beats/min/l/min, a normal value (<50 beats/min/l/min), indicating normal HRR to exercise. At E_{max} HR reserve is

$$(1 - [HR_{max}/\text{predicted } HR_{max}]) \times 100\% = (1 - [120/(220 - 60)]) \times 100\%$$

or 25%. In normal individuals and patients with cardiovascular disorders, HR reserve is <15%. This finding is consistent with limitation of E_{max} by factors other than cardiovascular response.

B. RESTRICTIVE PULMONARY DISEASE

The most common type of restrictive pulmonary disease referred for exercise testing is interstitial lung disease. In this condition, lung compliance is reduced and the elastic work of breathing is increased. Spirometry shows reduced FVC; FEV_1 is reduced in proportion to the reduction in FVC, resulting in normal values for FEV_1/FVC. The expected pattern of abnormality in arterial blood gases consists of hypoxemia at rest due to mismatching of ventilation and perfusion. Hypocapnia due to hypoxic stimulation of ventilation, as well as increased neurogenic ventilatory drive on the basis of reduced lung compliance, is frequently observed. Diffusing capacity is also low and results in exaggerated hypoxemia during exercise. Exercise is ventilatory limited. The pattern of ventilatory response during exercise is the rapid onset of excess tachypnea and a high degree of wasted ventilation.

C. CARDIAC DISEASE

Conditions which compromise myocardial function, such as valvular, hypertensive, or coronary artery disease, result in impaired left ventricular performance during exercise. Because of reduced pump proficiency, left ventricular filling is inadequate and cardiac output demands must be met by excessive tachycardia. Cardiac output is subnormal during submaximal exercise and at E_{max}. As a result of reduced O_2 delivery, AT and V_{O_2max} are decreased. The pattern of submaximal exercise reponse is a reduced AT, increased HRR (>50 beats/min/l/min), low HR reserve, and increased VR (>30%).[16]

REFERENCES

1. Snell, P. G. and Mitchell, J. H., The role of maximal oxygen uptake in exercise performance, *Clin. Chest Med.*, 5, 51, 1984.
2. Saltin, B. and Strange, S., Maximal oxygen uptake: "old" and "new" arguments for a cardiovascular limitation, *Med. Sci. Sports Exercise*, 24, 30, 1992.
3. Jones, N. L., Makrides, L., Hitchcock, C., Chypchar, T., and McCartney, N., Normal standards for an incremental progressive cycle ergometer test, *Am. Rev. Respir. Dis.*, 131, 700, 1985.
4. Gowda, K., Zintel, T., McParland, C., Orchard, R., and Gallagher, C. G., Diagnostic value of maximal exercise tidal volume, *Chest*, 98, 1351, 1990.
5. Younes, M. and Kivinen, G., Respiratory mechanics and breathing pattern during and following maximal exercise, *J. Appl. Physiol.*, 57, 1773, 1984.
6. Eschenbacher, W. L. and Mannina, A., An algorithm for the interpretation of cardiopulmonary exercise tests, *Chest*, 97, 263, 1990.
7. Warren, G. L., Cureton, K. J. Middendorf, W. F., Ray, C. A. and Warren, J. A. Red blood cell pulmonary capillary transit time during exercise in athletes, *Med. Sci. Sports Exercise*, 23, 1353, 1991.
8. Dempsey, J. A., Is the lung built for exercise? *Med. Sci. Sports Exercise*, 18, 143, 1986.
9. Higginbotham, M. B, Morris, K. G., Williams, R. S., McHale, P. A., Coleman, R. E., and Cobb, F. R., Regulation of stroke volume during submaximal and maximal upright exercise in normal man, *Circulation*, 58, 281, 1986.
10. Fleg, J. L., Tzankoff, S. P., and Lakatta, E. G., Age-related augmentation of plasma catecholamines during dynamic exercise in healthy males, *J. Appl. Physiol.*, 59, 1033, 1985.
11. Shepherd, J. T., Circulatory response to exercise in health, *Circulation*, 76 (Suppl. VI), VI–3, 1987.
12. Wasserman, K., Beaver, W. L., and Whipp, B J., Gas exchange theory and the lactic acidosis (anaerobic) threshold, *Circulation*, 81 (Suppl. II), II–14, 1990.
13. Wilson, J. R., McCully, K. K., Mancini, D. M., Boden, B., and Chance, B., Relationship of muscular fatigue to pH and diprotonated P_i in humans: a ^{31}P-NMR study, *J. Appl. Physiol.*, 64, 2333, 1988.
14. Wasserman, K., Determinants and detection of anaerobic threshold and consequences of exercise above it, *Circulation*, 76 (Suppl. VI), VI–29, 1987.
15. Coyle, E. F., Coggan, A. R., Hopper, M. K., and Walters, T. J., Determinants of endurance in well-trained cyclists, *J. Appl. Physiol.*, 64, 2622, 1988.
16. Neuberg, G. W., Friedman, S. H., Weiss, M. B., and Herman, M. V., Cardiopulmonary exercise testing. The clinical value of gas exchange data, *Arch. Intern. Med.*, 148, 2221, 1988.
17. Schneider, D. A., Lacroix, K. A., Atkinson, G. R., Troped, P. J., and Pollack, J., Ventilatory threshold and maximal oxygen uptake during cycling and running in triathletes, *Med. Sci. Sports Exercise*, 22, 257, 1990.

18. Fairshter, R. D., Walters, J., Fox, M., Minh, V.-D., and Wilson, A. F., A comparison of intrumental exercise tests during cycle and treadmill ergometry, *Med. Sci. Sports Exercise,* 15, 549, 1974.
19. Zhang, Y-Y., Johnson, M. C., Chow, N., and Wasserman, K., Effect of exercise testing protocol on parameters of aerobic function, *Med. Sci. Sports Exercise,* 23, 625, 1991.
20. Brischetto, M. J., Millman, R. P., Peterson, D. D., Silage, D. A., and Pack, A. I., Effect of aging on ventilatory response to exercise and CO_2, *J. Appl. Physiol.,* 56, 1143, 1984.
21. Schulman, S. P. and Gerstenblith, G., Cardiovascular changes with aging: the response to exercise, *J. Cardiopulm. Rehabil.,* 9, 12, 1989.
22. Fleg, J. L. and Lakatta, E. G., Role of muscle loss in the age-associated reduction in V_{O_2max}, *J. Appl. Physiol.,* 65, 1147, 1988.
23. Sparling, P. B. A., A meta-analysis of studies comparing maximal oxygen uptake in men and women, *Res. Q. Exercise Sport,* 51, 542, 1980.
24. Cureton, K., Bishop, P., Hutchinson, P., Newland, H., Vickery, S., and Zwiren, L., Sex difference in maximal oxygen uptake. Effect of equating haemoglobin concentration, *Eur. J. Appl. Physiol.,* 54, 656, 1986.
25. Dillard, T. A., Piantadosi, S., and Rajagopal, K. R., Prediction of ventilation at maximal exercise in chronic obstructive air-flow obstruction, *Am. Rev. Respir. Dis.,* 132, 230, 1985.
26. Loke, J., Mahler, D. A., Man, S. F. P., Wiedemann, H. P., and Matthay, R. A., Exercise impairment in chronic obstructive pulmonary disease, Clin. Chest Med., 5, 121, 1984.
27. Sue, D. Y., Wasserman, K., Moricca, R. B., and Casaburi, R., Metabolic acidosis during exercise in patients with chronic obstructive pulmonary disease. Use of the V-slope method for anaerobic threshold determination, *Chest,* 94, 931, 1988.
28. Light, R. W., Mintz, H. M., Linden, G. S., and Brown, S. E., Hemodynamics of patients with severe chronic obstructive pulmonary disease during progressive upright exercise, *Am. Rev. Respir. Dis.,* 130, 391, 1984.

Chapter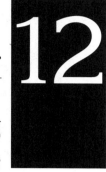

Principles of Prescribing Exercise

Scott O. Roberts

CONTENTS

0-8493-4593-6/97/$0.00+$.50

I. INTRODUCTION

The benefits of regular physical activity and exercise are becoming increasingly clear. Individuals that choose to be more physically active, in both their leisure and work activities, statistically lower their risk for developing certain degenerative diseases, such as osteoporosis, diabetes, obesity, and cardiovascular disease, to name a few. Despite the mounting evidence of the benefits of regular exercise, only 22% of adults engage in leisure-time activities at or above the level recommended for health benefits in the U.S. Public Health Service's health and disease prevention goals and objectives for the nation.[54]

　The number of Americans who do not participate in regular exercise has been called an epidemic. Some of these sedentary individuals should be encouraged to learn that recent research has shown one may not need to exercise as much as one thought to gain health-related benefits. The term "health-related fitness" now appears frequently in exercise literature to describe the health benefits of exercise. Instead of defining physical fitness in terms of one's athletic abilities (speed, power, balance, etc.), health-related

Figure 1 Physical Activity Readiness Questionnaire (PAR-Q)

If a person answers yes to any questions, vigorous exercise or exercise testing should be postponed. Medical clearance may be necessary.

1. Has your doctor ever said you have heart trouble?
2. Do you frequently suffer from pains in your chest?
3. Do you often feel faint or have spells of severe dizziness?
4. Has a doctor ever told you your blood pressure was too high?
5. Has a doctor ever told you that you have a bone or joint problem such as arthritis that has been aggravated by exercise, or might be made worse with exercise?
6. Is there a good physical reason not mentioned here why you should not follow an activity program even if you wanted to?
7. Are you over age 65 years and not accustomed to vigorous exercise?

(From *PAR-Q Validation Report*. British Columbia Department of Health, June 1975. With permission.)

physical fitness defines an individual's fitness status based on cardiorespiratory fitness, muscular strength, muscular endurance, flexibility, and body composition.

The simplest definition of health-related physical fitness is *the ability of the systems of the body (heart, lungs, blood vessels, and muscles) to function efficiently, as to resist disease and to be able to participate in a variety of activities without undue fatigue.* The five components of health-related physical fitness are *muscular strength, muscular endurance, cardiorespiratory endurance, flexibility,* and *body composition.* A comprehensive fitness program should have activities which develop and maintain each of the five components.

II. GETTING STARTED

Before designing an exercise program, several things need to be considered. First and foremost, one needs to know if there are any physical or medical problems that would place individuals at risk if they exercise. Second, fitness testing may provide valuable information which can be used to set specific goals and training limits. And third, an interview with a client will help establish clear goals and objectives for the exercise program. Neglecting any one of the three components mentioned can affect the safety and effectiveness of an exercise program.

A. PREEXERCISE HEALTH SCREENING

The potential benefits of exercise must outweigh the potential risks. For most healthy individuals, the risks associated with exercise are extremely low. It is estimated that death occurs in 1 in 15,000 to 20,000 adult exercisers as a result of vigorous exercise. In individuals with a known or unknown medical condition, exercise may cause serious injury or even death. Thus, an individual's health status needs to be evaluated prior to designing an exercise program.

A preexercise health screening can take many forms, including (1) a self-administered questionnaire, such as the Physical Readiness Questionnaire (PAR-Q) (Figure 1), (2) a complete physical exam, (3) a diagnostic exercise test, or (4) some combination of the three. Deciding on which health screening procedure to use will depend on (1) the age, sex, and health status of the individual (Table 1), (2) at what level of exercise intensity an individual wants to start (Table 1), and (3) available resources and trained personnel. An easy, quick, and reliable way to prescreen individuals for exercise is to administer the PAR-Q. The PAR-Q has been found to have a sensitivity of 100% and specificity of 80% for detecting medical conditions which would preclude an individual from exercising.

A health appraisal can provide valuable information which can be used to (1) design a safe exercise program, (2) identify risk factors for cardiovascular disease, and (3) design an appropriate exercise program, based on the needs of the individual. More-specific medical information regarding a client's past and present medical status can be obtained by reviewing a medical history. A medical history is generally obtained from a physician or nurse and, in most cases, can be made available upon request. The purpose of the health appraisal establishes the current health status of an individual and provides fitness professionals with baseline information which will be used to design an exercise program; it is not intended to screen for *all* health conditions that could affect the safety and effectiveness of an exercise program. A good motto to follow is "when in doubt about individuals readiness to exercise, they should consult with their physician."

Table 1 ACSM Recommendations for (1) Medical Examination and Exercise Testing Prior to Participation and (2) Physician Supervision of Exercise Testing

	Apparently Healthy		Higher Risk[b]		With Disease[c]
	Younger[a]	Older	No Symptoms	Symptoms	
Medical exam and diagnostic exercise test recommended prior to:					
Moderate exercise[d]	No[f]	No	No	Yes	Yes
Vigorous exercise[e]	No	Yes[g]	Yes	Yes	Yes
Physician supervision recommended during exercise test:					
Submaximal testing	No	No	No	Yes	Yes
Maximal testing	No	Yes	Yes	Yes	Yes

[a] Younger = ≤40 years (men), ≤50 years (women).

[b] Persons with two or more risk factors (see Table 3) or symptoms (Table 4).

[c] Persons with known cardiac, pulmonary, or metabolic disease.

[d] Moderate exercise (exercise intensity 40 to 60% $\dot{V}O_{2max}$) — Exercise intensity well within the individual's current capacity and can be comfortably sustained for a prolonged period of time, i.e., 60 min, slow progression, and generally noncompetitive.

[e] Vigorous exercise (exercise intensity >60% $\dot{V}O_{2max}$) — Exercise intense enough to represent a substantial challenge and which would ordinarily result in fatigue within 20 min.

[f] The "no" responses in this table mean that an item is "not necessary." The "no" response does *not* mean that the item should not be done.

[g] A "yes" response means that an item is recommended.

From Kenney, W. L. (Editor). *ACSM's Guidelines for Exercise Testing and Prescription,* 5th edition. Philadelphia, PA: Williams & Wilkins, p. 25, 1995. With permission.

B. FITNESS TESTING/ASSESSMENT

Fitness testing generally falls into two categories: field tests and laboratory tests. There are simple field tests and sophisticated laboratory tests which are used to measure the five components of physical fitness. Baseline data collected from fitness tests can be used to (1) plan safe and effective exercise, (2) motivate a client, and (3) change or modify an exercise program. The same criteria apply to fitness testing, as with health screening, as far as deciding on which one to use (field or laboratory). For a more detailed description of exercise testing procedures the reader is encouraged to read the American College of Sports Medicine's *ACSM's Guidelines for Exercise Testing and Prescription,* 5th edition, Philadelphia: Williams & Wilkins, 1995. Some form of initial fitness evaluation should be used to establish baseline measurements of body composition, muscular strength, aerobic capacity, flexibility, and muscular endurance.

C. CLIENT INTERVIEW

The goals of the client should be thoroughly explored. The *art* of designing an exercise program becomes important during the actual design of the program. The most thorough health screening and fitness test mean very little when designing an exercise program, if the client's needs are not discussed. A preexercise interview should discuss topics such as (1) past exercise experiences, (2) specific health goals, (3) time constraints, (4) equipment needs, and (5) perhaps personal reasons for exercising. Individuals generally adhere to an exercise program better, if clear, measurable, and concise goals have been identified.

III. PROGRAM DESIGN FOR APPARENTLY HEALTHY INDIVIDUALS

The American College of Sports Medicine defines *apparently healthy* as individuals who are asymptomatic and apparently healthy with no more than one major coronary risk factor (see Tables 2, 3, and 4). Individuals who have symptoms suggestive of cardiac, pulmonary, or metabolic disease, who have two or more coronary risk factors, or who have known disease should have a complete medical evaluation with a diagnostic exercise test prior to exercise. Safety should always be the primary factor dictating the readiness of an individual to exercise.

Table 2 ACSM Initial Risk Stratification

Apparently healthy	Individuals who are asymptomatic and apparently healthy with no more than one major coronary risk factor (see Table 3)
Increased risk	Individuals who have signs and symptoms suggestive of possible cardiopulmonary disease (Table 4) or metabolic disease and/or two or more major coronary risk factors (Table 3)
Known disease	Individuals with known cardiac, pulmonary, or metabolic disease

From Kenney, W. L. (Editor). *ACSM's Guidelines for Exercise Testing and Prescription,* 5th edition. Philadelphia, PA: Williams & Wilkins, p. 19, 1995. With permission.

Table 3 Coronary Artery Disease Risk Factors

1.	Age	Men >45 years; women >55 years or with premature menopause without estrogen replacement therapy
2.	Family history	Myocardial infarction or sudden death before 55 years of age in father or other male first-degree relative, or before 65 years of age in mother or other female first-degree relative
3.	Current cigarette smoking	
4.	Hypertension	Blood pressure ≥140/90 mmHg, confirmed by measurement on at least two separate occasions, or on antihypertension medication
5.	Hypercholesterolemia	Total serum cholesterol > 200 mg/dl or high-density lipoprotein cholesterol < 35 mg/dl
6.	Diabetes mellitus	Persons with IDDM who are >30 years of age, or have had IDDM for >15 years, and persons with NIDDM who are >35 years of age
7.	Sedentary life-style	Persons comprising the least-active 25% of the population, as defined by the combination of sedentary jobs involving sitting for a large part of the day and no regular exercise or active recreational pursuits

From Kenney, W. L. (Editor). *ACSM's Guidelines for Exercise Testing and Prescription,* 5th edition. Philadelphia, PA: Williams & Wilkins, p. 25, 1995. With permission.

Table 4 Major Symptoms or Signs Suggestive of Cardiopulmonary Disease

1. Pain, discomfort (or other anginal equivalent) in the chest, neck, jaw, arms, or other areas that may be ischemic in nature
2. Shortness of breath at rest or with mild exertion
3. Dizziness or syncope
4. Orthopnea or paroxysmal nocturnal dyspnea
5. Ankle edema
6. Palpitations or tachycardia
7. Intermittent claudication
8. Known heart murmur
9. Unusual fatigue or shortness of breath with usual activities

From Kenney, W. L. (Editor). ACSM's Guidelines for *Exercise Testing and Prescription,* 5th edition. Philadelphia, PA: Williams & Wilkins, p. 17, 1995. With permission.

The ACSM, in conjunction with the Centers for Disease Control and Prevention (CDC) and the President's Council on Physical Fitness and Sports, recently issued a new recommendation on increased physical activity for Americans. The recommendation states that: "Every American adult should accumulate 30 minutes or more of moderate-intensity physical activity over the course of most days of the week. Because most Americans do not presently meet the standard described above, almost all should strive to increase their participation in moderate and/or vigorous physical activity."

The ACSM/CDC Position Statement on Exercise is perhaps the most powerful single event to have occurred in the last decade in the field of sports medicine and exercise physiology. The consensus statement means that a little bit of daily physical activity results in health-related benefits. Examples of activities that can contribute to the 30-min total are walking up stairs (instead of taking the elevator), gardening, raking leaves, walking at lunch. In addition, more-typical forms of exercise are also encouraged, such as running, swimming, cycling, working out at a health club, and playing tennis. Individuals should strive to participate in activities that improve and maintain the key components of health-related fitness.

IV. EXERCISE PROGRAM DESIGN COMPONENTS

An exercise program is based on five key principles. These key principles include (1) mode, (2) intensity, (3) frequency, (4) duration, and (5) rate of progression.

A. WARM-UP PERIOD

The purpose of the warm-up period is to prepare the body for more-vigorous activity and to reduce the chance of injury. A gradual warm-up period gradually increases the blood flow to the muscles, which actually "warms the muscles" so they can function more effectively, and the enzyme activity of the muscles. The warm-up period consists of a light aerobic period, followed by some flexibility exercises. The light aerobic period might consist of some light calisthenics, jogging in place, or 5 to 10 min on some stationary aerobic exercise equipment. An adequate warm-up period should last at least 10 min.

B. COOL-DOWN PERIOD

The purpose of the cool-down period is to allow the body to gradually return to the resting state before exercise, or homeostasis. A gradual cool-down period or rhythmic exercise also facilitates return of blood to the heart, thus reducing the risk of venous pooling. The cool-down period basically consists of the same exercises as the warm-up period. The cool-down period should last between 10 and 15 min. The same types of activities and stretches can be performed during the cool-down period.

C. MODE

Mode refers to the type of activity performed during the exercise session. Various modes of exercise affect the components of fitness in different ways. For example, aerobic exercise affects aerobic capacity and body composition, but has little effect on muscular strength, flexibility, and muscular endurance. Choosing the correct mode of exercise is important because it has a direct effect on the outcome. The mode of activities that improve cardiorespiratory endurance must use large muscle groups, rhythmically, for a continuous period of time (i.e., running, swimming, cycling, etc.). The mode of activities that develop muscular strength requires activities that work large and small muscle groups, for brief periods of time (i.e., weight training).

D. INTENSITY

Intensity refers to the level of stress achieved during the exercise period. Exercise sessions can be low intensity or high intensity. Intensity is most often regulated by heart rate. However, other methods include breathing rate, METs, an estimated percentage of VO_2max, or by rate of perceived exertion (RPE). In order to determine training heart rate (THR), an individual's maximal heart rate (MHR) must first be determined. An individual's MHR can be directly determined from a submaximal or maximal exercise test, or it can be indirectly determined by subtracting one's age from 220. For example, an estimated MHR for a 20-year-old is 200.

Low-intensity exercise would be equal to 50 to 60% of an individual's MHR, whereas 85 to 90% would related to high-intensity exercise. When beginning an exercise program, it is best to start out at a low intensity and gradually increase the intensity over time. THR can either be taken as a direct percentage of the MHR obtained from an exercise test, or it can be estimated from using a percentage of an individual's heart rate reserve (HRR).

MHR	180
RHR	−60
HRR	120
Desired Intensity	× .60
	72
RHR	+60
THR	132

Another common method used to monitor exercise intensity is based on an individual's RPE (Table 5). RPE is derived from the Borg Scale. At rating of 12 to 13 (using the 15-point scale) corresponds to approximately 60% of the heart rate range. Using the RPE scale is an easy and reliable way to monitor

Table 5 Rating of Perceived Exertion (RPE)

6	
7	Very, very light
8	
9	Very light
10	
11	Fairly light
12	
13	Somewhat hard
14	
15	Hard
16	
17	Very hard
18	
19	Very, very hard
20	

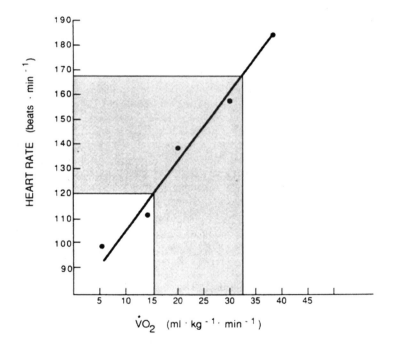

Figure 2 Heart rate, exercise intensity, and oxygen consumption relationship.

exercise intensity. The RPE scale is underutilized compared with heart rate when monitoring exercise intensity. One of the simplest ways to monitor an individual's stress during exercise is the old "talk test." During light and comfortable exercise, you should be able to carry on a normal conversation with your exercise partner. If not, you are probably exercising at too high of an intensity.

If an individual's maximal oxygen uptake was known, a training intensity based on a percentage of the predicted of obtained maximal oxygen uptake can be used to plan an exercise program (Figure 2). Since VO_2 and the rise in heart rate are usually linear, a THR can be determined from a percentage of the VO_2 vs. HR slope line. The last way to monitor exercise intensity is to convert predicted or obtained VO_2 to METs and prescribe an exercise program based a particular MET level.

E. FREQUENCY

Frequency refers to the number of training sessions per week. It is recommended that individuals try and exercise 4 to 5 days/week. The frequency of exercise depends on (1) the type of exercise performed,

(2) the fitness status of the individual, and (3) the goals of the individual. For sedentary individuals or individuals with medical and/or health limitations, the frequency of exercise may be daily, since their ability to exercise at a high intensity or duration is limited. For apparently healthy individuals, greater frequency generally results in greater fitness benefits. However, exercise frequency needs to be carefully monitored and adjusted if injuries result. The type of exercise performed also affects frequency. The components of fitness (flexibility, muscular strength and endurance, body composition, and cardiorespiratory endurance) need to be equally balanced. Too much aerobic exercise often makes one too tired to lift weights, and vice versa.

F. DURATION

Duration refers to the length of the training session. Duration and intensity are inversely related. That is, if the intensity of the exercise is high, the duration is generally low, and vice versa. Approximately 30 to 40 min of continuous (aerobic) exercise is recommended per exercise session. In addition, additional time must be dedicated to flexibility and muscular training. The duration of the exercise session can be affected by environmental factors (heat, humidity, altitude, etc.). It can also be affected by the present fitness level and/or energy supply of an individual.

G. RATE OF PROGRESSION

Rate of progression refers to how fast an individual progresses. Rate of progression is directly related to such factors as fatigue and drop-out rate, that is, the faster the rate of progression, the greater the fatigue and probability of drop-out. The intensity, duration, and frequency should all be gradually increased over time (weeks to months, not days). Rate of progression can be affected by chronic injury or illness. Rate of progression will need to be modified (reduced) if an injury or illness persists. As individuals adapt to training, the rate of progression can be increased.

H. REST

The amount of rest between workouts is just as important as the amount of time spent in workouts. Rest is needed between workouts to replace the energy stores in muscles (glycogen) and to let the overall body systems recover from training. If you push too hard, too long, your body will eventually break down. Individuals need to be instructed to take at least 1 day off between training sessions. In addition, always take at least 1 or 2 min to rest between resistance-training exercise sets. Certain training systems have recommended that you take as little as time as possible between sets to get the most out of your training; however, this technique is not recommended for young or sedentary individuals.

V. EXERCISE PROGRAM DESIGN CONSIDERATIONS FOR SELECTED SPECIAL CASES

Exercise is also becoming increasingly recognized as an important therapeutic modality in the treatment and rehabilitation of certain acute and chronic health conditions. For example, aerobic exercise is now widely recommended and supported as an adjunct treatment for individuals recovering from coronary heart disease. Several recent studies have shown that exercise combined with risk-factor modification can significantly decrease morbidity and mortality in individuals with known coronary heart disease. Even a modest amount of physical activity, such as daily brisk walking, can reduce the risk of developing heart disease.

VI. PHYSICAL ACTIVITY, HEALTH, AND DISEASE

Today, few would debate the benefits of physical activity. With the plethora of literature available, it appears that individuals who choose to be more physically active, in both their leisure and work activities, lower their risk for developing certain degenerative diseases, such as osteoporosis, diabetes, obesity, and cardiovascular disease.

Many organizations have realized the importance of regular exercise and have published major policy statements. In 1989, the U.S. Preventive Services Task Force concluded that the evidence linking exercise and health was strong enough to issue recommendations for physicians to be better able to counsel their patients.[25] Other major policy statements are presented in earlier chapters.

The epidemiology of the study of physical activity and morbidity and mortality had its origins in London, England. In the 1950s and 1960s, Dr. Jeremy Morris began to look at the association between physical activity during work and the rate of cardiovascular disease. Dr. Morris began by comparing the rate and severity of cardiovascular disease between London bus conductors, who had to walk up and down the stairs and aisles of double-decker buses collecting tickets, and the bus driver who sat most of day. Dr. Morris found that the conductors, who were more physically fit, had a lower incidence of coronary heart disease, a reduced fatality rate, and a lower rate of early mortality from the disease than did the bus drivers.[31] Dr. Morris found similar findings when comparing the leisure-time exercise habits of civil servants.[32] Based on his early findings, Dr. Morris concluded that:

> Physical activity of work is a protection against ischaemic heart disease. Men in physically active jobs have less ischaemic heart disease during middle age, what disease they have is less severe, and they tend to develop it later than similar men in physically inactive jobs.[33]

Between the years of 1951 and 1972, Paffenbarger and colleagues[36] followed the work activity levels and coronary heart disease records of San Francisco longshoremen. Paffenbarger and colleagues found that the men who expended 8500 or more kilocalories per week at work had significantly less risk of fatal coronary heart disease at any age than men whose jobs required less energy expenditure.[36] Paffenbarger and Wing[37] later looked at leisure-time physical activity vs. work-related physical activity and risk for coronary heart disease. They compared the levels of habitual and leisure physical activity of 16,936 Harvard University alumni between the years of 1962 and 1972. Once again, a clear pattern of age-specific rates of coronary heart disease was seen with an increase in energy expenditure, especially in the group expending more than 2000 kcal/week.[37]

Since the studies of London bus conductors in the early 1950s and the work of Paffenbarger in the 1960s and 1970s, the epidemiology of leisure and occupational activity, health, and disease has been investigated in hundreds of locations and occupations around the world. The consensus of the evidence from these studies is that physical activity has a protective effect against disease. More recently, Blair and colleagues[9] studied the association between physical fitness and risk of all-cause and cause-specific mortality in 10,224 men and 3120 women. After an 8 year follow-up, higher levels of physical fitness delayed all-cause mortality, primarily because of lowered rates of cardiovascular disease and cancer[9] (Figure 3).

The study of the association between regular physical activity and health and disease has continued to be expanded upon in recent years to include various chronic diseases, besides cardiovascular disease and cancer. There currently exists substantial evidence demonstrating the protective effect of exercise against various chronic diseases (Table 6).[30] The promotion of regular physical activity, including exercise, has truly become a national public health priority. The potential impact of an increase in the number of Americans who are habitually physically active on disease reduction and prevention, savings in health care costs, and reduced morbidity and mortality from chronic diseases could be staggering.

VII. CARDIOVASCULAR DISEASE

The association of physical activity and prevention of coronary artery disease (CAD) was discussed previously. Recently, Powell and colleagues[41] reviewed 43 epidemiological studies involving physical activity and CAD and found that two thirds of the studies had a significant inverse relationship. As Morris, Paffenbarger, Blair, and others have discovered in their studies, the greater the physical level, expressed by total kilocalories expended per week, the less the risk for CAD. The exact mechanisms relating to a decreased CAD morbidity and mortality with exercise are not entirely clear, but are probably related to the favorable effects exercise has on blood pressure, obesity, diabetes, hypercholesterolemia, and fibrinolytic activity.

A. THE ROLE OF EXERCISE AND CORONARY ARTERY DISEASE

Clearly, regular physical activity reduces the risk of CAD. How effective is exercise at treating CAD? Initially, extended bed rest was recommended for patients recovering from a myocardial infarction. The thinking at that time was that the heart takes approximately 6 weeks to heal after a heart attack and that any undue stress might compromise that healing process. Although the heart may be healing satisfactorily, the rest of the body is slowly deteriorating. Bed rest results in (1) a decrease in work capacity, (2) a decreased adaptability to changes in position, (3) a decrease in blood volume, (4) a decrease in muscle mass, (5) an increase in risk for thromboembolism, and (6) a decrease in respiratory and pulmonary function.

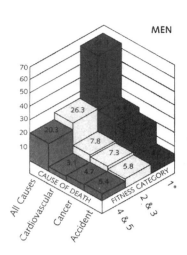
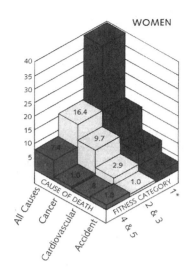

Figure 3   Age-adjusted cause-specific death rates per 10,000 person-years of follow-up (1970–1985) by physical fitness groups. (From Blair, S. N., Kohl, H. W., Paffenbarger, R. S., Clark, D. G., Cooper, K. H. and L. W. Gibbons. *J. Am. Med. Assoc.* 262: 2395–2401, 1989. With permission.)

Table 6   Summary of Selected Health Benefits Associated with Regular Exercise

Reduces the risk of cardiovascular disease
1. Increases high-density lipoprotein cholesterol (HDL-C)
2. Decreases low-density lipoprotein cholesterol (LDL-C)
3. Favorably changes the ratios between total cholesterol and HDL-C, and between LDL-C and HDL-C
4. Decreases triglyceride levels
5. Promotes relaxation; relieves stress and tension
6. Decreases body fat and favorably changes body composition
7. Reduces blood pressure especially if it is high
8. Blood platelets are less sticky
9. Fewer cardiac arrhythmias
10. Increases myocardial efficiency
    a. Lowers resting heart rate
    b. Increases stroke volume
11. Increases oxygen-carrying capacity of the blood

Helps control diabetes
1. Cells are less resistant to insulin
2. Reduces body fat

Develops stronger bones that are less susceptible to injury

Promotes joint stability
1. Increases muscular strength
2. Increases strength in the ligaments, tendons, cartilage, and connective tissue

Contributes to fewer low-back problems

Acts as a stimulus for other life-style changes

Improves self-concept

From Anspaugh, D. J., Hamrick, M. H., and Rosato, F. D. *Concepts and Applications Wellness.* St. Louis, MO: Mosby-Year Book, p. 143, 1991. With permission.

In the early 1940s, physicians began experimenting with early mobilization after a cardiac event, and the results were favorable. Early mobilization of cardiac patients resulted in fewer complications, a faster recovery, and a reduction in many of the other related complications of bed rest mentioned above. Today, exercise is a standard therapeutic modality in the treatment of cardiac disease. In almost all cases,

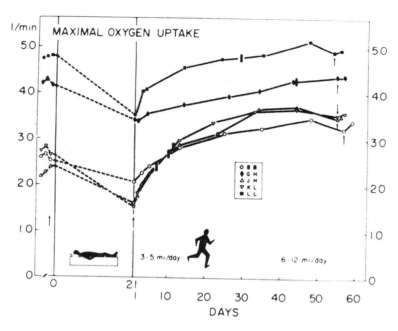

Figure 4 Changes in maximal oxygen uptake with bed rest and training. (From Saltin, B., Blomqvist, G., Mitchell, J. H., et al. *Circulation.* 37–38 (Suppl. 7): 1, 1968. With permission.)

individuals recovering from a myocardial infarction, cardiac surgery, or other cardiac procedure should benefit from a supervised cardiac rehabilitation program.

B. OVERVIEW OF CARDIAC REHABILITATION

The comprehensive rehabilitation of cardiac patients is collectively referred to as "cardiac rehabilitation." *Cardiac rehabilitation* is defined as "the process by which the person with cardiovascular disease, including but not limited to patients with coronary heart disease, is restored to and maintained at his or her optimal physiological, psychological, social, vocational, and emotional status."[1] It is typically divided into three or four phases. Phase 1 is the period directly following the event up until the patient leaves the hospital. During this period the focus is on overcoming deconditioning from bed rest, some education, and recovering from open heart surgery or other event or procedure. During Phase 2 the patient attends regular exercise and education classes. During exercise, the patient is usually continually monitored via electrocardiographic (ECG) telemeter. Phases 3 and 4 are maintenance phases.

C. EXERCISE GUIDELINES AND RECOMMENDATIONS

Exercise guidelines are based on the clinical status of the patient. The reader is referred to more detailed descriptions of setting up an exercise program for all levels of cardiac patients elsewhere.[30] Low–risk cardiac patients should have established stable cardiovascular and physiological responses to exercise. Low-risk is generally classified as those patients who (1) had an uncomplicated clinical course in the hospital, (2) have no evidence of resting or exercise-induced ischemia (ST segment depression), (3) have functional capacities >6 to 8 METs 3 weeks following the clinical event, (4) have normal ventricular function EF > 50%, and (5) do not have any significant resting or exercise-induced ventricular arrhythmias.

Individuals identified with cardiac risk factors need to have a physician release and referral to exercise. Ideally, low-risk cardiac patients should have a treadmill test to determine their functional capacity and cardiovascular status. The treadmill results can then be used to establish a safe exercise level. The exact exercise prescription should be based on the medical history, clinical status, and symptoms of the patients. General guidelines for cardiac patients have been developed by the ACSM.[30]

Intensity: RPE < 13 (6–20 scale)
Post-myocardial infarction: HR < 120 beats/min or HR_{rest} + 20 beats/min
Postsurgery: HR_{rest} + 30beats/min
To tolerance if asymptomatic

Duration: Intermittent bouts lasting 3–5 min

Rest periods (1) at patient's discretion, (2) lasting 1–2 min, (3) shorter than exercise
   bout duration

Total duration up to 20 min

Frequency: Early mobilization: 3–4 times per day (days 1–3)

Later mobilization: 2 times per day (starting day 3)

Progression: Initially increase duration to 10–15 min of continuous exercise, then increase intensity.

VIII. HYPERTENSION

Hypertension is one of the most prevalent chronic diseases in the United States. Hypertensives are individuals classified with chronically elevated blood pressures greater than 140/90 mmHg. As many as 50 million Americans have chronically elevated blood pressure or are taking antihypertensive medication (source: The Fifth Report of the Joint National Committee on Detection, Evaluation, and Treatment of High Blood Pressure). Hypertension is related to the development of CAD, increased severity of atherosclerosis, stroke, congestive heart failure, left ventricular hypertrophy, aortic aneurysms, and peripheral vascular disease (PVD). Hypertension is a serious medical problem if left untreated. Hypertensive individuals have a three to four times risk of developing CAD and up to seven times the risk of having a stroke.[3]

A. ROLE OF EXERCISE AND HYPERTENSION

Exercise training is now recognized as an important part of therapy for controlling hypertension, although the antihypertensive effects of exercise have yielded conflicting results.[22] Regular aerobic exercise appears to reduce both systolic and diastolic blood pressure by an average of 10 mmHg.[2,27,53] Although the exact mechanisms responsible for the reduction in blood pressure following endurance training are not completely understood, it appears that an exercise training–induced reduction in blood pressure can be caused by a reduction in cardiac output and total peripheral resistance at rest[48] and/or reduced sympathetic activity via a reduced plasma norepinephrine secretion.[16,27] Thus, exercise training appears to have an antihypertensive effect via a combination of elevated total resting plasma catecholamine levels and a reduction in cardiac output and total peripheral resistance (via resetting baroreceptors, altered blood volume distribution, changes in the renin–angiotensin axis, and a reduction in sympathetic nervous system activity)[22]

Recently, Hagberg[23] reviewed 33 exercise training studies involving individuals with hypotension. Approximately two thirds of these studies showed an average reduction in resting systolic blood pressure of about 10 mmHg, and 70% of the studies reported a similar drop in diastolic blood pressure. Based on the available literature, the ACSM has recently released a position statement on exercise and hypertension.

> The available evidence indicates that endurance exercise training by individuals at high risk for developing hypertension will reduce the rise in blood pressure that occurs with time. Thus, it is the position of the American College of Sports Medicine that endurance exercise training is recommended as a nonpharmacological strategy to reduce the incidence of hypertension in susceptible individuals. The exercise recommendations to achieve this effect are generally the same as those prescribed for developing and maintaining cardiovascular fitness in healthy adults. However, exercise training at somewhat lower intensities appears to lower blood pressure as much, or more, than exercise at higher intensities, which may be more important in specific hypertensive populations. (Portions adapted from American College of Sports Medicine, *Med. Sci. Sports Exercise*, 25(10), i–x, 1993. With permission.)

B. EXERCISE GUIDELINES AND RECOMMENDATIONS

Since many hypertensive individuals have several CAD risk factors, including obesity, nondrug therapy is usually the first line of treatment. A combination of weight reduction, salt restriction, and increased physical activity has been recommended as treatment for reducing and controlling high blood pressure.[49] Factors to be considered when recommending exercise for hypertensive individuals include (1) clinical status, (2) medications, (3) the frequency, duration, intensity, and mode of exercise the individual is currently participating in, and (4) how well the individual manages his or her hypertension.

1. Exercise Guidelines for Hypertension

1. All hypertensive individuals should be instructed to avoid holding their breath and straining during exercise (Valsalva maneuver).
2. Weight training should be used as a supplement to endurance training, not as the primary exercise. Circuit training is preferred over free weights. The resistance should be kept low and the repetitions high.
3. Exercise intensity may need to be monitored by the RPE scale, since medications can alter the accuracy of the THR during exercise.
4. Any changes in medications and/or any abnormal signs or symptoms before, during, or immediately following exercise should be reported and documented.
5. Physicians will often have patients with documented hypertension record their blood pressures before and after exercise.
6. Individuals with hypertension should be instructed to move slowly when transitioning from the floor to standing, since they are more susceptible to orthostatic hypotension if taking antihypertensive medication.
7. Both hypertensive and hypotensive responses are possible during and after exercise for individuals with hypertension.
8. Individuals with severe hypertension need to be carefully monitored during exercise initially, and possibly long term. Such individuals will likely be taking one or more hypertensive medications which can affect their response to exercise. A detailed treatment plan, including specific exercise guidelines and blood pressure cutoff points, should be developed with the patient's physician and exercise staff so that the exercise training is both safe and effective.
9. Individuals with hypertension may have multiple CAD risk factors, which should be considered when developing the exercise prescription.

2. Sample Exercise Prescription for Hypertension

Mode: The overall exercise training recommendations for mildly to moderately hypertensive individuals are basically the same as for apparently healthy individuals. Endurance exercise, such as low-impact aerobics, walking, and swimming, should be the primary exercise mode. Exercises with an isometric component should be avoided. Weight training can be prescribed and should use low resistance and high repetitions.

Intensity: Low-intensity dynamic exercise vs. high-intensity, high-impact exercise is recommended. The exercise intensity level should should be near the lower end of the heart rate range (40 to 65%).

Frequency: Hypertensives should be encouraged to exercise at least four times per week. Daily exercise may be appropriate for certain individuals with an initial low functional capacity or for elderly persons.

Duration: A longer and more gradual warm-up and cool-down period (>5 min) is recommended. Total exercise duration should be gradually increased, possibly to as high as 30 to 60 min per session, depending on the medical history and clinical status of the individual.

IX. STROKE

Stroke-related events were the third leading cause of death in 1990.[8] Strokes are also referred to as cerebrovascular accidents (CVA). Similar to a myocardial infarction, a stroke affects the arteries of the nervous system, instead of the heart. When nerve cells are deprived of oxygen because of a blockage or rupture of a blood vessel supplying blood to the brain, those cells die within minutes. The results of a stroke can be devastating. Strokes can affect speech, thought patterns and memory, behavioral patterns, sight, and sometimes they paralyze a part of the body. The risk factors for stroke include high blood pressure, heart disease, cigarette smoking, high red blood cell count, and transient ischemic attacks (TIAs).

A. THE ROLE OF EXERCISE AND STROKE

Very little data exist on the role of exercise and stroke. Most of the studies looking at exercise and stroke showed equivocal findings.[10] In general, since the risk factors for stroke are the same as for CAD, exercise may help reduce overall CAD risk and thus lessen the risk for stroke. Since hypertension is the major

Figure 5   Claudication Pain Scale

Grade I	Definite discomfort or pain, but only of initial of modest level (established but minimal)
Grade II	Moderate discomfort or pain from which the patient's attention can be diverted, for example, by conversation
Grade III	Intense pain (short of Grade IV) from which the patient's attention cannot be diverted
Grade IV	Excruciating and unbearable pain

modifiable risk factor for preventing strokes, exercise should be recommended for hypertensive individuals at risk for stroke or for those recovering from a stroke. Approximately 70 to 80% of strokes are caused by a thrombosis. Exercise may also help reduce blood clots via enhanced fibrinolytic activity.[47] Follow the guidelines and recommendations for coronary heart disease and hypertension.

X. PERIPHERAL VASCULAR DISEASE

PVD is caused by atherosclerotic lesions in one or more peripheral (usually in the legs) arterial and/or venous blood vessel. Most PVD patients are older and have long-established CAD risk factors. Common sites for atherosclerotic lesions include the illiac, femoral, and poplital arteries. PVD is 20 times more common in diabetic individuals than in nondiabetic individuals.[8] PVD is a painful and often debilitating disease.

The major symptom of PVD is muscular pain caused by ischemia to the working muscles. This type of ischemia is referred to as claudication. The ischemic pain caused by PVD can be the result of spasms or of occlusive blockages. Some PVD patients experience chronic claudication and pain even at rest. When pain results from physical activity, such as walking, cycling or stair climbing, it is referred to as intermittent claudication. Intermittent claudication is usually relieved by immediate rest. Most PVD patients describe claudication as a dull aching, cramping pain. The claudication pain scale (Figure 5) is a subjective rating of discomfort that can be used to regulate exercise intensity/duration and frequency.[30]

A. ROLE OF EXERCISE AND PERIPHERAL VASCULAR DISEASE

The treatment for PVD usually includes a combination of medication (vasodilating agents), exercise (to improve blood flow and functional capacity), medical procedures (angioplasty, atherorectomy, stents), or surgery (artery bypass). One of the primary benefits of exercise for PVD is to help lower overall CAD risk (hypertension, hypercholesterolemia, etc.). The other principal benefit of exercise for PVD appears to be improved blood flow and overall cardiovascular endurance. Exercise training studies have been shown to improve peak work capacity on exercise testing[26] and walking duration[42] in individuals with PVD.

B. EXERCISE GUIDELINES AND RECOMMENDATIONS

Individuals with PVD should undergo a complete medical evaluation before embarking on an exercise program. Initially, low-intensity, non-weight-bearing activities should be stressed. Individuals with PVD often have a high anxiety level when starting out, because of their chronic pain. As confidence builds with gradual progress, additional activities can be added. Most individuals with PVD don't particularly want to be able to run a marathon; they just want to be able to go shopping, climb stairs, and go for a walk without a great deal of pain. In addition to exercise, other life-style modifications should be stressed in an effort to lower overall CAD risk.

1. Exercise Guidelines for Peripheral Vascular Disease

1. Daily exercise should be encouraged to allow for maximal exercise tolerance, with frequent rest periods.
2. Low-impact, non-weight-bearing activities such as swimming, and cycling are recommended initially. Weight-bearing activities can be added as exercise tolerance improves.
3. Warm water and warm weather exercise and bathing vs. cold is recommended to avoid vasoconstriction.
4. Interval training may be appropriate for some PVD patients initially. This schedule might include one to three bouts of exercise each day (5 to 10 min).
5. Since many PVD patients are also diabetic, they need to take excellent care of their feet.
6. Initially, individuals with PVD should be closely supervised, such as in a cardiac rehabilitation program.
7. PVD patients should be instructed to gradually increase their exercise frequency, duration, and intensity. The degree of progress (absence of pain) will dictate how often and how much to increase these variables.

8. Since walking is the most common form of physical activity most people participate in, PVD patients are encouraged to walk as much and as often as tolerated.
9. As functional capacity improves, the exercise intensity, duration, and frequency can be increased.

2. Sample Exercise Prescription

Mode: Nonimpact endurance exercise, such as swimming and cycling, may allow for longer duration and higher-intensity exercise. Weight-bearing activities are also recommended, but may have to be shorter in duration, and lower in intensity, with more frequent rest periods.

Intensity: Low-intensity vs. high-intensity, high-impact exercise is recommended. PVD patients should exercise to the point of moderate-to-intense pain (Grade II to Grade III on the claudication pain scale). As functional capacity improves, the intensity can be gradually increased.

Frequency: Daily exercise is recommended initially. As functional capacity improves, the frequency can be reduced to 3 to 4 days/week.

Duration: A longer and more gradual warm-up and cool-down (>10 min) is recommended. Total exercise duration should be gradually increased to 30 to 40 min.

XI. DIABETES

Diabetes mellitus is characterized by diminished secretion of insulin by the pancreatic beta cells and/or reduced sensitivity of insulin target cells to insulin. Diabetes mellitus causes abnormalities in the metabolism of carbohydrates, protein, and fat. Diabetes mellitus is a serious disease if left untreated; unfortunately, diabetes mellitus is often asymptomatic in the early stages. Diabetic patients are at greater risk for numerous health problems, including kidney failure, nerve disorders, eye problems, and heart disease.[4] Prolonged and frequent elevation of blood sugar can lead to microangiopathy, a term that refers to damaged capillaries, which in turn leads to poor circulation. In addition, diabetic patients are at greater risk for developing neuropathy, a term referring to damaged nerves, which in turn can lead to permanent nerve damage.

There are two main types of diabetes, insulin-dependent diabetes mellitus (IDDM) and non-insulin-dependent diabetes mellitus (NIDDM). IDDM is caused by destruction of the insulin-producing beta cells in the pancreas, which leads to little or no insulin secretion. IDDM generally occurs in childhood, and regular insulin injections are required to regulate blood glucose levels. NIDDM is the most common form of diabetes, affecting 90% of all diabetic patients. NIDDM typically occurs in adults who are overweight. NIDDM is characterized by a reduced sensitivity of insulin target cells to available insulin. Treatment of NIDDM varies and may include a change in diet, medication, and exercise therapy.

The typical symptoms of IDDM include excessive thirst and hunger, frequent urination, weight loss, blurred vision, and recurrent infections. During periods of insulin deficiency, a higher than normal level of glucose remains in the blood because of decreased uptake and storage. A portion of the excess glucose is excreted in the urine, which leads to increased thirst, weight loss, and increased appetite. During periods of hyperglycemia, normal carbohydrate metabolism is altered, and the body relies on the catabolism of lipids and proteins in an effort to provide energy. The increased catabolism of fats and proteins produces high levels of triglycerides and free fatty acids in the plasma which can eventually lead to acidosis and the production of ketone bodies. Ketone bodies are a group of compounds (acetoacetic acid, beta-hydroxybutyric acid, and acetone) produced during the oxidation of fatty acids. The presence of ketosis can be detected easily by the fruity odor of breath. Frequent states of ketosis take a toll on the body because of the breakdown of lean tissue.

NIDDM is also characterized by frequent states of hyperglycemia, but without the increased catabolism of fats and protein. Typical NIDDM individuals are over 30 years of age, obese, and present with few, if any, classic symptoms of diabetes. They are not prone to ketoacidosis. Because 75% of NIDDM individuals are obese, or have a history of obesity, NIDDM is often reversible with permanent weight loss.

A. EFFECTIVE DIABETIC CONTROL

Effective diabetic control is based on long-term regulation of blood glucose levels. Glucose regulation in IDDM is achieved through regular glucose assessment, proper diet, exercise, and appropriate insulin medication. For NIDDM, glucose regulation is achieved through a change in life-style centered around proper diet, weight loss/control, exercise, and insulin or oral agents if needed.[5] A combined diet and exercise regimen results in weight loss and weight control, improvement in cardiorespiratory fitness, reduced need for insulin, improved self-image, and better ability to deal with stress.

B. ROLE OF EXERCISE AND DIABETES
1. IDDM
A complete understanding of the benefits of exercise training for individuals with IDDM is still unclear. While it has been shown that individuals with IDDM can improve their functional capacity, reduce their risk for CAD, and improve insulin receptor sensitivity and receptor number, the role of exercise in improving glucose control has not been well demonstrated.[51] The American Diabetes Association position stand on exercise for IDDM states that:

> Exercise programs have not been exclusively shown to improve glycemic control in people with IDDM. However, IDDM individuals should be encouraged to exercise because of the potential to improve cardiovascular fitness and psychological well-being and for social interaction and recreation. (From Position Statement on Diabetes Mellitus and Exercise. American Diabetes Association, 1993.)

2. NIDDM
The understanding of exercise and NIDDM is much clearer. Exercise plays an important role in control of diabetes for those with NIDDM. The primary benefit of exercise for individuals with NIDDM is the effect it has on reducing cholesterol levels and weight. With excessive blood glucose elevation, blood fats rise to become the primary energy source for the body. Since diabetic individuals are prone to having higher than normal blood fat levels, they are also at higher risk for heart disease. The American Diabetes Association position stand on exercise for NIDDM states that:

> An appropriate exercise program should be an adjunct to diet/or drug therapy to improve glycemic control, reduce certain cardiovascular risk factors, and increase psychological well-being in individuals with NIDDM. Patients who are most likely to respond favorably are those with mildly to moderately impaired glucose tolerance and hyperinsulinemia. This recommendation is based on the premise that the benefits of exercise outweigh the risks. (From Position Statement on Diabetes Mellitus and Exercise. American Diabetes Association, 1993.)

C. EXERCISE PROGRAM DESIGN CONSIDERATIONS
Before beginning an exercise program, diabetic individuals should speak with their physician or diabetes educator to develop a program of diet, exercise, and medications. The primary goal of exercise for individuals with IDDM should be better glucose regulation and reduced heart disease risk. For IDDM the timing of exercise, the amount of insulin injected, and the injection site are important considerations before exercising. Exercise should be performed daily so that a regular pattern of diet and insulin dosage can be maintained. Since the frequency and duration of exercise are lower for the IDDM patient, the intensity can be slightly higher than for the NIDDM patient.

The primary goal of exercise for the NIDDM patient is weight loss and control. Approximately 80% of NIDDM patients are overweight. By losing weight through the combined effect of diet and exercise, NIDDM patients will reduce the amount of oral insulin medication needed. The primary objective during exercise for the NIDDM patient is caloric expenditure. Maximizing caloric expenditure is best achieved by low–intensity, long–duration exercise. Since the frequency and duration of exercise are high for NIDDM patients, the intensity of exercise should be kept low.

1. Exercise Guidelines for Diabetes
1. Individuals with diabetes requiring insulin injections should not be injected in primary muscle groups that will be used during exercise. This regimen can cause the insulin to be absorbed too quickly, resulting in hypoglycemia.
2. Individuals with diabetes need to check their blood glucose levels frequently. Individuals with diabetes need to work closely with their physician to determine the right insulin dosage, based in part on the blood glucose levels before and after exercise.
3. Individuals with diabetes should be encouraged to always carry a rapid-acting carbohydrate (such as juice or candy) to correct for hypoglycemia.
4. Individuals with diabetes should be encouraged to exercise at the same time of day for better control.
5. Exercise should be avoided during peak insulin activity.
6. Carbohydrate snacks should be consumed before and during prolonged exercise.

7. Individuals with diabetes need to take very good care of their feet. Feet should be regularly checked for any cuts, blisters, or signs of infection. Good-quality exercise shoes are also very important.

2. Sample Exercise Prescription

Mode: Endurance activities, such as walking, swimming and cycling

Intensity: 50–60% VO$_2$max gradually working up to 60–70% VO$_2$max

Frequency: 5–7 days/week for IDDM, and 4–5 days/week for NIDDM; may need to start out with several daily sessions

Duration: IDDM should gradually work up to 20–30 min per session. For NIDDM, 40–60 min is recommended. The goal of individuals with NIDDM is caloric expenditure if they are obese.

D. SPECIAL PRECAUTIONS FOR EXERCISE AND DIABETES

For the individual with IDDM, two potential problems can occur during or following exercise. First, lack of insulin may cause a hyperglycemic effect. Hyperglycemia occurs when there is insufficient insulin to mobilize glucose, and glucose levels become elevated to dangerous levels. A second potential problem that can occur is when insulin is mobilized too quickly, thus leading to lowering of the blood glucose to a dangerous level. A low blood glucose level is referred to as hypoglycemia. One of the first rules for the insulin-dependent diabetic individual is to either reduce insulin intake or increase carbohydrate intake before exercise. For both types of diabetes, exercise should begin 1 to 2 h after a meal and before peak insulin activity. Usually insulin dosages must be decreased prior to exercise, since exercise has an insulin-like effect. The golden rules of glucose regulation during exercise are to check blood glucose levels frequently when starting an exercise program and to be aware of any unusual symptoms prior to, during, or after exercise.

XII. ASTHMA

Asthma is a reactive airway disease characterized by shortness of breath, coughing, and wheezing. It is due to (1) constriction of the smooth muscle around the airways, (2) a swelling of the mucosal cells, and/or (3) increased secretion of mucus. Asthma can be caused by an allergic reaction, exercise, infections, emotion, or other environmental irritants, such as pollens, inhalants, cigarette smoke, and air pollution. Asthma is one of the most common respiratory disorders, affecting as many as 1 to 2% of adults and 5 to 7% of children.[50]

Approximately 80% of individuals with asthma experience asthma attacks during exercise testing, a term referred to as exercise induced asthma (EIA).[6] EIA is defined as 15% or greater postexercise reduction of either FEV$_1$ or peak expiratory flow rate on preexercise values after exercise testing.[35] EIA attacks are typically characterized by moderate obstruction and are not life threatening. The severity of an EIA attack is related to the intensity of exercise and the ventilatory requirement of the task, as well as the environmental conditions. Breathing in cold, dry air vs. warm, moist air seems to cause greater airway obstruction.

The exact cause of EIA is not well understood, but it is believed to be caused by drying of the airways as moisture is absorbed from the air as it passes from the nose to the alveolar regions. As the airways become dryer, the osmolarity of the periciliary fluid changes, causing a release of bronchoactive mediators and risk of an EIA increase.[24] Asthma is not a contraindication to exercise; however, before starting an exercise program, individuals with asthma should develop a plan for exercise with their physician. Several studies have shown that regular exercise can reduce the number and severity of asthma attacks during exercise.[19,20]

A. ROLE OF EXERCISE AND ASTHMA

Individuals with controlled asthma should benefit from regular exercise. Although individuals with asthma are more more likely to experience breathlessness during exercise, this should not stop them from exercising. During exercise, some individuals with asthma will get short of breath because of the cooling effect in the airways caused by the large volumes of inspired air and also because of the evaporation of water in the respiratory tract. Exercise may help to reduce the ventilatory requirement for various tasks, making it easier for individuals with asthma to participate in normal daily activities with less shortness of breath, and possibly fewer asthma attacks.

B. EXERCISE GUIDELINES AND RECOMMENDATIONS
1. Exercise Guidelines for Asthma

1. Before starting an exercise program, individuals with asthma must have a medication/treatment plan to prevent EIA attacks.
2. Individuals with asthma should have a bronchodilating inhaler with them at all times and be instructed to use it at the first sign of wheezing.
3. The exercise intensity should be kept low to begin, and gradually increased over time. Intensity of exercise is directly linked to the severity and frequency of EIA.
4. The exercise intensity should be reduced if asthma symptoms occur.
5. Using an inhaler several minutes before exercise may reduce the possibility of an EIA attack.
6. The results of pulmonary exercise testing should be used to design the appropriate exercise prescription.
7. Individuals with asthma should drink plenty of fluids before and during exercise.
8. An extended warm-up and cool-down period should be encouraged with individuals with asthma.
9. Individuals with respiratory disorders will often experience more symptoms of respiratory distress when exercising in extreme environmental conditions (high or low temperature, high pollen count, and heavy air pollution).
10. Individuals with respiratory disorders need to be carefully followed by their physician.
11. Only individuals with stable asthma should exercise.
12. If an asthma attack is not relieved by medication, the individuals with asthma should be transported to a medical facility immediately or an ambulance should be called.
13. Wearing a face mask during exercise helps in maintaining a warmer and moister inspired air and can minimize asthmatic responses during exercise.

2. Sample Exercise Prescription

Mode: Dynamic exercise, walking, cycling, and swimming. Upper-body exercises such as arm cranking, rowing, and cross-country skiing may not be appropriate because of the higher ventilation demands. Swimming may be particularly beneficial because it allows individuals with asthma to inhale moist air above the surface of the water.

Intensity: Low-intensity dynamic exercise vs. high-intensity, high-impact exercise is recommended. The exercise intensity should be prescribed based on the client's fitness status and limitations.

Frequency: Individuals with asthma should be encouraged to exercise at least three to four times per week. Those with low functional capacities or those who experience shortness of breath during prolonged exercise may benefit from intermittent exercise (two 10-min sessions).

Duration: Encourage a longer and more gradual warm-up and cool down (>10 min). Total exercise duration should be gradually increased to 20 to 45 min.

XIII. BRONCHITIS AND EMPHYSEMA

Bronchitis is a form of obstructive pulmonary disease. Bronchitis is a chronic inflammation of the bronchial tubes. The major cause is due to cigarette smoking, whereas air pollution and occupational exposure play lesser roles. Acute bronchitis is an inflammation of the mucous membranes of the bronchial tubes, as well. However, an acute bout of bronchitis can develop following a cold or exposure to certain dust particles or fumes and can resolve in several days or weeks. Chronic bronchitis persists for a lifetime in most cases. Emphysema is another form of chronic pulmonary disease caused by overinflation of the alveoli. The overinflation results from a breakdown of the walls of the alveoli, which causes a significant decrease in respiratory function. The classic signs of emphysema are chronic breathlessness and coughing. Bronchitis and emphysema are collectively referred to as chronic obstructive pulmonary diseases, or COPD.

A. ROLE OF EXERCISE AND COPD

Individuals with chronic bronchitis and emphysema "may" benefit from mild exercise training. However, individuals with COPD may not receive any benefits from aerobic exercise, because of the severity of their disease. Individuals with COPD need to be carefully screened and followed by a physician. Most individuals with COPD do not improve their pulmonary function. However, other benefits such as reduced anxiety, body weight, and stress and an improved ability to perform in normal daily activities can be realized through exercise in patients suffering from COPD. The primary goals of exercise training for individuals with COPD are (1) increased functional capacity, (2) increased functional status, (3) decreased severity of dyspnea, and (4) improved quality of life.[43]

Individuals with COPD who are stable, and who have obtained all the potential benefits from a medically supervised exercise program, should benefit from participating in nonmedically supervised exercise. Individuals with COPD should be encouraged to "do the best they can," because every little bit of exercise they do can result in potential health benefits.

B. EXERCISE GUIDELINES AND RECOMMENDATIONS
1. Exercise Guidelines for COPD

1. Before starting an exercise program, individuals with COPD need to have extensive pulmonary tests completed.
2. Only stable COPD patients should be allowed to participate in a nonmedical setting.
3. The exercise intensity and type of exercise should be carefully chosen to avoid developing shortness of breath. For a complete review of strategies for setting exercise intensity for pulmonary patients see ACSM, *Guidelines for Exercise Testing and Prescription*, 5th edition, pp. 196–197.
4. The guidelines for working with asthmatic patients should also be considered.
5. Only individuals who are fully recovered from an acute bout of bronchitis should exercise.
6. Individuals with COPD should have a bronchodilating inhaler with them at all times and be instructed to use it at the first sign of wheezing.
7. Individuals with COPD should also perform their breathing exercises to help strengthen their respiratory muscles.
8. Upper-body exercises such as arm cranking or rowing should be avoided initially because of the increased strain on the pulmonary system. Upper-body resistance training should, however, be gradually added to a comprehensive exercise program.
9. Some individuals with COPD may require supplemental oxygen during exercise. Generally, supplemental oxygen is recommended for patients with a $P_aO_2 < 55$ mmHg or $S_aO_2 < 88\%$ while breathing room air.
10. COPD clients must not smoke.
11. The type and dose of medications should be reviewed with the client's physician, based on the client's response to exercise.
12. If COPD clients' performance in a nonmedical supervised program worsens, they should be encouraged to participate in a pulmonary rehabilitation program, until such time as their signs and symptoms have improved.

2. Sample Exercise Prescription

Mode: Dynamic exercise, walking, and stationary cycling. Upper-body exercises such as arm cranking, rowing, and cross-country skiing may not be appropriate initially because of the higher ventilation demands. Gradually, upper resistance exercises should be added.

Intensity: Low-intensity dynamic exercise vs. high-intensity, high-impact exercise is generally recommended. The exercise intensity should be carefully prescribed based on the client's breathing responses to exercise. The exercise intensity should be kept below the point where any difficulty in breathing is experienced.

Frequency: Individuals should be encouraged to exercise at least four to five times per week. COPD clients usually benefit from intermittent exercise sessions.

Duration: Encourage a longer and more gradual warm-up and cool-down (>10 min). Total exercise duration should be gradually increased to 20 to 30 min.

XIV. CANCER

Cancer affects one out of every four people in the United States. In 1990 more than 1 million Americans were diagnosed as having cancer, and about half that number of cancer deaths were recorded. It has been estimated that 80% of all cancers may be avoided by life-style choices and changes. For example, regular exercise, a low-fat/high-fiber diet, and the avoidance of smoking all help reduce the risk of developing cancer. The role of diet and exercise appears to be particularly important in reducing the risk for cancer. Dietary changes can reduce the risk of developing bowel cancer, the second most common cause of cancer overall. The leading cause of lung cancer in the United States is cigarette smoking. Thus, it appears that many types of cancers are highly preventable.

A. ROLE OF EXERCISE AND CANCER

In general, physically inactive people have greater rates of cancer. Paffenbarger et al.[38] found in their Harvard alumni study that cancer mortality was the highest in those who exercised least, even after age and cigarette smoking were considered. Sternfeld[46] recently found that of the 12 studies he reviewed, 7 demonstrated an inverse relationship between physical activity and all-cause mortality. A recent study by Blair et al.[9] revealed a relative risk for all-cancer mortality of 4.3 for men and 16.3 for women when least-fit individuals were compared with the most fit based on maximal treadmill testing.

Bartram and Wynder[7] recently reviewed the evidence linking physical activity and colon cancer. Physical activity decreases the transit time in the colon, thus possibly decreasing the exposure of the colon to potential carcinogens. Physical activity has also been shown to increase secretion of prostaglandins which have a protective effect against colon cancer.[7] There is also evidence to suggest that breast cancer and cancers of the reproductive system in women appear to be inversely related with physical activity.[46] Another mechanism by which exercise may have a protective effect against cancer is through the strengthening of the immune system. Several studies have shown an improvement in immune function following exercise.[17,44,45]

B. EXERCISE GUIDELINES AND RECOMMENDATIONS

No specific guidelines for exercise and cancer are available. Winningham[52] recommends asking six questions before designing an exercise program for cancer patients:

- Are there limitations to activity based on preexisting conditions?
- Are there limitations to activity based on medical procedures undergone by the patient?
- Are there limitations in mobility as a result of disease or treatment?
- Are there limitations in oxygen delivery as a result of disease or treatment?
- Are there limitations in activity as a result of nutritional and fluid deficits?
- Are there limitations based on risk for anemia, bleeding, and infections?

If individuals have any limitations based on the conditions listed above, the exercise prescription should be adjusted accordingly.

XV. OSTEOPOROSIS

Osteoporosis is a major public health problem. Osteoporosis is age related, but not gender specific. Osteoporosis in men has not been as widely investigated, as has postmenopausal osteoporosis in women. Osteoporosis is characterized by decreased bone mass and increased susceptibility to fractures. Fractures occur more commonly in men than women before 45 years of age and more commonly in women than men after 45 years or age.[28] Osteoporosis affects anywhere from 15 to 20 million Americans resulting in an estimated cost of $3.8 billion a year due primarily to hip fractures.[12]

Osteoporosis is primarily caused by decreased bone mass which increases the susceptibility of individuals to fractures. After reaching its peak, bone mass declines throughout life because of an imbalance of "remodeling" of the bone. Remodeling refers to the replacement of old bone with new bone. Osteoclasts reabsorb bone in microscopic cavities; osteoblasts then reform the bone surfaces, filling the cavities. Bone remodeling serves to keep the skeletal system in peak form and to help maintain Ca^{2+} homeostasis. Mechanical and electrical factors, hormones, and local regulatory factors influence remodeling.

A. ROLE OF EXERCISE AND OSTEOPOROSIS

The treatment for osteoporosis tries to prevent or retard bone mineral loss. Estrogen replacement is highly effective in preventing osteoporosis in women. Estrogen reduces bone resorption and retards or halts postmenopausal bone loss. Premenopausal women should consume 1000 to 1500 mg/day of calcium. High dietary calcium intake suppresses age-related bone loss. The importance of exercise in prevention and treatment of osteoprosis remains unclear. However, it is known that physical stress determines the strength of bone. Physical inactivity is a known risk factor for osteoporosis; thus, exercise is recommended for the prevention and treatment of osteoporosis. Weight-bearing exercise either retards loss or increases bone mass. Even individuals who have led sedentary lives can increase bone mass by becoming more active. The greater the physical stress and compression on a bone, the greater the rate of bone deposition (this is why weight bearing exercise is recommended).

XVI. LOW-BACK PAIN

Back injuries, including sprains and strains, are the number one disability for people under age 45 years. It has been estimated that 80% of the population will experience an episode of low-back pain (LBP) some time in their lives. Of the 80%, 5% will go on to develop chronic LBP.[21] LBP accounts for 10% of all chronic health conditions in the United States and 25% of days lost from work. LBP has been referred to by medical experts as the most expensive benign health condition in the United States.[40]

Back injuries translate into millions of lost work days every year and cost billions for medical care, disability payments, and legal payments. Reducing back injury rates is a top priority for all employers. In fact, the most common type of workers' compensation claim is a back strain/sprain, which accounts for up to 25% of all claims, representing annual payments of $2.5 to 7 billion, including one half of all disability compensation payments annually! In addition, nearly 2% of the U.S. work force files compensation claims for back problems.

The causes of LBP are often elusive, but four common causes are herniated disk (rupture of the outer layers of fibers which surround the gelatinous portion of the disk), spondylolisthesis (forward sliding of the body of one vertebra on the vertebra below it), trauma to the back (accident), and degenerative disk disease (progressive structural degeneration of the intervertebral disk). Lower-back problems are often associated with an imbalance of strength and flexibility of the lower back and abdominal muscle groups. Poor flexibility of the hamstring and hip flexor muscles has also been linked to LBP.

A. ROLE OF EXERCISE AND LBP

It appears that physical fitness combined with a healthy life-style may help prevent LBP. In fact, many physicians feel that the major cause of chronic LBP is simply physical deconditioning. More specifically, low endurance of large muscle groups, particularly the back extensors, seems to put one at a greater risk of developing LBP. Exercises for the low back should be performed on a regular basis to gain maximal benefits. Aerobic conditioning has also been found to be important in the treatment and prevention of LBP.[11] In addition, a strong correlation exists between body weight, smoking, and decreased physical activity and LBP.[15] Regular exercise appears important in the prevention and treatment of LBP.

B. PROGRAM DESIGN CONSIDERATIONS

Exercise participants should be screened for low-back risk factors. Prevention is the key to avoiding LBP. Listed below are some commonsense tips that are helpful in the prevention LBP. If someone has experienced a recent low-back strain or injury, they should be cleared by a physician before starting an exercise program. In addition, basic core back exercise should be performed on a regular basis, as well as a regular program of aerobic and resistance training.

1. Exercise Guidelines for LBP

1. Always be aware of proper form and alignment.
2. Always maintain pelvic neutral alignment and an erect torso during any exercise movements.
3. Avoid head-forward positions in which the chin is tilted up.
4. When leaning forward, lifting, or lowering an object, always bend at the knees.
5. Avoid hyperextending the spine in an unsupported position.
6. Allow for an adequate warm-up and cool-down period during all exercise classes.
7. Most LBP is caused by muscle weaknesses and imbalances, including tight hamstring and lower-back muscle groups, tight hip flexor muscles, and weak abdominal and lower-back muscles. Exercises should be routinely performed to improve muscle strength and flexibility.
8. Individuals who experience LBP or have a history of chronic LBP should be advised to consult with a physician and get specific recommendations for exercises.
9. If someone complains of LBP following an exercise class, have him or her sit or lie down in a comfortable position and apply ice to the affected area. Following a mild back strain, individuals should be encouraged to take several days off from exercise.

2. Exercises for the Low Back

Position: Supine with knees bent
Activity: Slowly pull one knee to chest and hold for 5 s; then do the same with the other knee.
Position: Supine, with knees bent and legs together
Activity: Slowly rotate knees from side to side while keeping them together.
Position: Hands and knees
Activity: Arch your back up like a cat, hold 5 s and relax.
Position: Hands and knees
Activity: Slowly sit back between your knees and then return to hands and knees.
Position: Hands and knees
Activity: Slowly bring one knee to the chest; then extend the leg straight out behind you. Repeat on the other side.
Position: Standing against the wall
Activity: Squat down so that your lower back is pressed against the wall. Move your feet out from the wall and bend your legs to a "half-squat" and hold. Gradually straighten legs out and repeat.
Position: Lying on your stomach, legs and arms straight out
Activity: Lift one arm, hold, and relax. Alternate arms.
Lift one leg, hold, and relax. Alternate legs.
Lift one arm and one leg on opposite sides, hold, and relax. Alternate sides.
Position: Supine, with knees slightly bent
Activity: Flatten your back against the floor by contracting your stomach muscles and rotating your hips backward.

Additional activities: side stretches, sit-ups, modified push-ups, lateral leg raises, groin stretches, hamstring stretches, calf stretches, and quadriceps stretches.

XVII. ARTHRITIS

Although there are different forms of arthritis, the most common forms are rheumatoid and osteoarthritis. Osteoarthritis, also referred to as degenerative joint disease, is a degenerative process caused by the wearing away of cartilage, leaving two surfaces of bone in contact with each other. Osteoarthritis is very common in older individuals affecting 85% of all people in the United States over the age of 70 years. Rheumatoid arthritis is caused by an inflammation of the membrane surrounding joints. It is often associated with pain and swelling in one or more joints. Rheumatoid arthritis affects about 3% of all women and 1% of all men in the United States.

The treatment for arthritis depends on the severity and specific form of arthritis. Individuals with arthritis can be classified in four categories of functional capacity (Table 7). Individuals in class 1 and 2 often are able to carry out their normal activities of daily living (ADLs) with little discomfort, while those in class 3 and 4 typically have serious limitations in what they can do. The treatment for arthritis often involves medicine (gold-based drugs, such as penicillamine, and steroids, such as corticosteroids), physical therapy, physiotherapy (TENS and hot packs), occupational therapy (improve ADLs), and, lastly, surgery (joint replacement). The benefits of exercise include stronger muscles and bones, improved cardiorespiratory fitness, and improved psychosocial well-being.[39] Exercise is contraindicated during inflammatory periods because exercise can worsen the process.

A. ROLE OF EXERCISE AND ARTHRITIS

Exercise is recommended for clients with arthritis to help preserve muscle strength and joint mobility, to improve functional capabilities, to relieve pain and stiffness, to prevent further deformities, to improve overall physical conditioning, to reestablish neuromuscular coordination, and to mobilize stiff or contracted joints. Improvement of function and pain relief are the ultimate goals.

Fitness programs should be carefully designed by the physician or physical therapist. The exercise prescription needs to be developed based on the functional status of the individual. For example, someone in functional class 1 should be able to perform most activities that a typical healthy person can. For those in functional class 2, initially non-weight-bearing activities are recommended, such as cycling,

Table 7 Classification of Functional Capacity for Arthritis

Class 1	Complete ability to carry on all usual duties without handicaps
Class 2	Adequate ability for normal activities despite handicap, discomfort, or limited motion at one or more joints
Class 3	Ability limited to little or none of the duties of usual occupational or to self-care
Class 4	Incapacitated, largely or wholly. Bedridden or confined to a wheelchair; little or no self-care

From Kelley, W. N., Harris, E. D., Ruddy, S. and Siedre, C. B., Eds., *Textbook of Rheumatism, 4th ed.,* Philadelphia, PA: Saunders, 1993. With permission.

heated pool exercise, and eventually walking.[14,18,29,34] Individuals in functional class 3 should benefit from a cycling or swimming program. Exercise should be avoided during an acute arthritic flare. Individuals with arthritis often report fatigue and some discomfort as common complaints following exercise. Exercise programs need to balance rest, immobilization of affected joints, and exercise to reduce the severity of the inflammatory joint disease.

B. EXERCISE GUIDELINES AND RECOMMENDATIONS
1. Exercise Guidelines for Arthritis

1. Individuals with arthritis should be encouraged to participate in classes where quick or excessive movement can be avoided, such as low-impact or water exercise classes.
2. Exercise session should begin at a low intensity with frequent sessions.
3. Exercise intensity and duration should be reduced during periods of inflammation or pain.
4. Individuals with arthritis may need an extended warm-up and cool-down period.
5. The exercise session should be modified in terms of intensity and duration according to how well the client responds, changes in medication, and the disease and pain levels.
6. Try to tailor the stretching portion of the exercise class to focus on the arthritic joints.
7. Have individuals take a day or two of rest if they continue to complain about pain during or following an exercise session.
8. Individuals with arthritis are encouraged to participate in different forms of aerobic exercise such as swimming, cycling, and walking.
9. Proper body alignment during exercise is important.
10. Poor posture can predispose clients to muscle aches and pains, which will limit the amount of exercise they can perform.
11. Pain is quite normal in people with arthritis. Individuals should be instructed to work just up to the point of pain, but not past it. Simple movements for healthy people can be quite painful for individuals with arthritis.
12. If certain movements are too difficult, isometric exercises should be encouraged. Rubber tubing can also be used to add resistance.
13. It is essential to put all joints through a range of motion at least once a day to maintain mobility.
14. Individuals with arthritis need to report any changes in their medications, medical plan, or response to exercise.
15. Individuals with rheumatoid arthritis should not exercise during periods of inflammation.
16. Proper body mechanics should always be taught and reinforced.
17. Regular rest periods should be stressed during exercise sessions.
18. If severe pain persists following exercise, have the client consult with a physician.

2. Sample Exercise Prescription

Mode: Non-weight-bearing activities such as cycling and swimming are preferred because they reduce joint stress.

Intensity: Low-intensity dynamic exercise vs. high-intensity, high-impact exercise is recommended. The exercise intensity should be carefully prescribed based on the client's pain tolerance before, during, and after exercise.

Frequency: Arthritic individuals should be encouraged to exercise at least four to five times per week. Arthritic clients usually benefit from frequent exercise sessions (daily).

Duration: Encourage a longer and more gradual warm-up and cool-down (>10 min). Total exercise duration should start out short, 10 to 15 min.

Table 8   Effects of Exercise and Aging on Select Body Systems

Body System	Exercise	Aging
Circulatory/cardiovascular		
Maximal oxygen consumption	Increase	Decrease
Maximal heart rate	Increase	Decrease
Cardiac output	Increase	Decrease
Blood pressure	Same or decrease	Increase
Vascular resistance	Decrease	Increase
Blood components		
Serum lipids		
Total cholesterol	?[a]	Increase
Triglycerides	Decrease	Increase
LDL-C	?	Increase?
HDL-C	Increase	Decrease?
Immune system	Increase	Decrease
Musculoskeletal		
Muscles		
Strength	Increase	Decrease
Endurance	Increase	Unchanged
Flexibility	Increase	Decrease
Bony structures		
Bone mineral content	Increase	Decrease
Body composition		
Lean body mass	Increase	Decrease
Adipose tissue	Decrease	Increase
Regulatory system		
Metabolic		
BMR	Increase	Decrease
Heat gain	Increase	Decrease
Heat loss	Increase	Decrease
Nervous		
Sleep	Increase?	Decrease
Anxiety/depression	Decrease?	Increase?
Cognitive functioning	Increase	Decrease

[a]   ? = Inconclusive or inadequate evidence.

XVIII. EXERCISE PRESCRIPTION CONSIDERATIONS FOR THE ELDERLY

Before starting an exercise program, elderly individuals should first see their physician. Although Table 8 lists some of the effects of exercise and aging on selected body systems, many of the effects are inconclusive. Further research needs to validate these, as well as other effects of exercise on aging. Although many of the principles of prescribing exercise to the elderly are the same as for any group, special care should be given when setting up a fitness program for older participants. A preexercise evaluation may involve a complete medical history, a physical, and a treadmill test. The results of the treadmill test can be used to develop the exercise prescription. For most elderly patients, low-impact exercise is advisable. Exercise programs should be tailored to combine endurance, muscle strength, and joint mobilization in the exercise sessions. Older individuals should be encouraged to become more physically active in all of their daily activities (use the stairs, walk to the store, etc.). Older individuals should be encouraged to bend, move and stretch in order to keep joints flexible.

A. GROUP EXERCISE GUIDELINES FOR SENIORS

1. All movement should be slow to moderately paced. For choreographed routines, steps should be simple and repeated often. Fast transitions from one type of movement to another should be avoided to prevent postural hypotension and subsequent dizziness, falling, or fainting.
2. Several modes and positions of exercise should be used. Some positions include standing, sitting, standing with a chair for balance, and floor exercise using a mat. Prior to initiating floor exercise, feedback should be solicited from the group on whether or not the exercise is desirable. Some adults feel awkward or embarrassed if they have difficulty getting up from the floor in front of their peers. Instruction in how to get up from the floor may be necessary.

3. A variety of equipment should be used to achieve program objectives and sustain motivation. Examples include wands or dowels, surgical tubing, towels, or rubber strips for flexibility and range of motion; Frisbees and low walking beams for balance and coordination; and 1-lb weights for strength.
4. The pressor reflex should be avoided by keeping the overhead position of the arms to a minimum.
5. Special precaution should be taken for all participants who take medications. These include cardiovascular drugs, such as beta blockers, calcium channel blockers, and diuretics, which affect exercise tolerance. Hypotension may develop if a participant exercises soon after taking nitroglycerin. The dose, type, and time of administration of insulin may need to be changed to prevent hypoglycemia. Medical approval and ongoing medical consultation for those on prescription drugs are recommended.
6. The exertion level of all participants should be continually monitored. Heart rate monitoring should be taught using the radial or carotid pulse. Permission to rest and get a drink of water should be given throughout the exercise class. Participants should be told frequently to progress at their own rate.
7. In addition to the instructor, one additional staff member should always be present to observe participants' physical reactions and to assist with any major or minor emergency.
8. The use of layered clothing should be suggested to prevent overheating or cooling. Older adults are less tolerant of the heat and cold.
9. A microphone should be used when conducting a program in a large area if the acoustics are poor. Lower tones can be more readily heard by the older adult.
10. For visual charts viewed from a distance, colors such as yellow, orange, and red are seen more clearly.
11. The instructor should be certified in CPR, and a well-defined emergency plan should exist.

B. SPECIAL PRECAUTIONS
Particular care should be given when prescribing weight-lifting exercises to those with high blood pressure, heart disease, or arthritis. Encourage an extended cool-down period, approximately 10 to 15 min. Elderly individuals often have a more difficult time when exercising in extreme environmental conditions. Avoid exercising in these conditions if possible. Some elderly individuals with arthritis or poor joint mobility may have to participate in non-weight-bearing activities, such as cycling, swimming, and chair and floor exercises.

REFERENCES

1. American Association of Cardiovascular and Pulmonary Rehabilitation. *Guidelines for Cardiac Rehabilitation Programs,* 2nd edition. Champaign, IL: Human Kinetics, 1995.
2. American College of Sports Medicine. Position stand "physical activity, physical fitness, and hypertension." *Med. Sci. Sports Exercise.* 25(10): i–x, 1993.
3. American Heart Association. *1993 Heart and Stroke Facts Statistics.* Dallas, TX: American Heart Association, 1992.
4. American Diabetes Association. *Physician's Guide to Non-Insulin-Dependent (Type II) Diabetes: Diagnosis and Treatment.* Alexandria, VA: American Diabetes Association, 1988.
5. American Diabetes Association. *Standards of Medical Care for Patients with Diabetes Mellitus. 1992–93 Clinical Practice Recommendations.* Alexandria, VA: American Diabetes Association, 1993.
6. Anderson, S. D., M. Silverman, P. Konig, and S. Godfrey. Exercise-induced asthma: a review. *Br. J. Dis. Chest.* 69: 1, 1975.
7. Bartram, H. P. and E. L. Wynder. Physical activity and colon cancer risk? Physiological consideration. *Am. J. Gastroenterol.* 84: 109, 1989.
8. Beach, K. W., G. R. Bedford, R. O. Berlin, et al. Progression of lower extremity arterial occlusion disease in type II diabetes mellitus. *Diabetes Care.* 11: 464–472, 1988.
9. Blair, S. N., H. W. Kohl, R. S. Pafffenbarger, D. G. Clark, K. H. Cooper, and L. W. Gibbons. Physical fitness and all-causes mortality: a prospective study of healthy men and women. *J. Am. Med. Assoc.* 262: 2395, 1989.
10. Blair, S. N., H. W. Kohl, N. F. Gordon and R. S. Paffenbarger. How much physical activity is good for health? *Ann. Rev. Public Health.* 13: 99, 1992.
11. Cady, L. D., D. P. Bischoff, E. R. O'Connell, P. C. Thomas, and J. K. Allan. Strength and fitness and subsequent back injuries in fire-fighters. *J. Occup. Med.* 21: 269–275, 1979.
12. Christiansen, C. Consensus Development Conference on Osteoporosis. *Am J. Med.* 95(5A), 1993.
13. Dail, D. H. and S. P. Hammar (editors). *Pulmonary Pathology.* New York: Springer-Verlag, 1988.
14. Danneskiold-Samsoe, B., K. Lyngberg, T. Risum and M. Telling. The effect of water exercise therapy given to patients with rheumatoid arthritis. *Scand. J. Rehabil. Med.* 19: 31–35, 1987.
15. Deyo, R. A. and J. E. Bass. Lifestyle and low back pain: the influence of smoking, exercise and obesity. *Clin. Res.* 35: 577A, 1987.

16. Duncan, J. J., J. E. Farr, J. Upton, R. D. Hagan, M. E. Oglesby and S. N. Blair. The effects of aerobic exercise on plasma catecholamines and blood pressure in patients with mild hypertension. *J. Am. Med. Assoc.* 254: 2609–2613, 1985.

17. Edwards, A. J., T. H. Bacon, C. A. Elms, R. Verardi, M. Felder and S. C. Knight. Changes in the populations of lymphoid cells in human peripheral blood following physical exercise. *Clin. Exp. Immunol.* 58: 420, 1984.

18. Ekdahl, C., S. I. Andersson, U. Mortiz and B. Svensson. Dynamic versus static training in patients with rheumatoid arthritis. *Scand. J. Rheumatol.* 19: 17–26, 1990.

19. Fitch, K. D., et al. Effect of swimming training on children with asthma. *Arch. Disabled Child.* 51: 190, 1976.

20. Fitch, K. D., et al. The effect of running training on exercise-induced asthma. *Ann. Allerg.* 57: 90, 1986.

21. Frymoyer, J. W., M. H. Pope, M. C. Contanza, et al. Epidemiologic studies of low back pain. *Spine.* 5: 419–423, 1980.

22. Gordon, N. F. and C. B. Scott. *Exercise and mild essential hypertension.* In Boone, J. L. (Ed.) *Primary Care: Hypertension.* Philadelphia: W.B. Saunders, pp. 683–695, 1991.

23. Hagberg, J. M. Exercise, fitness, and hypertention. In Bouchard, C., R. J. Shepard, T. Stephens, J. R. Sutton and B. D. McPherson (Eds.). *Exercise, Fitness and Health: A Consensus of Current Knowledge.* Champaign, IL: Human Kinetics, pp. 455–466, 1991.

24. Hahn, A., et al. A re-interpretation of the effect of temperature and water content of the inspired air in exercise-induced asthma. *Am. Rev. Respir. Dis.* 130: 575, 1984.

25. Harris, S. S., C. J. Casperson, G. H. DeFriese and H. Estes. Physical activity counseling for healthy adults as a primary prevention intervention in the clinical setting. Report for the U.S. Preventive Services Task Force. *J. Am. Med. Assoc.* 261: 3590–3608, 1989.

26. Hiatt, W. R., J. G. Regensteiner, M. E. Hargarten, E. E. Wolfel, and E. P. Brass. Benefit of exercise conditioning for patients with peripheral arterial disease. *Circulation.* 81: 602–609, 1990.

27. Jennings, G., L. Nelson, P. Nestel, et al. The effects of changes in physical activity on major cardiovascular risk factors, hemodynamics, sympathetic function, and glucose utilization in man: a controlled study of four levels of activity. *Circulation.* 73(1): 30–40, 1986.

28. Kanis, J. A. and F. A. Pitt. Epidemiology of osteoporosis. *Bone.* 13: S7–S15, 1992.

29. Karper, W. B. and B. W. Evans. Cycling program effects on one rheumatoid arthritic. *Am. J. Phys. Med.* 65: 167–172, 1986.

30. Kenney, W. L. *ACSM's Guidelines for Exercise Testing and Prescription,* 5th edition. Philadelphia: Williams & Wilkins, 1995.

31. Morris, J. N., J. Heady, P. A. Raffle, et al. Coronary heart disease and physical activity of work. *Lancet.* 2: 1053–1057; 1111–1120, 1953.

32. Morris, J. N., S. P. W. Clave, C. Adam, et al. Vigorous exercise in leisure-time and the incidence of coronary heart disease. *Lancet.* 1: 333–339, 1973.

33. Morris, J. N. *Uses of Epidemiology,* 3rd edition. New York: Churchill Livingstone, 1975.

34. Nordemar, R., et al. Physical training in rheumatoid arthritis — a controlled long-term study. *Scand. J. Rheumatol.* 10: 17, 1981.

35. Orenstein, D. M., M. E. Reed, F. T. Grogan and L. V. Crawford. Exercise conditioning in children with asthma. *J. Pediatr.* 106: 556, 1985.

36. Paffenbarger, R. S., A. S. Gima, M. E. Laughlin, et al. Characteristics of longshoremen related to fatal coronary heart disease and stroke. *Am. J. Public Health.* 61: 1362–1370, 1971.

37. Paffenbarger, R. S. and A. L. Wing. Chronic disease in former college students. XVI. Physical activity as an index of heart attack risk in college alumni. *Am. J. Epidemiol.* 108: 161–175, 1978.

38. Paffenbarger, R. S., et al. A natural history of athleticism and cardiovascular health. *J. Am. Med. Assoc.* 252: 491, 1984.

39. Panush, R. S. and D. G. Brown. Exercise, the musculoskeletal system, and arthritis. *Postgrad. Adv. Rheumato.* 2: 1–20, 1987.

40. Pope, M. H. and B. Flemming. Biomechanics of low back pain. *Surg. Rounds Orthopaed.* 21(5), 35–42, 1990.

41. Powell, K. E., P. D. Thompson, C. J. Caspersen and J. S. Kendrick. Physical activity and the incidence of heart disease. *Ann. Rev. Public Health.* 8: 253, 1987.

42. Regensteiner, J. G., J. F. Steiner, R. J. Panzer and W. R. Hiatt. Evaluation of walking impairment by questionnaire in patients with peripheral arterial disease. *J. Vasc. Med. Biol.* 2: 142, 1990.

43. Report of the European Respiratory Society Rehabilitation and Chronic Care Scientific Group. Pulmonary rehabilitation in chronic obstruction pulmonary disease (COPD) with recommendations for its use. *Eur. Respir. J.* 5: 266–275, 1992.

44. Robertson, A. J., K. C. Ramesar, R. C. Potts, J. H. Gibbs, M. C. Browning, R. A. Brown, P. C. Hayes, and J. Swanson-Buck. The effect of strenuous physical exercise on circulating blood lymphocytes and serum cortisol levels. *J. Clin. Lab. Immunol.* 5: 53, 1981.

45. Shephard, R. J. *Body Composition in Biological Anthropology.* London: Cambridge University Press, 1991.

46. Sternfeld, B. Cancer and the protective effect of physical activity: the epidemiological evidence. *Med. Sci. Sports Exercise.* 24: 1195, 1992.

47. Stratton, J. R., W. L. Chandler, R. S. Schwartz, et al. Effects of physical conditioning of fibrinolytic variables and fibrinogen in young and old healthy adults. *Circulation.* 83: 1692, 1991.

48. Tipton, C. M. Exercise, training, and hypertension: an update. In *Exercise and Sport Science Reviews*. Vol. 19, J. O. Hollozy (Ed.). Baltimore: Williams and Wilkins, pp. 447–505, 1991.

49. Trials of Hypertension Prevention Collaborative Research Group. The effects of nonpharmacologic interventions of blood pressure of persons with high normal levels: results of the Trials of Hypertension Prevention, Phase I. *J. Am. Med. Assoc.* 267: 1213–1220, 1992.

50. U.S. Department of Health and Human Services. *Asthma Statistics*. Washington, D.C.: U.S. Government Printing Office, 1989.

51. Vitug, A., S. H. Schneider and N. B. Ruderman. Exercise and type I diabetes mellitus. *Exercise Sport Sci. Rev.* 16: 285–304, 1988.

52. Winningham, M. L. The role of exercise in cancer therapy. In Watson, R. R. and Eisinger, M., Eds. *Exercise and Disease*. Boca Raton, FL: CRC Press, 1992.

53. World Hypertension League. Physical exercise in the management of hypertension: a consensus statement by the World Hypertension League. *J. Hypertension.* 9: 283–287, 1991.

54. Healthy People 2000. DHHS Publication No. (PHS) 91-50212. Washington, D.C.: U.S. Government Printing Office, 1990.

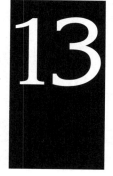

Chapter

Principles of Health Behavior Change

Douglas R. Southard and David Lombard

CONTENTS

0-8493-4593-6/97/$0.00+$.50

I. CLINICAL INTERVENTIONS FOR CHANGING HEALTH BEHAVIOR

A. INTRODUCTION

In most health care settings, a cardiovascular health assessment consists of a medical history, physical examination, blood chemistries, and one or more assessments of cardiovascular functional capacity. Recognizing the importance of life-style in the development of coronary heart disease (CHD), practitioners are also likely to inquire about dietary habits, physical activity, and smoking. It is unusual, however, for more than scant attention to be given to understanding *how* patients develop and maintain these disease-promoting behaviors and why they find it so difficult to change. This is an unfortunate omission as one of the greatest challenges health care practitioners face is promoting long-term life-style changes in their patients.

This chapter will provide an introduction to cognitive/behavior modification theory and techniques that are useful in facilitating health behavior change. It should be understood, however, that such techniques are not as effective in isolation as they are when integrated into the context of a true counseling relationship. A practitioner's prescription for behavior change is rarely as powerful as a patient's commitment to behavior change. To facilitate such a commitment, patients should be active participants in the interview, and practitioners must learn to listen as much as they speak. Patients need to feel that their perspective and values are an important part of treatment planning. This is particularly true when setting goals and making decisions regarding specific treatment modalities. Patient involvement in the planning process is also essential in promoting ownership of the plan and assumption of responsibility for their own health-related behaviors. Establishing the patient as an active partner in the behavior change process is a prerequisite for achieving long-term success.

B. READINESS FOR CHANGE

A fairly recent conceptual advance in the area of behavior change has been the concept that behavior change is a dynamic, ongoing process rather than a simple description of the patient as ready or not ready. Prochasta and DiClemente (1983) have suggested a stages-of-change model which seems to describe the basic change process regardless of the specific behavior examined. This has led to a revision in approach away from treating all individuals as if they were at the same level of readiness and toward stage-appropriate interventions. Four stages of change are described below. The reader should note, however, that this is not a linear model. Individuals clearly move back and forth between stages over the course of time between beginning a behavior change effort and a successful conclusion.

1. Precontemplation

This initial stage is characterized by a lack of awareness of the importance of behavior change, denial of its importance, or a decision that the costs of change outweigh the benefits. In any case, the patient is not actively contemplating behavior change. During assessment, the practitioner must be wary not to assume that all patients understand the relationship between their behaviors and various disease risks. This is particularly true among the less-educated and medically underserved populations. Verbal discussion and the use of visually engaging educational materials are both useful in enhancing understanding.

More frequent, perhaps, are the individuals who are knowledgeable regarding the general health risks involved but attempt to minimize them through a distortion of their severity or the likelihood that the adverse consequence will occur. The "I know someone who's smoked two packs a day for 45 years and is doing just fine" comparison is often used in this regard. Such comparisons are used to justify continuance of a behavior. When gently confronted, most patients will concede that they are rationalizing in order to avoid the anxiety associated with contemplating the loss of a valued habit. In such cases, the practitioner may facilitate movement to the next stage of readiness by reviewing the patient's general perception of the costs and benefits associated with behavior change. Such perceptions are usually based upon previous experiences, often negative, in attempting behavior change. In identifying and validating these fears and negative experiences, the practitioner is demonstrating empathy for the patient's concerns, which is essential in developing a counseling relationship. The patient is actively reviewing his rationale for maintaining a current habit, and the practitioner is well positioned to gently confront such rationalizations.

2. Contemplation

In addition to practitioner-initiated discussions, patients may experience "cues" that stimulate contemplation from a variety of sources. Illness of a family member (particularly a disease relevant to their risky behavior), onset of a new or troublesome side effect of the behavior (e.g., coughing up blood associated with smoking), a media release regarding new research, or a major life event such as the birth of a child may also initiate contemplation. Such cues, however, may or may not result in any action to change the behavior.

Practitioners can assist individuals in the contemplation stage by reviewing the specific costs and benefits of change in an open and rational manner. All likely costs including discomfort, financial, emotional, and logistical should be noted and an attempt made both by the patient and practitioner to develop ways of minimizing their impact. This is particularly important for adverse effects that are likely to occur immediately after behavior change has begun. Gentle confrontation regarding irrational beliefs may also be indicated. Such beliefs often emerge based upon the patient's negative experience with previous behavior change attempts and generalization to future attempts. The practitioner should note significant differences between past efforts and what could be done to improve the outcome of future efforts.

When promoting behavior change, practitioners often appeal to improved health as the desired outcome. While this is of importance to most people, a general appeal to good health may not be powerful enough to overcome the negative consequences associated with behavior change. Given all of the costs involved, what specific benefits would there be? Salesmen long ago discovered that it is extremely difficult to sell a product that the customer doesn't want or doesn't see as serving an important need. The practitioner should therefore first seek to identify activities that the patient (not the practitioner!) highly values and then relate participation in those activities to good health. For example, being able to play golf again, hunt with friends, comfortably walk around the mall, play outside with the children, etc. may be patient-valued activities; activities perceived by the patient as worthy of working toward. The metabolic, flexibility, and strength requirements of these activities should be explicitly identified and incorporated into the treatment plan.

Such discussions provide an excellent opportunity to develop a contract describing the patient's commitment to behavior change. This may be a verbal or written agreement between practitioner and patient. In either case, the practitioner would be wise to explicitly elicit the patients' agreement to change specific behaviors and their expectations for what that change might bring in terms of health/activity benefits. It should also include a contingency statement indicating what actions the patient agrees that the practitioner should take given the patient's performance or nonperformance of the new behavior. For example, should the practitioner call the patient if he/she misses more than one exercise session? In addition, some practitioners identify a portion of their professional fee as refundable if the patient performs the required behaviors.

3. Action

Having appealed to patient motivators and received a commitment for behavior change, the next step is to facilitate the patient's initial efforts. This necessitates:

1. setting reasonable expectations for short- and long-term achievement,
2. tailoring the intervention to the patient's medical needs and personal preferences,
3. utilizing a shaping process to promote early successes and reduce risk of adverse consequences (such as injury or extreme withdrawal effects),
4. insuring that the patient has the cognitive and behavioral skills necessary to perform the behavior change (e.g., assertiveness, pulse taking, dietary fat percentage calculations, problem solving, etc.),
5. designing home and work environments to facilitate the new behavior and extinguish the old behavior (e.g., remove ashtrays and cigarettes from the home, etc.),
6. establishing an adequate support system including a "buddy" system if needed,
7. developing a reward system (e.g., social, monetary, etc.) to reinforce new behavior, and
8. setting up a schedule for professional follow-up.

As one can see from the above outline, there is a fairly broad range of cognitive/behavioral interventions that target this stage of patient readiness. It is, therefore, not surprising that getting the committed patient started is generally what most programs and practitioners do best. However, when patients drop out early, as so many do, it may suggest that the treatment plan was not based upon a sufficient assessment of patient needs or that there was incomplete attention to detail in utilizing the techniques noted above.

4. Maintenance

Recognition that the majority of individuals undergoing behavior change efforts return to their original behaviors has led to an emphasis on relapse prevention. Although commonly referred to as if it were a singular maintenance technique, it is more aptly described as a process beginning at the initial interview and continuing for the duration of the clinical contact. During this process two themes are generally emphasized, ownership and flexibility.

Patients must appreciate that only they can change their life-styles and that professional assistance is just that — assistance. Thus, patients need to be empowered to take control of their own lives. This can be enhanced by identifying patient strengths (e.g., social skills) as well as achievements in other areas of their lives (e.g., successful business woman). Empowerment can also be advanced by having the patient successfully complete small steps in self-management (e.g., taking pulse, recording blood pressure, removing ash trays from house, etc.) from the very beginning of the intervention program. In contrast, oral persuasion in the form of "you can do it" may be of minimal value.

Intervention plans also need to be flexible. Rigid treatment plans often suit structured environments (e.g., supervised exercise programs) but may be very difficult to maintain as an ongoing life-style. For instance, if patients are led to believe that the *only* way to exercise is by walking 30 min on a track, they will be severely limited in their exercise options when a track is not available. Working with the patient to plan for alternate behaviors in situations in which there is a high risk of failure is also important (e.g., resuming smoking at an office party). Of course, there is no way that the practitioner or the patient can foresee all of the possible high-risk situations. It is often helpful, therefore, to have the patient practice problem solving for difficult situations during the initial program with empowering feedback provided by the practitioner. Finally, relapse prevention efforts often incorporate a series of follow-up visits designed to maintain motivation, assist problem solving, and monitor progress.

C. MULTIPLE RISK FACTOR INTERVENTION

Although patients often have more than one behavior modification need, it is generally unwise to recommend substantial changes in more than two areas at a time. For instance, the overweight, sedentary smoker may do well to first begin an exercise program. This would serve both as a weight maintenance mechanism and stress management tool during a subsequent smoking cessation effort. After smoking cessation has been well established, a more rigorous fat reduction diet may be implemented. Behavior change priorities are usually established based upon the practitioner's assessment of the health risk of the behavior and the patient's perception of its changeability. Such efforts may also be sequenced in the manner illustrated above. It is of particular import in such sequencing to provide opportunities for early successes to enhance patients' self-efficacy.

Prioritizing of behavior modification efforts is generally well accepted as reasonable and prudent for the average patient. There has been speculation, however, that some individuals may actually find sudden, intensive changes in diet, exercise, and general lifestyle easier to tolerate than gradual, systematic changes (Ornish, 1990). Although this may be true for some highly motivated patients in fairly structured therapeutic contexts, it remains to be seen if this is a successful strategy in general patient populations.

D. LEVEL OF SERVICE DELIVERY

Successful modification of health-related behaviors can occur in a variety of contexts ranging from one-on-one sessions to small-group work. Individual therapy is generally most helpful in developing a valid assessment and when working with some types of psychologically distressed individuals. It is also the most expensive modality. Small groups are cost-effective formats for conveying information both from the practitioner and from patient to patient. However, the greatest value of small groups lies in the potential for social support which lessens the sense of isolation during this often challenging period. Small groups also offer an excellent environment for modeling and practicing assertiveness and problem-solving skills.

E. DEALING WITH THE PATIENT IN DISTRESS

Individuals recently diagnosed as having a chronic and potentially debilitating disease such as CHD often develop feelings of anxiety, anger, and depression. In addition to the stressful nature of the diagnostic and treatment procedures, they may also be asked to make major life-style changes. The level of distress that an individual experiences will be determined by their previous level of psychological health, adequacy of their social support system, and the presence of other financial, employment, health, and social stressors.

Considerable anxiety often derives from fears regarding the return of chest pain, upcoming surgery, or the lingering possibility of sudden death. Anger is also frequent as patients ask, why me? This anger and irritability can be free-floating and directed at health care practitioners as well as other individuals in their life. The presence of irritability is often revealed by the patient's spouse rather than reported by the patient. Other distressed patients tend to experience depressive symptoms and may require pharmacological as well as psychological assistance. The objective of treatment in these patients is to elevate mood and restore sleep, appetite, energy, and general interest in life. A brief screening for emotional distress, particularly depression, is recommended for all patients experiencing chronic disease. Those identified should be referred to their family physician for further evaluation.

II. STRESS MANAGEMENT

A. PATIENT ASSESSMENT

Current literature in the behavioral and medical sciences is replete with observations that stress is a precipitating or aggravating factor in the development of many medical conditions including cardiovascular disorders. This is consistent with the clinical impressions of many professionals working with heart disease patients. Stress as a causal agent, however, has been very difficult to empirically demonstrate. What is clear is that individuals suffering from stress-related disorders may benefit from counseling, enhanced social support, and specific stress management techniques. This is particularly true for heart disease patients.

Stress may be best conceptualized as a state of psychophysiological imbalance in which individuals perceive that the magnitude of the demands facing them exceeds their ability to successfully cope with those demands. Stress can also be experienced when resources greatly exceed demands as so often occurs when a highly skilled and dedicated employee retires. Such a conceptualization emphasizes two basic principles of stress management. First, it is the individual's perceptions of the stressor, not necessarily the nature of the stressor itself, which influences the response. Second, stress is likely to occur only when individuals perceive that they lack the resources to adequately respond to the demand or that their resources greatly exceed the demand. Such a definition is also "user friendly" in that it avoids highly technical terms, and it is consistent with the Western medical concept of homeostasis as well as many Eastern philosophies regarding life management. In addition, it provides a convenient lead-in to a discussion of the various demands (work, family, financial) and resources (skills, money, social support, etc.) that the individual possesses.

In the assessment of the distressed patient, it is important to review the wide range of stressors (demands) as well as coping resources which might be influential. This includes family relationships, employment and career-related concerns, and the recent occurrence of multiple major life events. Past and present health concerns resulting in hospitalization, operations, functional impairment, and financial loss are particularly important. Characterological strengths (hardiness, etc.) and weakness (e.g., Type A or coronary-prone behavior, chronic depressive tendencies, etc.) may be present. Finally, the clinician will wish to inquire regarding previous attempts at managing stress. How does the individual cope on a day-to-day basis and how did he or she respond to major stressors in the past?

Given that the stress response is quite generic, it is not surprising that individuals may present with a multitude of affective, behavioral, cognitive, and physiological symptomatology. Affective manifestations generally include dysphoria, anxiety/fear, irritability, and anger. Maladaptive health behaviors, such as the ingestion of alcohol, caffeine, tranquilizers, and high-fat/sugar foods, as well as cigarette smoking, often increase. In contrast, health-enhancing physical activities tend to diminish. Individuals may also begin to exhibit polyphasic activity in an effort to accomplish more and more in less and less time. Interpersonal relationships may suffer as the individual either withdraws socially or overburdens his or her support system. Insomnia, changes in appetite, decreased libido, and anhedonia also occur. Cognitive manifestations include obsessive thinking about failure ("I can't ..."; "I never will ..."), loss of concentration and short-term memory, and at the extreme — suicidal ideation. Physiological markers often include elevated blood pressure at rest or excessive blood pressure response to relevant stressors (including the white coat hypertension syndrome); both migraine and musculoskeletal headaches, bruxism, and shoulder/back pain; gastrointestinal discomfort, heartburn, and irritable bowel syndrome; and nervous mannerisms and "tics."

Although most of these markers can be established during the patient interview, family members can be invaluable in providing another (and often quite different) perspective. Brief questionnaires such as the Beck Depression Inventory (Beck et al., 1961), the State-Trait Anxiety Inventory (Spielberger, Gorsuch et al., 1970), and the SCL-90 (Derogatis, 1977) are excellent supplements to the clinical interview and enhance the sensitivity of the assessment. In addition, repeated monitoring of blood pressure and heart rate at rest and during the diagnostic interview may reveal the presence of excessive cardiovascular reactivity.

The link between Type A or coronary-prone behavior and the development of CHD remains a controversial issue. During the 1970s and early 1980s, there was considerable evidence to support a significant, causal role between Type A behavior and CHD (Review Panel, 1981). Most importantly, the Recurrent Coronary Prevention Program demonstrated that Type A behavior can be modified in CHD patients and that such modification results in a reduction in secondary cardiac events (Friedman et al., 1984). However, a number of recent epidemiological and clinical studies have found negative and even inverse findings. This has prompted a reconceptualization of the coronary-prone behavior construct (Haynes and Matthews, 1988). While originally conceived to include two primary constructs (time urgency and free-floating hostility), the current consensus is that hostility may be the only component that is pathogenic for CHD. While time urgency, competitiveness, and overcommitment to work-related activities may be a stress management issue, these factors may not be influential in the development of CHD. Hence, current research and the exploration for a treatment for coronary-prone behavior primarily centers on reducing hostility and cynicism.

It should also be noted that excessive cardiovascular reactivity is generally hypothesized to be a mediating variable in the relationship between coronary-prone behavior and CHD risk. Several authors have suggested that rather than rely solely on affective and behavioral measures of coronary proneness, we should also include an assessment of the cardiovascular system response to a variety of mental stressors (Elliot and Breo, 1984). Although Elliot and Breo describe a variety of assessment protocols, an informal assessment for excessive reactivity can be performed by simply placing an automated blood pressure monitor cuff on the patient and measuring blood pressure throughout the clinical interview. A more sensitive assessment can be accomplished through 24-h ambulatory blood pressure monitoring as the individual pursues normal daily activities (Brunner and Waeber, 1992).

B. CURRENT THERAPEUTICS

1. Determining Treatment

Clinicians should offer interventions appropriate to the severity and chronicity of the individual's presentation and the individual's stage of readiness. As with other health behaviors, individuals may be at any point along the readiness continuum. Those not even aware of their stress management needs may first need to develop a better awareness of their signs and symptoms of stress before moving on to specific stress management techniques. Individuals in this precontemplation stage are often exemplified by the male with excessive blood pressure response to specific stressors who is unaware of any emotional, cognitive, or behavioral stress markers. Hence, measuring his cardiovascular response during a clinical interview may increase his awareness of the need for change.

Those with mild-to-moderate symptomatology and who are contemplating stress management training may benefit most by enhancing their awareness that stress is manageable and by discussing the definition of stress as the need to rebalance resources and demands. This can be done during the course of general clinical interactions or through a group stress management presentation. The availability of more-intensive stress management training may also encourage their movement to the action stage. Those actively seeking stress management training should be cautioned to develop realistic expectations for change as well as advised of the availability of formal training opportunities which may exist in their community. Finally, maintenance of stress management skills is best reinforced by the success patients experience in using them, as well as by the development of a social support network, either informally at work or home, or in a more formal support-group setting.

Although most individuals with excessive stress levels can be adequately treated in a general stress management setting, some may require more-intensive psychotherapy and/or pharmacological therapy.

Practitioners providing stress management training are advised to consult with a mental health practitioner to establish subjective and objective criteria for determining which patients might need referral.

2. Essential Components

The initial step in stress management is to enhance awareness of the individual's signs and symptoms of stress, provide a general definition of stress as noted above, and describe how stress can occur as the cumulative result of multiple life stressors. Individuals diagnosed with CHD should also be reassured that their emotional reaction to illness onset, although unique in quality, is a natural reaction shared by all who have experienced the trauma of CHD.

Two general stress management strategies are particularly useful.

1. Using the definition of stress reviewed above, the clinician can assist the individual in restoring a sense of balance to his or her life. Usually, this means increasing resources and/or decreasing demands. It should be clear, however, that it is unrealistic and unhealthy to totally eliminate all life demands in order to manage stress. Rather, the level of demands should be commensurate with resources.

2. The "tool box" approach emphasizes the need to develop an assortment of stress management resources or tools that can be used in stressful situations. The key issue is that an individual should use the stress management tool that is most effective for the specific situation. For instance, it would be inappropriate to only use a relaxation technique when the demands of the particular situation could be reduced through assertive behavior. Individuals, therefore, are encouraged to develop and refine their skills by utilizing a wide assortment of stress management tools and to develop an appreciation of when to use each. A brief review of common stress management resources and skills is presented below.

Relaxation has been described as a natural response designed to counterbalance the stress response. A wide assortment of techniques is available to facilitate relaxation. These techniques include autogenic training, yoga, imagery, progressive muscle relaxation, meditation, massage, hot tubs (for individuals without cardiac disease), deep-breathing exercises, biofeedback, etc. All of these techniques can be effective; the individual's challenge is to find the relaxation training exercise which is most appealing. Essential elements in learning a relaxation exercise are (1) quiet environment, (2) comfortable position, (3) mental focus, and (4) passive attitude (Benson, 1994). Most difficult is the development of a passive attitude. Some individuals try too hard and tend to actively concentrate on the relaxation activity rather than using a passive focus and sense of letting go. Some may actually experience anxiety rather than relaxation during such training, presumably because letting go decreases their perception of control.

The critical issue in relaxation training is generalization. Most people do not continue daily or b.i.d. relaxation training because they can't seem to "find the time." There is also the problem of becoming tense all day long and then having the greater task of relaxing at night. An alternative is to integrate relaxation procedures throughout the day. This approach has been coined the "quieting response" by Charles Stroebel and includes frequent (20 to 30 times per hour) but brief (3 to 5 s) relaxation exercises including deep breathing, scanning for muscle tension, and a pleasing mental focus.

Additional stress management tools include anger control techniques (Williams and Williams, 1993), assertiveness training, a quality social support system, time management training, the development of realistic self-talk, and guidelines for a stress-reducing diet and exercise plan (Davis et al., 1988). In addition, most programs will incorporate some attention to philosophical aspects of stress management. This is particularly salient when working with individuals exhibiting Type A behavior, as there is often an associated belief system emphasizing performance as the only measure of self-worth (Price, 1982; Watkins et al., 1987).

C. BARRIERS TO SUCCESS

Stress management training requires a strong commitment on the part of the individual to develop and refine coping skills and to practice them in everyday settings. Such training takes time and patience which are difficult elements to achieve if the individual is already overwhelmed by various demands. A realistic expectation is that the individual will be capable of reducing but not eliminating stress and that the individual would see stress management as truly a lifelong growth process. Success in managing stress in some specific and highly troublesome situations may be a reasonable preliminary goal.

D. PROGRAMMATIC CONSIDERATIONS

There are numerous self-help books, audio and videotapes, seminars, and workshops available in most communities. Most formats are useful in increasing awareness of stress-related symptoms and the basic issues in stress management. The variety of formats available provides the individual the opportunity to select one that best matches his or her interests and financial abilities. To maximize the chance of truly enhancing one's stress management repertoire, however, it is generally helpful to attend a workshop entailing a 6 to 8 week series of 1 to 2 h presentations, discussions, and skill-building exercises. This format provides the opportunity to practice skills between sessions and to receive feedback and support from the instructor and group regarding this practice.

Clinicians wishing to offer stress management presentations on their own can avail themselves of these same materials. It is strongly suggested, however, that clinicians wishing to provide intensive stress management workshops should first receive training both in stress management and in group therapy techniques.

III. SMOKING CESSATION

A. PATIENT ASSESSMENT

For most individuals, cigarette smoking cessation is a major challenge as it is often perpetuated by both psychological dependency and nicotine addiction. Psychological assessment should include a thorough examination of the patient's smoking history, smoking pattern, and any past attempts to quit smoking. A patient's smoking history can be obtained through structured questionnaires, a short interview, and self-monitoring of smoking behavior. A minimum of the following information should be obtained: how many years smoking, what times of day and where the patient smokes, the type of tobacco smoked, how many cigarettes a day, what prompts the patient to smoke, what the patient finds reinforcing about smoking, and whether or not the patient smokes to relax. Not unexpectedly, those individuals who believe that they do not have control over their own behaviors and who have a low level of confidence that they can quit have a poor prognosis. In contrast, those with high self-confidence and who previously have been able to stop smoking for more than a day have higher success rates (Coelho, 1985).

Assessment of the patient's social environment should include family, friends, and co-workers as they can exert a strong influence on smoking behavior. When one member of a social group stops smoking, other smokers may be threatened by the implication that they should stop as well. It is not unusual in such circumstances for there to be subtle pressure on the member who stopped smoking to resume smoking or risk losing friends. This is particularly troublesome as the patient struggling with smoking cessation needs increased not decreased social support. It is therefore useful to inquire whether or not family, friends, and co-workers smoke and whether or not they would be supportive of the patient's cessation attempt. Methods to enhance social support and minimize social sabotage also need to be built into the treatment plan.

Significant nicotine addition is suggested by:

1. High-nicotine cigarettes (greater than 0.6 m) which can be identified by finding the patient's cigarette brand in nicotine/tar content tables available from the American Lung Association and other professional groups,
2. Smoking ≥ one pack per day,
3. Smoking within 5 to 10 min after arising in the morning, and
4. Irritability if unable to smoke for 1 to 2 h because of environmental restrictions (Coelho, 1985).

The assessment should also identify any personal or family history of CHD, lung and throat cancer, chronic obstructive lung disease, chronic cough, or high blood pressure. Such a review will give you information about possible motivators for change and rule out some treatment options. For example, the use of transdermal patch systems may be contraindicated in patients with uncontrolled hypertension. Finally, measurement of height and weight is useful for body composition calculations and provides an opportunity to discuss the possibility of weight gain with smoking cessation. The patient needs to be aware that even if there is some weight gain, the cardiovascular benefits of smoking cessation are greater than any increased risk associated with mild to moderate weight gains (Coelho, 1985). Weight gain can also be minimized by the addition of stress management, dietary modification, and physical activity components in the overall treatment plan.

B. CURRENT THERAPEUTICS

Smoking cessation research and programs have been conducted for over 100 years. The average success rates for the present techniques used, 14% at 6 months, is not much better than those found 100 years ago (Coelho, 1985). Current approaches include replacement therapies (i.e., transdermal nicotine patches, nicotine gum), behavioral strategies (i.e., contingency contracting, self-monitoring, aversion therapy), self-help materials, hypnosis, acupuncture, and support groups. Although all these individual approaches have had some success, the most successful programs include a combination of nicotine replacement, behavior modification techniques, and social support (Coelho, 1985).

The rationalization for replacement therapy is to substitute either nicotine gum or a transdermal nicotine patch that provides low-to-moderate blood nicotine levels without the cancer-causing agents associated with tobacco use. Ideally, the dose of nicotine dispensed from the transdermal patch or nicotine gum is then reduced over a 1- to 3-month period resulting in a gradual reduction in blood nicotine levels and minimized withdrawal symptoms. Both replacement therapies get nicotine into the patient's system and reduce withdrawal symptoms, but they do not address the behavioral aspects of the addiction (i.e., the habit of smoking).

There is broad agreement among practitioners and pharmaceutical companies that nicotine replacement therapy must be combined with a behavior modification program to obtain maximum effectiveness. Reducing nicotine addiction without addressing the psychological dependency is not particularly effective. Patients using a replacement therapy note that they still experience craving for cigarettes and particularly miss the relatively large nicotine "jolt" associated with smoking. Many people also miss the familiar aspects of the smoking habit itself. It is not surprising, therefore, that the patches are often used improperly (i.e., patient smokes *and* uses the patch). The patches are also expensive, making it difficult for the low-income patient to purchase sufficient quantities. In addition, the patches are occasionally prescribed inappropriately. For example, it is probably not helpful to prescribe nicotine replacement therapy for a patient after he or she has already been abstinent for 3 weeks. By 3 weeks, all the nicotine is out of the patient's system and any cravings a patient feels are behavioral cravings, not a result of nicotine withdrawal. Using the patch at this point only puts nicotine in the patient when they were already nicotine free.

An alternative to using nicotine replacement therapy and to quitting "cold turkey" is the brand-switching method. Individuals using this technique gradually reduce nicotine addiction by switching from their current brand of cigarettes to one lower in nicotine. Switching is performed weekly with most individuals reaching cigarettes with the lowest level of nicotine in 1 to 3 weeks. In some cases, decreasing the number of cigarettes is also possible. Having greatly reduced nicotine addiction, the individual is then instructed to establish a quit date for total smoking cessation. Problems with this approach include patients increasing the number of cigarettes smoked or the amount of each cigarette smoked to compensate for decreased nicotine concentration. A second concern with the brand-switching and fading approach is that psychological dependency on cigarettes may be enhanced as the increasingly greater duration between cigarettes increases the perceived value of each one. Lastly, there is the concern that this method is simply delaying the patient's inevitable withdrawal experience.

A wide variety of behavioral strategies has been incorporated into smoking cessation programs, most with limited success. They include stimulus control, covert sensitization, systematic desensitization, self-monitoring, fear appeals, aversive conditioning, deep breathing, deep muscle relaxation, self-reinforcement, and contingency contracting, to name only a few. Although almost any of these techniques will, on average, result in a decrease in smoking levels by as much as 30 to 40% of baseline, the average 6-month relapse rate is 75% (Coelho, 1985). Nonetheless, there are a few behavioral techniques that appear more successful than the others — contingency contracting and aversive conditioning.

Aversive conditioning is any technique that pairs the behavior of smoking with a personally negative event for the patient. Successful treatments generally include 10 to 12 sessions of training. Some of the aversive conditioning techniques used include electric shock and rapid smoking. Rapid smoking, the most commonly utilized technique, is defined as having a patient inhale every 6 s until a cigarette is done, repeating this for three cigarettes or until the patient is nauseous. Some researchers have found a 100% initial abstinence rate with this technique (Lichtenstien and Rodrigues, 1977). Unfortunately, unless the rapid smoking sessions are continued, relapse is high. Furthermore, there are considerable concerns regarding the health risk, particularly for the patient with cardiopulmonary disease.

Of the behavioral strategies used, contingency contracting, when done correctly, has met with the most success. In using contingency contracting, the counselor and the patient draw up a contract specifying what the patient will receive for various behaviors the patient performs. For example, the patient may get a program T-shirt if he or she is abstinent for 3 weeks, or the patient may receive a 10% discount on the program fees for doing all the program's homework exercises. Problems some practitioners have had are mistakenly using contingencies the patient is not affected by. For example, offering a 10% discount on program fees to a wealthy patient may not motivate that patient as much as a financially limited client. Consequently, researchers and clinicians have found that if the target behavior is well defined and the contingency is personally relevant to the patient, 6-month abstinence rates are high.

Support groups or group smoking cessation meetings have been used predominately because they are expected to provide a sense of support for quitting smoking and offer group cohesiveness to induce compliance with program methods. Another, more practical reason groups are often used is to reduce the individual costs to the patient and the time required by the practitioner. When the group is supportive and cohesive, some data indicate groups can be an effective treatment delivery point.

C. BARRIERS TO SUCCESS

Despite two decades of heavy media campaigns against smoking and publicity about the many deadly health hazards of smoking, approximately 26% of Americans still smoke (Coelho, 1985). Barriers to smoking cessation include lack of a social support (home and work) for change, stage or readiness to quit smoking, concern about weight gain, and loss of identity as a smoker.

The social barriers appear to be the most difficult barriers for smoking cessation. For many smokers, their spouse, friends, and co-workers all smoke and the restaurants, bars, and other places where they go are generally filled with smokers. Thus, the smoker's social life is filled with prompts and social pressure not to quit smoking. This situation is not accidental. Many smokers noted they socialized with only those friends who smoked as they did not feel guilty smoking around them. Thus, smoking dictated their choice of friends and social activities. For the greatest chance of success, patients trying to quit smoking need to consider in advance how they will cope with social situations in which others may pressure them to smoke or to anticipate avoiding such situations altogether.

Being ready and prepared to change is recognized as so important in the smoking cessation area that most programs do not have the clients quit until the 2nd or 3rd week when they are more prepared. Furthermore, the majority of the work on the stages of behavior change model comes from work in the smoking cessation area, again reflecting the importance of the client's stage of readiness (Prochaska et al., 1994). As with the other behaviors discussed earlier, the client's stage will dictate what you should and should not do. If the patient is in precontemplation, information and education, not stimulus control strategies, are important. The patient has to want to change for it to be successful.

For many patients, concern regarding weight gain associated with smoking cessation keeps them from quitting. It is important to educate your patient that (1) not all quitters gain weight, (2) the average weight gain is in the 6- to 12-lb range (Spring et al., 1991; Nides et al., 1994), and (3) the weight gain tends to be due to an increased intake of carbohydrates (30 to 40%), not to changes in metabolism (Spring et al., 1991). Furthermore, a moderate diet or exercise program is usually enough to reduce the weight some people gain when they quit smoking. Some researchers recommend programs initiate an exercise program several weeks before the smoker's quit date (Marcus et al., 1992).

Boredom and loss of identity also affect many smokers once they quit. Smoking gave them something to do, a reason to take a break from work, an excuse to socialize with a friend. Once smokers quit, they sacrifice these activities and get bored. You can work with patients to fill in these missing activities with other activities they may enjoy. It is very important to remember that when smokers quit, they are giving up a part of their identity and life and this new void needs to be filled with something they enjoy or they will go right back to smoking because they enjoy it.

D. PROGRAMMATIC CONSIDERATIONS

Commercial smoking cessation programs generally consist of self-help books and/or a smoking cessation group. Both formats provide a general understanding of the addiction of smoking, where it comes from, and how to initiate quitting. They also teach people some strategies for long-term maintenance. These approaches are usually fairly inexpensive and do not require a lot of time on either the patient's or practitioner's part. Furthermore, the groups may offer greatly needed support that the patient gets nowhere else.

Unfortunately, there are some drawbacks to these commercial programs. Although the better self-help books are structured in a "read a chapter and learn a strategy a week" format, patients usually try to read and incorporate too many things at once or they only choose one technique and expect it to change their lives. Furthermore, patients may not like the idea of participating in a group either because they are shy or because they dislike the idea of having to attend meetings over several weeks. An individualized program may be more effective for these patients.

There are also several pros and cons for individualizing a program for a patient. On the pro side, individualized programs take into account the specific reinforcement the patient gets from smoking and can choose the correct tactics needed for that patient. Furthermore, individualized programs generally allow the patient to ask questions when problems occur or when a strategy fails to work. On the con side, individualized programs require more time from both the patient and the practitioner and may be more costly.

IV. PHYSICAL ACTIVITY PROMOTION

A. PATIENT ASSESSMENT

Areas for assessment include medical history, activity history, psychological factors affecting activity, and a graded exercise test. A full medical history is a key component in assessing the patient. The areas to assess include cardiovascular and pulmonary disease, orthopedic disorders, cerebrovascular impairments, back or other muscular problems, dizziness in reaction to exertion, and any present medications. Although reviewing these areas with the patient may illuminate a medical problem contraindicating strenuous exercise, generally, a physical activity program can be designed to meet almost any patient's unique medical needs.

The patient's exercise history data will identify the patient's past attempts, present type of activity, and intensity/duration/frequency levels. The clinician can obtain his data in a variety of ways. Some programs use an exercise history questionnaire that asks specific questions about various activities over the past week, month, or year. Other programs have patients complete 3 to 7-day physical activity logs, noting what, where, how much, and at what intensity they exercised (Lombard, 1993).

As many psychological variables affect one's adherence to an exercise program, psychological screening should be conducted for all potential patients wanting to exercise. The areas affecting adherence include self-efficacy (belief in one's ability) for change, depression, anxiety, stress, perceived difficulty of exercise, social support for activity, and Type A/coronary proneness (Dishman, 1988). As always, noting any past physical activity program attempts the patient has made is important to determine during assessment. Furthermore, what are the patient's motivation to exercise, activity preference, and logistical considerations? Does the patient desire to decrease fat, increase flexibility, strength or endurance, or just build aerobic capacity?

The graded exercise test will offer important information about a patient's aerobic capacity and form the basis for an exercise prescription. A variety of standardized formats for graded tests on treadmills and exercise bikes are available and reviewed elsewhere in this book. The practitioner should use this data along with activity goals, history, and preferences in choosing the initial prescribed activity levels. The graded exercise test will also warn of any cardiovascular complications (ischemia, arrhythmias, etc.) the patient may have that limit physical activity.

B. CURRENT THERAPEUTICS

The American College of Sports Medicine (ACSM) guidelines (1995) recommend individuals exercise at a moderate intensity between 50 to 85% of maximal capacity (VO_{2max}: maximal aerobic power or maximal oxygen uptake) or 60 to 90% of maximum heart rate (HR_{max}). The ACSM does recommend exercising at a moderate intensity for a long duration over exercising at a high intensity for a shorter duration mainly because of the increased risk for injury with high-intensity exercise (ACSM, 1995).

The guidelines also recommend that individuals exercise for a duration of 20 to 60 min of *continuous* aerobic activity for each exercise session (ACSM, 1995). Furthermore, the activity should use large muscle groups in a continuous, rhythmic, and aerobic manner. The ACSM guidelines describe a relationship between intensity and duration and their effects on fitness. For example, individuals who could not perform high-intensity exercise could perform a lower-intensity activity for a longer period of time to increase their aerobic power and for weight loss (Blair et al., 1989).

Finally, the guidelines recommend individuals exercise 3 to 5 days/week (ACSM, 1995). When exercise is performed less often than 3 days/week (unless the exercise is very strenuous), studies have found only minimal change in fitness. Furthermore, ACSM noted exercising more often than 5 days/week does not produce greater improvement in fitness than training 5 days/week.

In addition to aerobic training, the ACSM guidelines also recommended individuals perform resistance training of 8 to 12 repetitions for 8 to 10 exercises involving large muscle groups at least twice each week. Furthermore, exercise sessions should have appropriate warm-up and cool-down periods, including flexibility exercises (ACSM, 1995).

While supervised exercise programs are particularly well suited and necessary for high-risk patients, for most individuals organized but relatively unsupervised programs and "life-style" approaches appear to be the most promising as they relate to long-term maintenance of activity levels (Blair, 1991). For decades researchers have studied exercise in highly structured and supervised programs. These include cardiac rehabilitation programs, some work site interventions, aerobic classes, running groups, and supervised health club visits. Generally, these programs use trained facilitators to work with the patients while they exercise. The facilitators offer encouragement and feedback on progress. In the more successful programs, they also conduct goal setting with the patients. While these programs have had some success, the patient may become too dependent on the staff for guiding them through their workouts and for support. This is not a problem if patients can continue in the group program indefinitely or can afford a private trainer to work with them at home. Ideally, the program staff should work with the patient to make a good transition to an unsupervised program at some point.

Unsupervised programs have attempted to empower patients in their exercise program. The staff teaches strategies patients can use on their own such as self-monitoring, setting hard but achievable goals, stimulus control strategies, and prompting strategies. For example, the staff may suggest that patients place their workout bag on the front seat of their car so it will be the first thing they see after work. Thus, the bag acts as a prompt to exercise. Patients can learn to use these strategies very well. In some unsupervised programs, the staff may use a weekly or monthly follow-up call to the patient to strengthen the intervention (Lombard, 1993). As the cost for such telephone prompting is low, it could be a very cost-effective strategy.

A variety of self-help books in the exercise area is available. These books tend to slowly take the patient through the process of initiating an exercise program. Some contain self-monitoring forms and sheets for goal setting. Others contain posters for the patient to put up as prompts to exercise. Thus, some of these books use those strategies found most effective in the supervised and unsupervised programs.

There are two important caveats when using exercise self-help books. First, they tend to be written for the "average person" and use those strategies that are most successful on the average. They may not take into consideration the individual needs of the person. Second, most self-help books address exercise as a target behavior, not a life-style change. Fortunately, some self-help books take a life-style approach to physical activity (e.g., *Living with Exercise*, Blair, 1991). These books educate and offer strategies to include regular physical activity simply as a part of life. For example, they look at physical activity not just as the "workout," but also as making the more active choices in life (i.e., suggesting using the stairwell instead of the elevator and suggesting parking one's car in the back of the parking lot and then walk the extra yards). By teaching such strategies, these books can help clients increase their overall activity level without increasing their "workout sessions." This is consistent with the goal of weight management and enhancing general muscle tone, particularly for the formerly sedentary individual.

C. BARRIERS TO SUCCESS

There are numerous barriers to a patient's success in an exercise program. Some of the factors influencing adherence are stage of readiness to change, psychosocial factors, past failure attempts, and physical limitations. The staff needs to pay particular attention to these areas to aid the patient throughout the program.

Generally, the patient should be in the action stage of readiness when beginning a program. By using a stage-of-change questionnaire (Marcus et al., 1992), the practitioner can decide if the patient is ready to begin a program or not. If the patient is in precontemplation or contemplation, supportive counseling and education about the health benefits of exercising (i.e., weight reduction, lowered lipid levels, more energy, more muscle tone) are important to facilitate transition to the action stage. Once the patient has decided to become more physically active, the behavioral strategies such as prompting, feedback, goal setting, and contingency contracting will be more effective. By being sensitive to the stage of readiness, a program will use the appropriate strategies at the correct time to increase program success.

Several psychosocial factors are potential barriers to the success of a physical activity program. Lack of social support for exercise is a frequently encountered barrier. Those programs that incorporate social support (i.e., exercising in a group format or using a buddy program) can successfully deal with this problem. Stress, anxiety, and perceived time demands all can become barriers to success. Changes in routine or increases in time demands at work can end an otherwise successful attempt. Lastly, low self-efficacy, or the belief in one's ability, for change resulting from past failed attempts may influence the effectiveness of any intervention. Poor self-efficacy is most effectively treated by designing an initial program with very modest expectations for increases in physical activity. This facilitates early patient success, elevates self-efficacy, and forms the foundation for subsequent increases in a gradual, step-wise fashion.

Physical limitations can be a potential barrier in two ways. First, as noted earlier, some patients may have a physical condition that interferes with their ability to exercise (e.g., arthritis). But, with careful supervision and appropriate precautions, patients with almost any condition can be physically active and obtain benefit particularly if they focus not just on aerobic increases, but also on flexibility and strength. Second, as exercise does involve some risk for injury, a patient may become injured from their exercise program. In addition to routine exercise precautions, the risk of injury can be reduced by identifying the overly aggressive or "gung-ho" patient and providing appropriate counseling. This may entail education and exploration regarding the reasons the individual feels so compelled to exercise so intensely.

D. PROGRAMMATIC CONSIDERATIONS

In the physical activity promotion area there are many good commercial programs. These range from fitness centers with personal trainers to self-help books. The better commercial programs incorporate those strategies successful at initiation and maintenance of activity (e.g., stimulus control, goal setting, social support). Those commercial programs that include social support, either through group activities or enthusiastic and encouraging staff, tend to be more effective. Furthermore, if patients compare various books or programs, they can find a commercial program that fits best with their life-style.

The drawback of some commercial programs is the dependence they create between the patient and the staff. Therefore, a patient should look for commercial programs that teach the patient skills to exercise without continued formal guidance. Of course, self-help books do not have the same problem of dependence upon staff. But, these books do have the added problem of not being able to offer feedback or social support to the patient. Nonetheless, they are a good starting point for most novice exercisers.

Individualizing an exercise program for a patient can be very effective. By being able to individualize the program, the patient's stage of readiness, any psychosocial factors influencing adherence, and any medical problems can all be addressed in a patient's unique program. Furthermore, as the patient's needs change over time, the program can change to meet his or her specific needs.

The drawbacks to individualizing a program center on the time required to create and monitor the program. The assessment, designing, and monitoring of an individual patient's program requires a large amount of time. And, if there are several patients in the program, the overall time needed to monitor these patients is immense. Furthermore, as commercial programs have increasingly realized the need to tailor programs to their clients, patients may be able to get their unique needs met through such programs.

V. WEIGHT CONTROL

A. PATIENT ASSESSMENT

Patient assessment for weight control should include a medical examination, dietary and activity analyses, psychological assessment, review of past attempts to control weight, and body composition evaluation. As most weight control programs are going to ask patients to alter their diet and activity levels, the medical examination should be fairly comprehensive to rule out any medical problems that may interact with such treatments. The medical examination should also include assessment of disorders related to weight control problems such as hypothyroidism, hypoglycemia, and diabetes.

As weight is closely tied to both diet and activity level, a comprehensive diet and activity analysis is needed. To obtain the data for these analyses, the patient could fill out either prospective or retrospective food and exercise diaries. The dietary data are then analyzed to indicate daily calorie intake, calories from fat, grams of fiber and saturated fat, and other nutritional information. The exercise data give calories expended daily, daily MET levels, and the frequency, intensity, and duration of activities. Both the dietary and activity assessments will offer important information for assessment and subsequent prescription.

Psychological assessment is a priority for any weight control intervention as dieting can, in a small number of cases, lead to several types of eating disorders (i.e., anorexia and bulimia). Assess anxiety levels, depression, and stress because they are related to binge eating and low activity levels. Furthermore, assessment of social support for weight change is important because the more support a patient has for losing weight, the stronger the probability of a successful intervention. The desire to lose weight, however, must come from the patient. Pressure from others to lose weight in the absence of self-motivation is likely to lead to resentment and failure. Finally, as past dieting experiences will affect further attempts, assess past weight management attempts, successes, and failures the patient has had.

Determining whether the patient is overweight vs. over-fat is clearly important. Therefore, simply weighing and measuring a patient's height are not enough. This is why most exercise physiologists and weight management programs conduct a body fat assessment either through use of body submersion, body fat calipers, or the wrist-neck-waist measurement method to indicate if the patient is over-fat.

B. CURRENT THERAPEUTICS

Currently, there are two major therapeutic approaches to weight control, dietary vs. activity interventions. Within the dietary interventions there are also three different approaches — fat reduction, calorie reduction, and very low calorie diets. Lastly, there is the integrated approach using both dietary and exercise interventions.

Dietary interventions have a long history in the weight management area. For most of that history, the approach has been to reduce total daily caloric intake for the patient. This was generally done through initial dietary analysis, prescribed daily caloric intake, and extensive self-monitoring and feedback of the patient's diet. The dietary analysis was generally based on a 3- to 7-day diet diary which was used to generate initial feedback to the patient on present nutritional levels. Next, the patient was given a maximum daily caloric intake goal. This value was generally arrived at through examination of the patient's present and target weight, average caloric expenditure, and calculating a daily caloric intake that would put the patient in a caloric deficit. Historically, most of these programs have prescribed very large caloric deficits to maximize patient weight loss in the short run. Unfortunately, for most patients, such a large deficit is difficult to maintain, and they often drop out of the program. In contrast, many programs have reduced the caloric deficit to a level where the patient will lose weight, but do so more gradually. Still other programs offer the patient the choice between a range of caloric deficit programs to lose weight (e.g., Physician's Weight Loss Centers).

One concern commercial programs have had to deal with lately is the issue of the high fat content in the foods they recommend. Since gram for gram, fat has more calories than carbohydrates, and a high-fat diet is related to heart disease even when total caloric intake is controlled for, many patients and physicians found those interventions targeting only calorie reduction unacceptable. Therefore, some commercial programs have recently begun targeting dietary fat reduction and not just calorie reduction. These programs use diet diaries to analyze not only the total caloric intake, but also the percentage of intake from fats and the grams of saturated fat. Then, the dietary prescription is given in terms of reduction of caloric intake through reduction of daily percentage of calories from fat and reducing overall intake. As these interventions stress switching from high-fat to low-fat foods, not only do they help reduce weight, they also help reduce risk of those disease states related to a high-fat diet and result in lower lipid levels for some patients.

As two of the determinants of an individual's weight are the caloric intake and the caloric expenditure, exercise has been prescribed, increasingly, as an intervention strategy for weight loss. The reader is referred to the previous section on physical activity promotion to see those behavior change techniques most effective in achieving adherence to an exercise program.

In general, a weight loss program needs to focus on proper goal setting, feedback, and long-term support. Proper goal setting is conducted by working with each patient to choose goals that are challenging but reasonable for that patient. Feedback can be given to the patient in many forms (weekly dietary analysis, weekly or monthly body fat checks) as long as the feedback is personally relevant to the patient and is directly associated with the prescribed goal. However, for long-term success, feedback should be given on the goal behavior (i.e., eating lower-calorie/fat foods) vs. on a goal outcome (i.e., decrease in body fat) because behaviors are easier for the patient to control and see immediate change in. Lastly, ensuring the patient has long-term support for weight loss (i.e. support from spouse, family members) will increase the maintenance of any changes the patient makes.

Thus far, the dietary and exercise interventions have been referred to as weight *loss* programs because they generally are not weight *management* programs. To be truly a weight management program, the intervention should teach the patients strategies to maintain and integrate the dietary and physical activity changes into their life-style. Many programs do not teach these important skills. Cueing, reinforcement, feedback, contracting, goal-setting, self-monitoring, and stimulus control strategies have all been successful in the weight management area. Furthermore, those strategies patients can perform on their own are the most predictive of long-term weight maintenance (i.e., goal-setting, self-monitoring, and stimulus control strategies). Therefore, interventions, regardless of whether they are diet or exercise focused, will be more effective if they use these strategies.

C. BARRIERS TO SUCCESS

There are several factors affecting the success of weight management programs. They include past failed attempts, psychosocial factors, stage of readiness to change, and diet insensitivity. Addressing these areas could increase the effectiveness of an intervention and, it is hoped, reduce the usually high-drop out rate seen in most programs (60 to 90% after 6 months; Brownell, 1991).

Most of the patients in weight management programs have attempted to lose weight at one time or another in their past. These attempts, both successful and unsuccessful, will have an impact on the patient's present attempt. For the patients with failed past attempts, their belief in their ability to change their weight may be low and may affect the effort they put into the program. By being aware of this, the program staff may try to empower patients by showing them how they actually have complete control over what they eat and how much they exercise and by highlighting the patients' own modest successes.

Several psychosocial factors can have a large influence on the outcome of a program. Anxiety, depression, stress, and many other psychological states will take away a patient's ability to fully benefit from a program. By being aware of these states, program staff can direct the patient to get the psychological help necessary to benefit from the program. In the social area, lack of support for weight management, marital or family problems, change in work status, and restrictions of available food all affect the effectiveness of a program.

Just as with physical activity, stage of readiness to change one's weight is very important. If patients are in precontemplation or contemplation, they have not made the decision to actually commit the energy required to make such a large change in their life. Many individuals enter weight loss programs as a result of a physician's advise or the prodding of a loved one, not because the patient has decided to. Patients of this type will most likely not be successful unless the staff appeals to the factors that truly motivate them and they then actively decides that weight loss is important for them.

There are also physiological barriers to success in weight management. For example, for some patients weight appears to be relatively insensitive to dietary changes. Thus, a primarily diet-oriented program would not work for these patients. Addition of a physical activity regimen may lead to greater success. On the other hand, some patients have major physical limitations that exclude them from most types of exercise. Thus, a dietary intervention would be the major treatment modality for them. Being aware of a patient's unique situation will increase the probability of a successful experience for the patient and the staff.

D. PROGRAMMATIC CONSIDERATIONS

Commercial weight management programs range from intensive one-on-one, diet-centered programs, such as Jenny Craig™ and Weight Watchers®, to self-help life-style approaches, such as the LEARN program for weight control (Brownell, 1991). As there is a large variety of programs, there is large variability in the quality of commercial programs. The better programs include individualized treatment to ensure a program most fitting the individual patient's needs, a combination of exercise and dietary interventions, and emphasize those behavior change strategies that allow patients to take control of their weight management program (i.e., self-monitoring, goal setting, stimulus control, and education on what foods to keep in the home).

Unfortunately, some one-on-one commercial programs survive through their clients' continued reliance on the ongoing activities and products of the program. Thus, they do not always teach patients strategies that empower them to take control of their own weight management efforts. If patients leave the program, they may have few skills with which to maintain the weight loss. As an alternative, there is a variety of fairly effective self-help books that emphasize patients' ability to develop and maintain their own weight loss program. By promoting patient control, there is an increased probability of turning short-term efforts into long-term life-style changes. The major drawback to the self-help approach is that it lacks the goal setting–feedback loops and social support offered by most commercial programs.

VI. LIPID MANAGEMENT

A. PATIENT ASSESSMENT

Assessing a patient's lipid status should include medical and psychological information. Medical assessment includes a general physical, blood lipid assessments including total cholesterol, high density cholesterol (HDL), low density cholesterol (LDL), and dietary analysis. The National Cholesterol Education Program (NCEP) guidelines recommend lipid assessment preferably taken two or more times several days apart as lipid levels can vary significantly from day to day (NCEP, 1988). Furthermore, the patient should complete a 3- to 7-day food diary to obtain enough information to calculate nutritional intake averages and get important information on the patient's eating pattern. The dietary data are important as NCEP guidelines advise patients with high cholesterol levels to reduce their daily fat intake to 30% or less of total calories from fat and cholesterol consumption to 300 mg or less per day.

Psychological assessment should center on social support for change, any present stressors and reactions to these stressors, the patients' belief in their ability to change, and any past attempts at dietary change. Social support is an important consideration as changing diet or adding exercise or medications to one's life-style can be stressful. Social support can help reduce this stress. Furthermore, if there is little support for these changes at home, the patient's program will most likely be unsuccessful, especially if the nonsupportive person cooks the meals and is not willing to change the menu. Assessing for major stressors in the patient's life is important as stress has been linked to high cholesterol levels, possibly directly or indirectly by increasing behaviors such as drinking alcohol, eating fatty foods, and binge eating.

The last area of assessment is to review any past attempts at lipid management the patient has made. Any past failures will strongly influence the success of any present or future attempts. If patients were unsuccessful with dietary changes before, their confidence in their ability to change their dieting habits may be low. Self-confidence can be increased by designing a program in which the patient is likely to have early successes by implementing relatively small dietary changes.

B. CURRENT THERAPEUTICS

The National Heart, Lung, and Blood Institute, through the NCEP, has urged individuals to adopt a diet that reduces the percent of total calories from fat from a current average of 40% to less than 30%; reduces the saturated fat intake to less than 10% of total calories; and reduces the daily intake of dietary cholesterol to less than 300 mg (NCEP, 1988). It is estimated that adherence to this diet will reduce total cholesterol by 10 to 15% (NCEP, 1988).

NCEP guidelines offer goals to work toward, but do not offer much guidance about how to attain these goals. A number of different types of dietary interventions have been attempted, with the most successful interventions using a combination of education, dietary and lipid-level feedback, and goal setting. It is important to develop a plan for the patient's lifetime. The educational component of these interventions includes information on acceptable levels of cholesterol, HDL, LDL, and triglycerides, on how poor levels affect one's physiology and health, on how diet affects these levels, on what changes are good to make, and on how to measure the fat and soluble fiber content of a food. The target diet is generally less than 30% of daily calories from fat. Some programs also include calorie reduction as part of the program, but, generally, as patients reduce their daily percentage of calories from fat, their overall caloric intake usually is reduced. Thus, some lipid management diets are very similar to weight reduction diets.

In providing dietary intervention, the patient receives detailed dietary feedback before and during the program. The patient completes daily food diaries as data for feedback. The detailed feedback generally includes calories from fat, calories from saturated fat, and grams of dietary cholesterol and fiber. The advent of sophisticated dietary analysis programs allows for quick and accurate dietary feedback for both the clinician and the patient. Once the patient receives the detailed feedback, the patient and the clinician work on reasonable dietary change goals for the patient. Bandura (1986) indicated that for such goals to work it is important that the goals are clear, that they will result in some measurable change, that the patient understands the relationship between a change in dietary fat and in resulting lipid levels, and that the goals are hard, but attainable and linked in a sequential nature to the ultimate dietary and lipid-level goals.

Since the ultimate goal is to alter lipid levels, feedback on changes in lipid levels is important. With the invention of quick, accurate, low-cost, easy-to-use light spectrometry machines, such as Abott Vision, Kodak DT-60, and Reflotron, some interventions offer lipid feedback as frequently as once a week, while others only do so once every few months. The NCEP guidelines recommend measuring lipid levels and giving feedback once a month, as this is frequent enough and spaced out enough to show patients some progress if they truly have made progress.

C. BARRIERS TO SUCCESS

There are several types of barriers to success in lipid management. First, most programs primarily use dietary interventions to control lipid levels. Unfortunately, as with weight reduction, some patients appear to be diet insensitive. Changes in their dietary fat intake do not relate to changes in the lipid levels. For these individuals, lipid-controlling medications may be necessary. Second, stage of readiness to change is as important for lipid management as for any other area of behavior change.

There are several psychological factors that can influence the success of a lipid management intervention. First, self-efficacy for change, or patients' belief in their ability to make change, is very important. If patients believe they cannot change, they probably will not. But, the higher their self-efficacy for controlling their diet and lipid levels, the more successful your intervention will be. Second, lack of social support, especially at home, can eliminate the effects of any intervention. If your patient eats meals at home with someone else (e.g., a spouse or roommate), the other person may dislike the dietary changes and insist on a return to the earlier diet. Third, past failure experiences can block a patient's willingness to work with the intervention. Thus, program staff may want to focus on how this program is different from the last program and why this one will be more effective for the patient given a strong effort on the patient's part.

D. PROGRAMMATIC CONSIDERATIONS

Most of the commercial lipid management programs are self-help books. Many of these books offer good education on what lipid levels are, what are desirable levels, and what changes to make to control lipid levels. Some of the better books even offer recipes, menus, and ways to track progress over time. *Beyond Cholesterol* (Kwiterovich, 1989) and *Count Out Cholesterol* (Ulene, 1989) are two good examples of books that stress the need to integrate dietary changes and physical activity into one's life-style to truly achieve long-term control over lipid levels. These books are informative and relatively inexpensive when compared with the costs of individualized treatment.

A shortcoming of the commercial approaches is the lack of individualization of the program. These programs choose those strategies that work, on the average, fairly well. Individual needs, strengths, and weaknesses all affect the outcome of any intervention. Since these books are limited in how they can address these issues, they may not be sufficient for some patients. Furthermore, the commercial programs, when used in isolation, do not offer the feedback that is so rewarding for patients. Patients want and need to see progress toward their goals if they are to continue.

Although individualized programs address some of these issues, they do have several drawbacks. First, high monetary and time costs are associated with individualized programs for both the patient and the primary care giver. Second, highly individualized programs tend to rely too much on the interactions between the patient and the staff for feedback and support. When the intervention ends, these interactions end, leaving patients on their own to continue.

A combination of individualized and self-help approaches may be most successful. For example, a patient and a care giver could review the strategies suggested by a self-help book such as *Beyond Cholesterol* and choose the ones most appropriate to the patient's life-style. The patient could refer to the book for help and recommendations as he or she progresses. Feedback regarding the success of these strategies could be obtained by periodic dietary analysis and lipid profiles performed at the clinic. Such a combination of professional and self-help approaches reduces overall monetary and time costs and may offer an acceptable alternative to those individualized approaches requiring more extensive interactions between staff and the patient.

REFERENCES

American College of Sports Medicine (1995). *ACSM'S Guidelines for Exercise Testing and Prescription. Fifth Ed.* Baltimore: Williams and Wilkins.

Bandura, A. (1986). *Social Foundations of Thought and Action: A Social Cognitive Theory.* Englewood Cliffs, NJ: Prentice Hall.

Beck, A. T., Ward, C. H., Mendelson, M., Mock, J., and Erbaugh, J. (1961). An inventory for measuring depression. *Arch. Gen. Psychiatry*, 4, 561–571.

Benson, H. (1984). *Beyond the Relaxation Response.* New York: Times Books.

Blair, S. N. (1991). *Living with Exercise.* American Health, Dallas.

Blair, S. N., Kohl, H. W., Paffenbarger, R. S., Clark, D. G., Cooper, K. H., and Gibbons, L. W. (1989). Physical fitness and all-cause mortality: a prospective study of healthy men and women. *J. Am. Med. Assoc.*, 262, 2395–2401.

Brownell, K. D. (1991). *The LEARN Program for Weight Control.* American Health, Dallas.

Brunner, H. R. and Waeber, B. (Eds.; 1992). *Ambulatory Blood Pressure Monitoring.* New York: Raven Press.

Coelho, R. J. (1985). *Quitting Smoking: A Psychological Experiment Using Community Research.* New York: Peter Lang.

Davis, M., Eshelman, E. R., and McKay, M. (1988). *The Relaxation and Stress Reduction Workbook* (3rd ed.). Oakland, CA: New Harbinger Publications.

Derogatis, L. R. (1977). *SCL-90-R Manual — I*. Riderwood, MD: Clinical Psychometric Research.

Dishman, R. K. (1988). *Exercise Adherence: Its Impact on Public Health*. Champaign, IL: Kinetics Books.

Elliot, R. S. and Breo, D. L. (1984). *Is It Worth Dying For?* New York: Bantam Books.

Friedman, M., Thoresen, C. E., Gill, J. J., Powell, L. H., Ulmer, D., Thompson, L., Price, V. A., Rabin, D. D., Breall, W. S., Dixon, T., Levy, R., and Bourg, E., (1984). Alteration of Type A behavior and reduction in cardiac recurrences in post-myocardial infarction patients. *Am. Heart J.,* 108, 237–248.

Haynes, S. G. and Matthews, K. A. (1988). Coronary-prone behavior: Continuing evolution of the concept. *Ann. Behav. Med.,* 10, 47–59.

Kwiterovich, P. (1989). *The Johns Hopkins Complete Guide for Avoiding Heart Disease: Beyond Cholesterol*. Baltimore, MD: Johns Hopkins University Press.

Lichtenstien, E. and Rodrigues, M. R. P. (1977). Long-term effects of rapid smoking treatment for dependent cigarette smokers. *Addictive Behav.,* 2, 109–112.

Lombard, D. N. (1993). Walking to meet health guidelines: The effect of prompting frequency and feedback and goal setting. An unpublished manuscript. Virginia Polytechnic Institute and State University, Blacksburg, VA.

Marcus, B. H., Banspach, S. W., Lefebvre, R. C., Rossi, J. S., Carleton, R. A., and Abrams, D. B. (1992). Using the stages of change model to increase the adoption of physical activity among community participants. *Am. J. Health Promotion,* 6, 424–429.

National Cholesterol Education Program. (1988). *Report of the Expert Panel on Detection, Evaluation, and Treatment of High Blood Cholesterol in Adults*. NIH Publication no. 88-2925, National Institutes of Health.

Nides, M., Rand, C., Dolce, J., Murray, R., O'Hara, P., Voelker, H., and Connett, J. (1994). Weight gain as a function of smoking cessation and 2-mg nicotine gum use among middle-aged smokers with mild lung impairment in the first 2 years of the Lung Health Study. *Health Psychol.,* 13, 354–361.

Ornish, D. (1990). *Dr. Dean Ornish's Program for Reversing Heart Disease*. New York: Random House.

Price, V. A. (1982). *Type A Behavior Pattern: A Model for Research and Practice*. New York: Academic Press.

Prochaska, J. O. and DiClemente, C. C. (1983). Stage process of self-change of smoking: toward an integrative model of change. *J. Consult. Clin. Psychol.,* 51, 390–395.

Prochaska, J. O., Velicer, W. F., Rossi, J. S., Goldstein, M. G., Marcus, B. H., Rakowski, W., Fiore, C., Harlow, L. L., Redding, C. A., Rosenbloom, D., and Rossi, S. R. (1994). Stages of change and decisional balance for 12 problem behaviors. *Health Psychol.,* 13, 39–46.

Review Panel (1981). Coronary-prone behavior and coronary heart disease: a critical review. *Circulation,* 63, 1199–1215.

Spielberger, C. D., Gorsuch, R. L., and Lushene, R. E. (1970). *STAI Manual*. Palo Alto, CA: Consulting Psychologists Press.

Spring, B., Wurtman, J., Gleason, R., Wurtman, R., and Kessler, K. (1991). Weight gain and withdrawal symptoms after smoking cessation: a preventive intervention using d-fenfluramine. *Health Psychol.,* 10, 216–223.

Ulene, A. (1989). *Count Out Cholesterol*. New York: Random House.

Watkins, P. L., Ward, C. H., and Southard, D. R. (1987). Empirical support for a Type A belief system. *J. Psychopathol. Behav. Assessment,* 9, 119–134.

Williams, R. and Williams, V. (1993). *Anger Kills*. New York: Times Books.

Chapter 14

Exercise, Health, and Disease

Arthur S. Leon and Mark Richardson

CONTENTS

". . . modern humans are still hunter-gatherers metabolically and the sedentariness of civilization is regarded as a major environmental stress on an evolutionary legacy."[1]

I. INTRODUCTION

Few would dispute that for most of humankind's tenure on earth, survival was dictated, in large part, by the ability to sustain regular, prolonged physical exertion. However, due to profound technological changes, resulting in the modern mode of living, strenuous physical exertion has been eliminated from most occupations, and an abundance of leisure time created for most people in industrialized societies in the Western hemisphere is used for sedentary pursuits. The consequences of an evolutionary–genetic legacy, which resulted over millennia from selected pressures and now suddenly removed in the 20th century, are becoming apparent. Many major public health problems associated with the modern life-style are attributed in part to the marked reduction in physical activity. These include coronary or ischemic heart disease (IHD), hypertension, obesity, hyperlipidemias, non-insulin-dependent diabetes mellitus (NIDDM), osteoporosis, some forms of cancer (breast and colon) and possibly mental health problems.[2]

    Although exercise has been extolled since antiquity to promote health and well-being, the systematic study of the health consequences of physical inactivity is a rather recent phenomenon. The study of

London transport workers and later of British civil servants by Morris et al.[3,4] and of U.S. railroad workers by Taylor et al.[5] were pioneering observational epidemiological studies demonstrating the adverse health effects of inactivity. Over the past 30 years, research has markedly increased our understanding of the contributions of sedentary living to the etiology of several chronic degenerative disorders, particularly IHD, and recent excellent reviews are available on this topic.[6-8] This chapter provides an update on the status of knowledge on the relationship of physical activity habits to several important modern health problems, i.e., cardiovascular disorders (IHD, stroke, peripheral vascular disease, and hypertension), obesity, NIDDM, cancer, and osteoporosis.

II. CARDIOVASCULAR DISORDERS

A. ISCHEMIC HEART DISEASE

IHD is the consequence of severe atherosclerotic disease, which has its onset during childhood. This disease process has a multifactorial causation. There is now general agreement that the three major risk factors for this disease are above-optimal levels of serum total cholesterol generally related to a "rich" diet, blood pressure, and cigarette smoking.[9] Other contributing factors include diabetes mellitus (and hyperinsulinemia), obesity, and physical inactivity. Our understanding of the contributions of an inactive life-style and associated reduced fitness level is based primarily on epidemiological data, but is supported by post-mortem studies, animal research, and small-scale experimental studies in humans defining potential mechanisms.

More observational epidemiological studies (over 100) have been performed on the relationship between physical inactivity or reduced fitness levels and IHD than for any other medical condition. The results of this research has been previously reviewed.[10-15] The heterogeneity of the epidemiological approaches used should be appreciated.[16,17] They include cross-sectional comparisons of IHD prevalence in physically active vs. inactive men, case-control studies, and longitudinal or prospective cohort studies. Assessments of physical activity have been made through a variety of survey methods of occupational physical activity, leisure-time physical activity (LTPA), combined occupational and LTPA, or, less commonly, assessment of cardiorespiratory endurance. Likewise, the manifestations of IHD have been established by a variety of criteria. Similarly, sample selection procedures and statistical analyses varied among these studies. Thus, a simple interpretation of these results is not possible. Of these observational studies, several major prospective studies which included a careful assessment of habitual LTPA are of particular interest, since this is the main contributor to discretionary physical activity for most people. Morris et al.[4,18] followed about 9000 to 18,000 British executive male clerks and civil servants for almost 10 years. Paffenbarger et al.[19] followed almost 17,000 college alumni for more than 20 years. Slattery et al.[20] followed over 3000 U.S. railroad workers, originally studied by Taylor et al.[5] from 17 to 20 years. Leon et al.[21] and Leon and Connett[22] followed over 12,000 men with multiple risk factors for IHD participating in the Multiple Risk Factor Intervention Trial (MRFIT) for 10.5 years. Kannel and Sorlie[23] followed 4000 men and women participating in the Framingham Study for 14 years. Salonen et al.[24] followed over 15,000 men and women who constituted a population-based, representative sample of people in eastern Finland for 6 years. Garcia-Palmier et al.[25] followed almost 9000 Puerto Rican men for 8 years. Finally, Donahue et al.[26] followed over 8000 men of Japanese origin participating in the Honolulu Heart Study for 12 years. These studies employed a variety of LTPA survey methods representing varying periods of recall. All showed a significant inverse relationship between LTPA level and IHD. Relative risks for IHD for the least active compared with the most active ranged from 1.2 to 2.3, and the differences were statistically significant in all these studies ($p < 0.05$).

The report by Paffenbarger et al.[27] concerning the college alumni cohort and changes in their physical activity level is noteworthy. Men who did not engage in moderately vigorous sports activity in 1962 or 1966 but took up this type of activity by 1977 had a 41% lower risk of death from IHD over an 8-year follow-up period than those alumni who continued not to engage in such activity.

However, approximately one third of the observational studies reported in the literature do not support an inverse relationship between physical activity and manifestations of IHD.[11,13] In part to reconcile these difference, Powell and colleagues[13] performed in 1987 what is considered a classic summary of these observational studies on physical activity and IHD. These authors evaluated the literature with respect to criteria they developed regarding the adequacy of individual measurements of occupational and/or LTPA and incidence or prevalence of IHD and of several aspects (adherence, data collection methods, confounding variables, population representativeness, and loss to follow-up) of the epidemiological methods employed. Of an initial list of 121 articles representing 54 different studies found in the literature, only 43 met their selection criteria as "adequate" studies. Approximately two thirds of these showed an inverse relationship between physical activity and incidence of IHD, while three fourths of the subgroup of 27 studies judged to be "better" ones showed such a relationship. Finally, of the 19 studies which employed "adequate" individual measurements of physical activity, all showed an inverse relationship between physical activity and IHD. The 43 "adequate" studies demonstrated a median relative risk ratio for IHD of 1.9 for the least-active vs. most-active individuals. Furthermore, the median relative risk for IHD associated with inactivity was 2.4 in those studies judged to be of the highest quality. Adjustments for confounding risk factors and other factors only slightly weakened these relative-risk ratios.

A more recent critical analysis of the physical activity–IHD literature, employing meta-analysis, reported similar findings.[14] Pooled relative risk for IHD mortality was 1.9 for sedentary vs. highly active persons in occupational-based cohort studies. Similarly, in non-occupational-based cohort studies, the relative risk for IHD mortality, for the least-active vs. highly active individuals was 1.6. These authors also found that "methodologically stronger" studies tended to show higher relative risks than lower-quality studies. In fact, in regression analyses, study quality was the strongest predictor of relative risk for IHD.

Another approach utilized in a small number of observational studies was to assess physical fitness (more specifically, direct or indirect assessments of aerobic capacity or cardiovascular endurance) and compare this with risk for IHD.[28] Although a variety of measures of aerobic capacity were employed, all ten longitudinal studies recently reviewed by Blair et al.[28] demonstrated an inverse relationship between measures of aerobic fitness and future risk of IHD. One of the most recent and substantial of these was performed at the Aerobic Center in Dallas by Blair et al.[28] who followed over 13,000 men and women for more than 8 years. Physical work capacity was assessed by maximal treadmill testing. The considerably greater relative risk for IHD of low fitness than of low levels of physical activity is noteworthy. Risk ratios for men and women when the least fit were compared with the most fit ranged from 1.4 to approximately 5.0 for IHD (combined fatal and nonfatal manifestations) and from 1.5 to 8.5 for cardiovascular disease deaths. Furthermore, low fitness levels were independently associated with these relative risks when several other risk factors (singularly and combined) were statistically considered. The results of a recent study by Sandvik and co-workers[29] comparing initial fitness levels (determined from maximal bicycle ergometry) in 1960 healthy middle-aged Norwegian men with subsequent relative risk for cardiovascular and all-cause mortality over a 16-year follow-up period are consistent with these findings. The relative risk of cardiovascular-related death for the most fit (quartile 4) as compared with the least fit (quartile 1) was 0.41 after adjusting for conventional coronary risk factors. It should be appreciated, however, that aerobic capacity is only modestly related to exercise habits or habitual physical activity.[30,31] In addition, age, relative weight, cigarette smoking, as well as other variables, negatively impact upon physical work capacity. Finally, and most importantly, there appears to be a strong constitutional or genetic component to aerobic capacity[32] so self-selection for LTPA by the more physically fit may play a role.

1. Clinical Trials

Because of the inordinately large sample size required, potential major compliance problems, and immense cost, a rigorously controlled randomized clinical trial to determine the relationship between exercise training and IHD has not been (and likely will not be) performed.[1,16] A more-feasible, alternative approach is a controlled secondary prevention trial where individuals who have had a myocardial infarction are randomized into either an exercise or control group. The majority of these (there have been more than 20 randomized secondary prevention trials) have demonstrated a favorable trend toward decreased mortality in cardiac rehabilitation programs in the exercise compared with control groups.

However, none of these studies had sufficient sample size, duration of follow-up period, and/or study design to have the statistical power to demonstrate a possible independent protective effect of exercise on the recurrence of coronary heart disease events. For this reason, data have been pooled from these individual, randomized, secondary prevention trials which include an exercise component (usually in conjunction with other risk factor modification) and meta-analyses have been performed.[33,34] Results showed an approximately 20% to 25% decrease in 1- to 3-year rates of cardiovascular and total mortality for the intervention group compared with the control group. However, it is impossible to determine for certain the independent effect of exercise on subsequent mortality because the trials consisted of multiple risk factor management in addition to a structured exercise program or exercise advice. Interestingly, there was no apparent protective effect of intervention on the rate of nonfatal reinfarction. Additionally, when begun very early (within 8 weeks after myocardial infarction), there was actually a 32% increased risk of reinfarction which approached statistical significance.[1]

2. Mechanisms by Which Physical Activity May Reduce the Risk of IHD

The many anatomical, physiological, hormonal, and metabolic adaptations resulting from acute and chronic exercise provide several plausible mechanisms by which physical activity can reduce the risk of IHD. These include (1) reduced progression (and possibly regression) of coronary atherosclerosis; (2) reduced risk of coronary thrombosis; (3) improved balance between myocardial oxygen supply and demand; (4) reduced myocardial vulnerability to ventricular fibrillation; and (5) improved myocardial metabolic capacity and mechanical performance.[16]

a. Reduced Progression of Coronary Atherosclerosis

Regular exercise may have both direct and indirect effects on coronary atherosclerosis. The relatively few post-mortem studies of activity level and severity of coronary atherosclerosis generally have not indicated a lower prevalence of severe coronary atherosclerosis with increased activity level.[11,12] However, physically active men generally have larger coronary artery luminal diameters and a lower prevalence of complete or near complete occlusions of major coronary arteries on post-mortem examination. Animal experimental data suggesting that regular exercise can directly reduce the severity of coronary athero-sclerosis were provided in a classic study by Kramsch et al.[35] In this study, two groups of monkeys (an exercise and control group) were fed an atherogenic diet for several years. At autopsy, those that jogged on a treadmill for 30 min three times a week over the study period were found to have a substantial reduction in overall severity of coronary atherosclerosis and much larger diameters of the lumen of the main coronary arteries. Recently, Ornish et al.[36] performed a well-controlled, prospective, 1-year, ran-domized trial in patients with coronary artery disease of the effect of life-style changes (low-fat vegetarian diet, smoking cessation, stress management, and moderate exercise) on coronary atherosclerosis assessed by quantitative coronary angiography. Results showed that after 1 year, the intervention group demon-strated an average percentage coronary luminal diameter regression in stenosis from 61.1 to 55.8% for lesions causing greater than 50% narrowing of the luminal diameter. Conversely, the usual-care (control) group showed progression of atherosclerosis. However, in this study it is not possible to tease out the independent contribution of exercise training.

Probably the major contribution of exercise is through its effects on other risk factors for atheroscle-rosis and IHD. These include blood lipid and lipoprotein alterations, blood pressure and body weight reductions, correction of hyperinsulinemia, and reduced risk of NIDDM. Our discussion here will be limited to the effects of exercise on blood lipid and lipoprotein levels. The effects on blood pressure levels and on prevention of obesity and NIDDM are discussed elsewhere in this chapter.

i. Lipid and Lipoprotein Metabolism

The relationship between plasma lipid and lipoprotein concentrations and risk of atherosclerosis and IHD is well established.[37,38] Severity of atherosclerosis and risk of IHD progressively increase with levels of total cholesterol and low-density lipoprotein cholesterol exceeding 200 mg/dl and 130 mg/dl, respec-tively.[29,40] Conversely, the risk of IHD has been shown to be inversely related to plasma concentration of high-density lipoprotein cholesterol (HDL-C).[41-44] Risk of IHD progressively increases with levels of HDL-C below 35 mg/dl (i.e., 2 to 3% increased risk of IHD with every 1 mg/dl decrease in HDL-C). The significance of elevated plasma triglyceride and its principal lipoprotein carriers (very low density lipoproteins and chylomicrons) on the atherosclerotic process and risk of IHD remains uncertain.[37,39,45,46] However, there is evidence that supports a direct relationship between plasma triglyceride concentration and incidence of IHD.[47] Furthermore, plasma triglyceride is inversely related to HDL-C and directly associated with the atherogenic hyperapobeta-lipoproteinemia syndrome.[48]

The relationship between physical activity and lipid metabolism has been an active area of research over the last 30 years and has been extensively reviewed.[37,48-55] Exercise has been shown to have a beneficial effect on both plasma HDL-C and triglyceride concentrations, but little consistent effect on LDL-C and total cholesterol in the absence of weight loss. Cross-sectional studies report a dose–response association between habitual physical activity and HDL-C levels. This association is apparent through a full spectrum of physical activity levels ranging from the extreme inactivity associated with quadriplegia to the high volume of training required for marathon running.[56] Numerous studies have consistently demonstrated HDL-C values of 12 to 20 mg/dl or 20 to 35% higher in endurance-trained individuals than those found for matched inactive people.[37,57-59] Smaller, but significant increases in HDL-C have also been demonstrated for those participants in the Lipid Research Clinics Prevalence Study[60] and MRFIT[21] who reported greater amounts of habitual physical activity than their less-active counterparts.

Plasma triglyceride levels have also consistently been demonstrated by cross-sectional comparisons to be lower in endurance-trained vs. more-sedentary individuals.[37,58,61] In these studies, differences between active and inactive groups were often pronounced, with endurance athletes typically having plasma triglyceride levels below 100 mg/dl. It should be emphasized that there are many potential confounding variables (some of which are concomitant changes associated with increased physical activity) which can influence plasma lipoprotein concentrations, making interpretation of the cross-sectional data difficult. These include changes or differences in plasma volume, caloric intake, diet composition, body fat mass, fat distribution, coffee consumption, alcohol consumption, cigarette smoking, medications, and the use of oral contraceptives.[48,62,63]

An acute bout of endurance exercise of moderate-to-long duration has been shown to transiently increase HDL-C[64,65] and lower triglyceride levels.[64] Furthermore, endurance exercise conditioning has been relatively consistently shown to reduce elevated levels of fasting and postprandial plasma triglycerides, but not generally triglyceride levels in the normal range.[37,48,66-69] However, studies investigating the effect of chronic endurance exercise on HDL-C levels have not yielded consistent results. Approximately one half of these training studies have demonstrated a significant exercise-induced increase in HDL-C concentration.[37,67,70] When an exercise effect was present, increases in HDL-C levels generally ranged from 3 to 8 mg/dl or 5 to 16%.[62] Differences in the HDL-C response to exercise in these studies are probably related to failure to control some of the same variables mentioned in the discussion of the cross-sectional studies. One of the most important of these confounders is changes in body composition.[48,62] Sopko et al.[71] demonstrated an additive effect of exercise conditioning and weight reduction on HDL-C levels. Those previously sedentary and overweight men that exercised and lost weight showed increases in plasma HDL-C levels (22% above baseline levels) almost twice those observed in groups of men either performing a similar amount of exercise but maintaining body weight or losing a similar amount of body weight but not exercising.

Women do not appear as likely to increase HDL-C levels through endurance exercise training as men.[37,67,69,72,73] This may be due in part to the following: (1) a lower volume of exercise achievable in training studies in sedentary women compared with sedentary men; (2) the higher baseline HDL-C levels in sedentary women compared with sedentary men; (3) greater resistance to body weight and composition changes during exercise training in women compared with men; and (4) perhaps differences in body fat distribution and lipase activity between the sexes.[37]

The possible underlying mechanisms of exercise-induced changes in lipoprotein metabolism have recently been reviewed.[37,63] They are probably related in large part to increased energy needs in working muscles and include changes in several key enzymes involved in lipid metabolism. These include increased activity of lipoprotein lipase and lecithin cholesterol acyltransferase and decreased activity of hepatic lipase.

b. Reduced Risk of Coronary Thrombosis

There is now general agreement that most major IHD clinical events are accompanied by coronary thrombosis. Further evidence suggests that people with coronary artery disease have a disturbance in balance between blood coagulation and the ability to dissolve blood clots, that is, fibrinolysis.[74] Although controversy still exists, there is evidence to suggest that exercise training may reduce blood platelet adhesiveness and aggregability.[75,76] Moreover, acute exercise enhances fibrinolytic activity through an increase in plasminogen activator.[77] Plasminogen activator converts the proenzyme plasminogen to the active enzyme plasmin, which, in turn, digests fibrin to soluble degradation products. Furthermore, exercise training may augment this increased fibrinolytic activity seen with acute exercise while concomitantly attenuating the increased coagulation of the blood induced by physical exertion.[77,78] Finally, exercise training has recently been demonstrated to decrease plasminogen activator inhibitor type I activity and lower plasma fibrinogen concentration.[79] Increased plasma volume reducing blood viscosity may also play a role.

c. Improved Myocardial Oxygen Supply/Demand Balance

There are a number of mechanisms by which exercise training may improve the relative balance between myocardial oxygen supply and demand. A well-known training adaptation is the attenuated rate–pressure product elicited by a given submaximal work load.[80] This reflects a reduced myocardial oxygen demand

and thus a reduction in coronary blood flow requirements.[15,81,82] As a result of exercise conditioning, individuals with coronary artery disease can exercise at a greater absolute work load prior to attaining the myocardial oxygen threshold associated with ischemic manifestations (i.e., the ischemic threshold is higher). In addition, since the major portion of coronary blood flow occurs during diastole, slowing of the heart rate with training also serves to improve myocardial oxygen supply.

Whether or not exercise training results in an increase in myocardial vascularity in coronary artery disease patients remains controversial. Experimentally in animals, including nonhuman primates, exercise causes an enlargement of the main coronary arteries.[35,81,83,84] In humans, autopsy studies and, more recently, echocardiography have demonstrated similar changes in physically active men.[11,85-87] In addition, in animals, physical activity increases myocardial capillary density.[81,83-84] Although technology is not available to confirm such changes in humans, supporting evidence is the well-documented increase in skeletal muscle capillary density with exercise training. Pioneering work on the effects of chronic endurance exercise on the development of coronary collateral vessels in dogs with experimentally induced partial occlusions of a major coronary artery was performed by Eckstein.[88] More recently, similar findings were demonstrated in miniature swine trained by treadmill running.[89] However, this effect is not seen in these animal models in the absence of coronary occlusion.[15,81,90] Further, there is limited evidence in humans to confirm these findings. Serial coronary arteriography has been utilized on several occasions to demonstrate increased coronary collateral artery formation in coronary artery disease patients undergoing exercise training.[15,81-82] However, it cannot be excluded that the increase in coronary collateral vessels observed in these isolated cases was due to progression of the underlying coronary atherosclerosis rather than a beneficial effect of exercise. There is, however, indirect evidence that supports the hypothesis that exercise conditioning can increase maximal myocardial blood flow and, hence, myocardial oxygen supply. The ability to achieve a higher rate–pressure product prior to the development of angina or electrocardiographic evidence of myocardial ischemia with exercise training has been reported.[15,82] Additionally, Froelicher[15,82] reported improved myocardial perfusion as measured by thallium-201 myocardial scintigraphy in a heterogeneous group of IHD patients as a result of 1 year of exercise training.

d. Reduced Myocardial Vulnerability to Fibrillation

The increased risk of ventricular fibrillation during acute exercise in the presence of coronary artery disease has been well substantiated in both animals and humans.[10,91-93] Contributing factors undoubtedly include the increased sympathetic tone and associated catecholamine release and the increased myocardial oxygen requirements during physical exertion. Improvement in the myocardial oxygen supply–demand balance and a reduction in sympathetic tone and associated catecholamine release[94-95] resulting from endurance training should reduce the risk of ventricular fibrillation. Indirect evidence that exercise training may protect against lethal ventricular arrhythmias is provided by both primary and secondary IHD prevention studies,[21,33,34,92,93] which strongly suggest that chronic exercise conditioning reduces the overall risk of sudden death, which is due most often to ventricular fibrillation.

Experimental animal evidence has recently been reviewed by Blair et al.[6] The hearts of exercise-trained rats have been shown to be more resistant to ventricular fibrillation during acute regional myocardial ischemia, normoxia, and hypoxia.[96] More recently, it was demonstrated in previously infarcted isolated rat heart that exercise training increased the ventricular fibrillation threshold both before and after the onset of reinfarction.[97] These results strongly suggest that exercise training may have a direct effect on the myocardium in diminishing the likelihood of ventricular fibrillation.

e. Improved Myocardial Metabolic Capacity and Mechanical Performance

Increased metabolic capacity and improved mechanical performance of the myocardium are well-substantiated adaptations to endurance exercise training.[15,81,98] Specific contributory adaptations include increases in the following: coronary reserve, oxygen delivery to the myocardium, myocardial glycogen stores, utilization of fatty acids from endogenous stores, mitochondrial size, availability of intracellular calcium, and myosin ATPase activity. This last adaptation contributes to faster cardiac relaxation and is considered a biochemical correlate of enhanced contractile function.

Echocardiography has demonstrated an increase in end-diastolic volume as early as 1 week after initiating an endurance training program.[15] Prolonged ventricular filling time due to resting bradycardia contributes, in part, to this increase in end-diastolic dimensions. Eventually, increased hemodynamic diastolic loading of the myocardium results in the adaptive response of global hypertrophy of the heart. Conditioning exercise that repetitively causes volume overloading of the left ventricle results in a relatively greater increase in chamber size than left ventricular wall thickness. Associated with this type of hypertrophy is an increased myocardial vascularity (previously discussed) resulting in the maintenance of adequate blood flow to the hypertrophied myocyte.[99]

The physiologically hypertrophied heart is considered functionally superior to one that has not had to adapt to volume overloading. Indeed, measures of left ventricular function are primary considerations in determining the risk of morbidity and mortality following myocardial infarction. Because relatively less damage is incurred to the myocardium during a myocardial infarct in individuals with hypertrophied hearts, their prognosis may be improved.[100]

B. HYPERTENSION

High blood pressure is a major chronic health problem worldwide. In the United States alone, approximately 50 million people (15 to 20% of adult men and women) have elevated levels of diastolic and/or systolic blood pressure or are on antihypertensive drug therapy.[101] Hypertension is related to the development of IHD, severity of atherosclerosis, hemorrhagic and atherosclerotic stroke, nephropathy, peripheral vascular disease, dissecting aortic aneurysms, left ventricular hypertrophy, and congestive heart failure.[102] For at least 90% of the hypertensive population the underlying cause of this disorder is not completely understood. However, there are several known risk factors for this so-called idiopathic or essential hypertension. These include genetic predisposition, age, race, salt intake, alcohol ingestion, obesity (especially central and intra-abdominal excess body fat distribution), and, possibly, physical inactivity.[102] The relationship between physical activity and hypertension has been actively investigated for over 20 years and has been reviewed a number of times during the past decade.[103-105] However, in contrast to IHD, relatively few prospective longitudinal studies have been performed. Paffenbarger et al.[107] observed in almost 15,000 Harvard alumni, free of hypertension at baseline, and followed for 8 years, a relative risk for physician-diagnosed hypertension of 1.35 for the least-active alumni vs. the most active. This relationship was independent of other known risk factors for hypertension. Blair et al.[108] assessed aerobic fitness by maximal treadmill testing in 4820 men and 1219 women free of hypertension and followed these individuals for up to 8 years for the development of physician-diagnosed hypertension. The least-fit individuals exhibited a relative risk of 1.52 for the development of hypertension over this follow-up period compared with the most-fit individuals. These results were not affected by factors such as age, smoking habits, family history of hypertension, or body composition.

Numerous cross-sectional epidemiological comparisons of blood pressure levels in physically active vs. more-sedentary individuals have been reported.[103,104] The results have been equivocal when comparisons between men in physically demanding vs. light occupations have been made. However, approximately 60% of the cross-sectional comparisons assessing sport or LTPA participation found lower systolic and diastolic blood pressures (generally 5 to 15 mmHg lower) in active individuals vs. matched inactive subjects.[104]

Experimental endurance-training studies have been performed with both normotensive and hypertensive animals and humans. More than 70% of those trials involving normotensive rats or rats with genetically mediated, spontaneous hypertension demonstrated significantly lower blood pressures in the trained vs. untrained animals.[104]

Similar to the cross-sectional data, the results of endurance exercise training trials with normotensive and hypertensive individuals have been contradictory.[103,106] Many of these studies (particularly the earlier ones) were methodologically flawed (e.g. lack of a control group). Hagberg[106] reviewed 33 better quality exercise training studies involving individuals with hypertension. Approximately two thirds of these studies showed an average reduction in resting systolic blood pressure of about 10 mmHg, while a similar reduction in diastolic blood pressure was reported in 70% of these training studies. However, rarely did training completely normalize blood pressure levels. Fagard et al.[109] also reviewed the effects of regular endurance training on blood pressure in both normotensive as well as hypertensive individuals, considering only "controlled" studies in their review. They concluded that well-controlled studies provide evidence that regular endurance exercise can lower blood pressure levels. On average, normotensive and hypertensive subjects reduced their systolic and diastolic resting blood pressures by –4/–4 and –11/–6 mmHg, respectively.

The underlying mechanisms responsible for the apparent antihypertensive effect of increased physical activity are unclear at this time. However, a strong possibility is attenuation of sympathetic nervous system activity.[103-106,110] Conceivably, this would result in reduced renin-angiotensin system activity, a resetting of baroreflexes, arterial vasodilatation, and a reduction in elevated peripheral vascular resistance. Additionally, an associated exercise-induced improvement in glucose–insulin dynamics, with a reduction in circulating insulin levels, may contribute to a reduction in blood pressure by a number of physiological mechanisms.[111]

C. ATHEROTHROMBOTIC CEREBROVASCULAR DISEASE (STROKE)

Hypertension and cigarette smoking appear to be more important risk factors for stroke then hypercholesterolemia. Further, hypertension increases the risk of both atherothrombotic and hemorrhagic stroke. Limited data exist regarding the role (if any) physical activity plays in preventing stroke. Nine studies recently reviewed by Blair et al.[6] showed equivocal findings. Interpreting these data is difficult because stroke has multiple etiologies (atherothrombotic, hemorrhagic, and embolic).[6,17] Additionally, physical activity classification was determined by a variety of methods (e.g., participation in varsity college athletics, LTPA, and occupational physical activity assessment by survey, and job classification of physical activity at work). Nevertheless, three of the nine studies showed a significant inverse association between physical activity and risk of stroke after adjusting for confounders. It is conceivable that physical activity may favorably impact upon atherothrombotic stroke by reducing severity of atherosclerosis and risk of thrombosis in an analogous manner as postulated for IHD prevention. Additionally, since hypertension is considered one of the most prevalent risk factors for stroke, physical activity may decrease the risk of hemorrhagic stroke through its blood pressure–lowering effect.[6,17]

D. PERIPHERAL ARTERIAL DISEASE

Cigarette smoking and diabetes appear to be the major contributors to the etiology of atherosclerotic peripheral vascular disease. In contrast to the effects of physical activity on the clinical manifestations of coronary atherosclerosis, much less is known regarding the relationship between physical activity and peripheral arterial atherosclerosis. Kannel and Sorlie[23] followed middle-aged males from the Framingham cohort for the development of peripheral vascular disease over a 14-year period and found no association between physical activity level and this disorder.

Conceivably, physical activity may favorably impact upon several known risk factors (low HDL-C, hypertension, elevated triglycerides, risk of diabetes mellitus) for peripheral arterial disease.[17] Again, this has not been as extensively studied in patients with peripheral arterial disease as it has in IHD patients.[17] Finally, exercise training has been shown to improve peak work capacity on exercise testing[112] and walking duration[113] in patients with peripheral vascular disease.

III. CANCER

Cancer ranks second to cardiovascular disease as a cause of mortality in this country. However, in contrast to IHD and cardiovascular disease, the mortality rates from cancer have steadily risen over the past 20 years.[114]

As early as 70 years ago an inverse relationship between occupational physical activity and cancer mortality was demonstrated in an observational study.[6] Since this time, numerous epidemiological, as well as experimental, animal studies have been performed investigating the relationship between physical activity and a variety of forms of malignancies, and several detailed reviews of these studies are available.[6,114-116]

The epidemiological evidence in humans relating physical activity and total-cancer mortality is equivocal.[114] Seven of twelve studies recently reviewed by Sternfeld[114] demonstrated an inverse association between physical activity or physical fitness and all-cancer mortality, while five did not. A variety of methods was employed to assess physical activity in these studies which may explain some of the discrepancy. A recent study by Blair et al.,[28] employing an objective measure of aerobic capacity, revealed a relative risk for all-cancer mortality of 4.3 for men and 16.3 for women when least-fit individuals were compared were the most fit based on maximal treadmill testing. Because cancer is made up of a heterogeneous set of diseases, using all-cancer mortality as an end point may obscure site-specific effects.[114]

The site-specific malignancy most often studied in relation to physical activity has been colorectal cancer. In these studies, the incidence of colorectal cancer was compared with physical activity status as determined from job classification, self-reported occupational activity, LTPA or total activity, and previous college athletic activity. Epidemiological approaches have included retrospective, prospective, and case-control studies. Despite the variability in study methodology, results have consistently demonstrated an inverse relationship between physical activity and colon but not rectal cancer.[114] These studies reported increased risks of colon cancer associated with physical inactivity to range from 10 to 100%.[114] There are several postulated mechanisms by which physical activity may influence the biology of colon cancer.[114] Physical activity decreases transit time in the colon, thus perhaps decreasing the exposure of the colon to potential carcinogens.[117,118] This effect may be mediated through exercise-induced increased vagal tone.[119] Another potential mechanism by which physical activity may favorably affect colonic tissue physiology is through prostaglandin synthesis.[119] Vigorous exercise has been shown to increase secretion of a series of prostaglandins,[120] which decrease the rate of cell division in the colon[121] and increase gut motility.[122]

Although not as extensively studied as colorectal cancers, breast cancer and cancers of the female reproductive system (ovary, uterus, cervix, and vagina) also appear to be inversely associated with physical activity level.[114,115] The study most often cited was performed by Frisch et al.[123] in which more than 5000 athletic and nonathletic college alumnae were surveyed by mailed questionnaire regarding activity habits and cancer diagnoses. The relative risks for breast and reproductive cancers for the nonathletes was 1.8 and 2.5, respectively. Potential confounders (age, family history of cancer, age of menarche, number of pregnancies, use of oral contraceptives, use of estrogen during the menopausal period, and cigarette smoking) were adjusted for in this study. If a protective effect of physical activity does indeed exist with malignancies at these sites, the most plausible biological mechanism is probably related to exercise-induced changes in the secretion of estrogen and other sex hormones.[114-115] Through its ability to stimulate cell proliferation, estrogen activity has been strongly implicated in the pathogenesis of breast and reproductive cancers.[124,125]

Of the ten investigations recently reviewed by Sternfeld[114] of physical activity and prostrate cancer, four suggest an inverse relationship, three did not demonstrate an association of any type, and two suggested a direct relationship. Due to these inconsistent findings the effect (if any) of physical activity on the development of prostate cancer remains unclear. If there is a protective effect, it may be mediated through exercise-induced lowering of circulating testosterone levels.[126] Relatively little research has been devoted to the effect of physical activity on other site-specific neoplasms.

Experimentally, increased physical activity has been shown to retard the growth of various types of tumor in animals.[115] However, the extent to which these results can be extrapolated to humans is questionable.[115] For instance, as pointed out by Shephard[115] "If a rat is exercised for 12 weeks, beginning at an age of two years, is this equivalent to a human volunteer who exercises regularly from 50 to 60 years of age?"

IV. DIABETES MELLITUS AND ASSOCIATED GLUCOSE–INSULIN DYNAMICS

Diabetes mellitus is one of the oldest diseases known to man and currently ranks as the sixth leading cause of mortality in the United States.[127] This disease is best characterized as a group of metabolic disorders that have in common an actual or relative insufficiency of insulin. As there is evidence that diabetes is a heterogeneous syndrome, a number of systems for classification of individual types of diabetes mellitus have been developed.[128] A common distinction is that made between Type I, or insulin-dependent diabetes mellitus (IDDM), and Type II, or non-insulin-dependent diabetes mellitus (NIDDM). Although the etiology of NIDDM is not fully understood, two major risk factors appear to be obesity[129-132] and a genetic predisposition (positive family history) for NIDDM.[133,134] Along with weight loss, exercise has been recommended as part of the treatment for NIDDM and several reviews of the relationship between physical activity and glucose–insulin dynamics have been published.[127,135]

Exercise conditioning has been promoted since ancient times as a treatment for diabetes mellitus. Over 20 years ago it was demonstrated in an epidemiological cross-sectional comparison that increased levels of physical activity were associated with lower plasma insulin concentrations as well as enhanced insulin sensitivity.[136] Since this time, numerous cross-sectional studies have documented an increased insulin sensitivity with increased activity level.[62,127,135,137] Not surprisingly, physically inactive societies have demonstrated a higher incidence of NIDDM than more active societies.[138] Likewise, in several cross-sectional studies, the prevalence of NIDDM was inversely associated with physical activity level.[139,140] However, physical inactivity is often associated with obesity, the most potent risk factor for Type II diabetes, making the interpretation of the cross-sectional data difficult.

Helmrich et al.[141] followed almost 6000 male alumni of the University of Pennsylvania for up to 14 years for the development of NIDDM. Life-style habits and health status were assessed by questionnaire. Results showed steadily decreasing relative risks for NIDDM for every 500 kcal · week[-1] increment in LTPA. For example, those individuals expending >3500 kcal · week[-1] had approximately one half the relative risk for the development of NIDDM as individuals expending <500 kcal · week[-1]. Furthermore, the protective effect of physical activity was independent of the common risk factors for NIDDM (obesity, age, history of hypertension, and parental history of diabetes) and more apparent in individuals at high risk for NIDDM. Also, the performance of vigorous vs. more moderate intensity activity was associated with a greater protective effect. The relative risks of NIDDM for those individuals performing moderate sports only and vigorous sports only were 0.90 and 0.69, respectively.

The experimental data support the epidemiological findings suggesting a beneficial effect of physical activity on glucose–insulin dynamics. In a classic study with healthy young volunteers, physical inactivity due to bed rest resulted in insulin insensitivity, reduced glucose tolerance, and hyperinsulinemia after only a few days.[142,143] Additionally, an acute bout of endurance exercise has been shown to be accompanied by an accelerated rate of glucose utilization and increased insulin sensitivity.[106] This effect may persist up to 48 h after termination of exercise. Furthermore, numerous endurance exercise training studies have documented reduced insulin secretion in response to a glucose challenge in NIDDM patients as well as in healthy individuals.[127] Regular exercise training may potentiate the acute metabolic and hormonal adaptations occurring during acute exercise that contribute to reduced insulin requirements.

However, there is a paucity of controlled clinical studies involving either Type I or Type II diabetic individuals to determine whether or not there are chronic effects of exercise on glucose–insulin dynamics and glycemic control beyond those resulting from repeated bouts of acute exercise.[144] The few chronic exercise studies involving subjects with IDDM have yielded contradictory results.[135,145-151] In a similar fashion, studies evaluating the effects of exercise training on metabolic control of NIDDM have also yielded contradictory results.[144] Inconsistency in changes in glucose–insulin dynamics with endurance exercise conditioning in subjects with Type I or II diabetes mellitus or glucose intolerance may be related to a number of factors. These include (1) the heterogeneity of study populations; (2) baseline differences in disease severity; (3) differences in relative weight, body fatness, and initial physical fitness of study subjects; (4) the variability in control of diet composition; (5) the presence or absence of weight changes; (6) the type, intensity, frequency, and duration of exercise; (7) the magnitude of the resulting improvement in VO_{2max}; and (8) how long after the last exercise session the metabolic measurements were made. None of the studies reporting metabolic benefit with exercise training could exclude the possibility that the observed changes may have at least partially been due to the last bout of exercise, since most measurements were made 36 to 48 h after the last exercise session. Additional research is needed to clarify the discrepancies among exercise studies in diabetic individuals, taking the above variables into consideration.

There are several plausible mechanisms by which acute and possibly chronic physical activity enhance insulin sensitivity. The plasma membranes of skeletal muscle have been shown to have an increased number and activity of glucose transporter proteins after a single bout of exercise.[152] Furthermore, as a result of endurance training, both adipose and muscle tissue substantially increase glucose-transporter proteins and exhibit enhanced transport of glucose into these tissues in response to insulin stimulation.[153] Results of recent studies demonstrated that exercise training also increases cellular sensitivity to insulin in all people by significantly increasing the number of insulin receptors in proportion to the improvement in physical fitness.[154-157] Conversely, overeating and weight gain both in animals and humans have been demonstrated to cause insulin resistance, associated with a loss of insulin receptors in distended adipocytes.[158,159] Considering that approximately 80% of individuals with NIDDM are obese and that the incidence of this disease is extremely low in lean populations, physical activity can also reduce the susceptibility to diabetes mellitus by promoting proper weight maintenance. In particular, centralized or abdominal obesity is most closely associated with an increased incidence of hyperinsulinemia and disorders of glucose metabolism.[160,161] With exercise, body fat may be lost more rapidly from the central or abdominal region of the body.[162] Coupled with these changes, exercise conditioning also results in hemodynamic and metabolic adaptations in the working skeletal muscles (i.e., an increase in skeletal muscle mass, capillary density, and blood flow, and enhanced mitochondrial oxidative capacity) which theoretically should enhance glucose delivery and metabolism and glycogen synthesis and storage.[127,135,145,163] Thus, it appears that the major effect of physical training on insulin–glucose dynamics is to increase both glucose transport and storage into muscle and adipose tissue in response to insulin stimulation.[163]

V. OBESITY

The word "obesity" is derived from the Latin term meaning "to overeat" but has come to mean "overfat," that is, an excess accumulation of body adipose tissue. However, this reflects the age-old bias that obesity is simply due to gluttony and ignores the fact that body weight is determined by a balance between energy intake and energy expenditure.

Obesity is clearly a growing problem of major health concern in the United States[164] affecting about one of every three adults age 20 or older and is closely associated with physical inactivity. Indeed, reduction of obesity favorably impacts many of the same physiological and metabolic risk factors positively affected by exercise. These include favorable changes in lipid and lipoprotein values, reductions in elevated blood pressure levels, and improved glucose–insulin dynamics.[49,165]

Mass sedentariness coupled with easy access to high-caloric-density foods is generally considered the primary explanation for the high prevalence of obesity in the United States.[166] The relative roles of increased energy intake vs. decreased energy expenditure in the etiology of obesity has been extensively studied.[165] Observational data indicate that the prevalence of obesity has progressively increased in the United States during this century despite an apparent decline in per capita food energy intake.[165] Furthermore, the progressive weight gain common to many Americans from age 30 to 60 years is actually associated with a decline in energy intake.[167-169] Both cross-sectional and prospective observational epidemiological studies consistently have demonstrated an inverse relationship between activity level and obesity.[170-173] Similarly, in cross-sectional comparisons between endurance-trained athletes and sedentary controls it is well established that the athletes have lower levels of body fat.[174] In contrast, observational studies comparing physical activity levels in obese and nonobese individuals have yielded contradictory results. Some have reported less activity in obese individuals,[175,178] while others found obese and normal-weight subjects to be equally active.[179,180]

However, it should be emphasized that many of these observational studies have serious limitations. For example, many used small nonrepresentative study samples; failed to consider the severity of obesity; failed to account for dynamic vs. static phases of weight gain; used only a limited number of physical activity measurements; used physical activity assessment instruments with large measurement errors; and were not able to control for the possibility that habitual activity patterns may have been altered during the assessment period. Furthermore, because of the increased energy cost of dynamic activity associated with carrying excess weight, less-active obese subjects may actually expend the same or more energy during activity as their more-active, but leaner counterparts.[181] Finally, obesity may precede a reduction in physical activity rather than vice versa. Therefore, the observational data suggest an association between activity level and obesity, but do not prove a causal relationship. Large-scale, long-term, longitudinal studies employing better measures of physical activity are needed.

Despite the absence of proof of a cause–effect relationship, exercise is now widely accepted as being at least a component of a good treatment program for obesity.[181-186] Controlled studies of exercise or exercise in conjunction with caloric restriction have consistently resulted in weight and fat reduction in overweight individuals.[165] For example, the value of exercise for a weight reduction program was demonstrated by Sopko et al.[71] In this study, obese young men were subjected to a negative energy balance of 3500 kcal · week^{-1} provided by either treadmill exercise or caloric restriction over a 12-week period. Although the resulting weight loss was nearly identical (1.1 to 1.2 lb week^{-1}) for both regimens, the rate of body fat loss was significantly greater in the exercise group. Most other studies comparing fat loss by dietary restrictions and exercise alone or in combination with diet have shown similar results.[174,181,187-190] However the intervention periods for most of these studies ranged from only 8 to 17 weeks. The general consensus in the literature is that exercise alone is an ineffective, long-term treatment for obesity, but is a useful adjunct for weight reduction and maintenance when combined with a moderate reduction in energy intake.[182]

The metabolic mechanisms by which exercise contributes to weight loss and/or maintenance include increased energy expenditure associated with the performance of the physical activity (primary mechanism); enhanced fat mobilization by increasing adipose tissue activity; a transient small increase in postexercise resting metabolic rate; perhaps an increased thermogenic response to food if exercise is in proximity to a meal; attenuation of the decline in basal metabolic rate with dietary restrictions; and possibly better appetite control (at least for a short period after exercise).[165]

Recently, a great deal of scientific interest has been generated regarding the health implications of the regional distribution of body fat.[160] Several epidemiological studies have demonstrated an increased risk of cardiovascular disease and mortality associated with abdominal or upper body accumulation of fat (android-type obesity) compared with a concentration of fat around the thighs, hips, and buttocks or lower body (gynoid-type) obesity.[191-195] Additionally, abdominal obesity has been clearly shown to be related to disturbances in glucose homeostasis (insulin resistance, hyperinsulinemia, and glucose intolerance), dyslipoproteinemia (high plasma triglycerides and low concentrations of HDL-C), and hypertension.[160] Moreover, it appears to be mesenteric adipose tissue (sometimes called "portal" adipose tissue because it is drained by the portal vein) which exhibits unique characteristics that may lead to these adverse health effects.[160,196] Portal adipose tissue is highly sensitive to lipolysis because of a high concentration of beta-adrenergic receptors and little alpha-adrenergic inhibition. Coupled with this is a low concentration of insulin receptors in portal adipose tissue which reduces insulin uptake and associated inhibition of lipolysis. Thus, as a result of these two mechanisms, hepatic tissue is exposed to high concentrations of free fatty acids. The resulting effect on liver metabolism may ultimately be responsible for the metabolic alterations and subsequent morbidity and mortality previously mentioned. Recently, it has been shown that exercise training may alter body fat distribution by preferentially mobilizing abdominal subcutaneous fat.[162]

VI. OSTEOPOROSIS

Osteoporosis is a disorder characterized by a reduction in bone mass with subsequent increased susceptibility to fracture with little or no trauma.[197] As there appears to be a wide continuum of bone mass levels specific for age and gender, a more precise definition of osteoporosis is difficult.[198] This condition affects anywhere from 15 to 20 million Americans and is responsible for approximately 1.3 million fractures a year in individuals aged 45 years and older.[197] The resulting economic burden in the United States is an estimated $3.8 billion a year particularly due to morbidity/mortality from hip fractures.[197] Several excellent reviews are available which discuss the underlying pathogenesis of osteoporosis and the role of several preventative measures, including physical activity.[197-201] This condition is predominantly found in caucasian or Oriental postmenopausal women. Other contributing factors are a reduced bone mass at physical maturing, low calcium (dairy products) intake, slender body build, no postmenopausal estrogen replacement, and physical inactivity.

For over a century, it has been recognized that bone tissue responds to mechanical forces.[202] In the absence of these forces, immobility such as that due to bed rest, a gravity-free environment (astronauts), or paralysis clearly leads to a reduction in bone mass.[203-207]

Cross-sectional comparisons between athletes and healthy controls have consistently demonstrated an increased bone mass at various sites in the athletes,[197-201] particularly in the limbs primarily used in the activity.[201,208-212] In contrast to these data, cross-sectional comparisons in the general population between active vs. sedentary individuals have not produced consistent findings regarding the relationship between bone density and physical activity.[199,201] Problems with physical activity assessment methodology probably contribute in large part to a failure of some studies to demonstrate an increase in bone density with increasing levels of self-reported activity.[199,201] However, a fairly consistent relationship has been shown between various objective measures of physical fitness and bone mass.[201]

Numerous intervention exercise training studies have been performed to study the effects of an exercise program on bone mass. These have recently been reviewed by Smith et al.[201] In general, a period of endurance training either retards loss or actually increases bone mass. This effect has been noted in different age groups and for men and women, including postmenopausal women, a population at greatest risk for osteoporosis. Changes in bone mass were more likely to occur if the bone being measured was involved in the performance of the activity. However, the specific exercise prescription necessary for optimal results has yet to be determined.

VII. DOSE–RESPONSE — AN OVERALL RECOMMENDATION FOR HEALTH PROMOTION, DISEASE PREVENTION, AND GOALS FOR HEALTHY PEOPLE 2000

The foregoing discussion provides abundant evidence that physical activity is related to a variety of health benefits. However, emphasis has shifted recently to not only documenting associations and/or

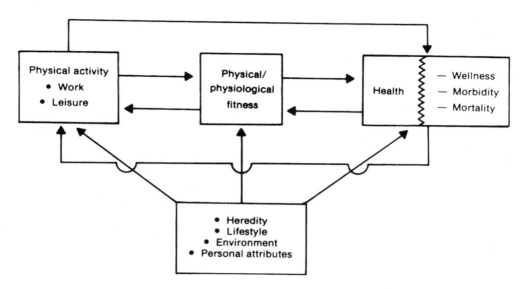

Figure 1 Interactions between physical activity, fitness, and health. (From Bouchard, C. and Shephard, R. J., 1994, Physical activity, fitness, and health: The model and key concepts, in *Physical Activity, Fitness, and Health: International Proceedings and Consensus Statement*, Bouchard, C., Shephard, R. J., and Stephens, T., eds., Human Kinetics Publishers, Champaign, IL, 79.)

causal pathways between physical activity and specific health outcomes, but to defining the dose–response relationship as well. As stated by Haskell[213] "The question is no longer, should a person exercise, but how much of what type of exercise is going to be most effective in providing specific benefits." The traditional approach for prescribing exercise to improve health was to prescribe that level of exercise which would lead to improvement in aerobic capacity.[6,213,214] That is, in order to receive the health benefits of exercise, the dose of exercise would have to be sufficient to result in an improvement in aerobic fitness. However, recent evidence suggests that this is not the case. Although this level of exertion may be necessary to attain the full gambit of the physiological and metabolic adaptations conveying health benefits, it does not appear to be a minimal requirement. A substantially reduced risk for several adverse health outcomes is related to the performance of regular physical exertion below the threshold of intensity required for improving aerobic capacity.

There are several possible relationships which may exist among physical activity, fitness, and health.[213] For instance, physical activity (1) may improve fitness thereby improving health; (2) may improve health and fitness through separate mechanisms; (3) may improve some aspect of health but not necessarily fitness; or (4) may improve fitness but not certain aspects of health. At the recent Consensus Symposium on Physical Activity, Fitness, and Health[215] a model (Figure 1) was developed specifying the relationships among physical activity, health-related fitness, and health. An important distinction was made between health-related and performance-related fitness. Health-related fitness is characterized by "... (a) an ability to perform daily activities with vigor and (b) demonstration of traits and capacities that are associated with a low risk of premature development of hypokinetic diseases and conditions."[215]

As Figure 1 depicts, the issue of the dose–response relationship concerning physical activity and health is a highly complex one. The model specifies that physical activity leads to health-related fitness which, in turn, favorably impacts on health. However, both health status and degree of health-related fitness can reciprocally impact on level of physical activity. Furthermore, other factors such as life-style behaviors, personal attributes, and the social and physical environment can influence each of these components of the model. Finally, genetic factors can influence not only the individual's level of physical activity, degree of health-related fitness, and health status, but also the interrelationships between each of these. Moreover, the dose of physical activity must be considered in relation to several factors.[213,215] These include not only the type, intensity, duration, and frequency of exercise, but also whether a particular health-related benefit results from an acute bout of exercise, chronic exercise training, or through an interaction between acute and chronic exercise. Following is a brief overview of the dose–response relationship between physical activity and several health outcomes.

Early studies of the occupational activity of longshoremen[216] and of LTPA of British executive-class civil servants[4,18] suggested that hard physical labor and vigorous LTPA were required to reduce the risk of IHD. However, several recent studies suggest that moderate levels of lower-intensity activity, performed on a regular basis, are related to a reduced risk of IHD, as well as to all-cause mortality.[12,13,19-26,28,100,207] For instance, those college alumni studied by Paffenbarger et al.[12,19] who expended as little as 500 kcal·week^{-1} in a combination of walking, stair climbing, and sports play demonstrated a reduction in the risk of IHD. The lowest age-adjusted incidence rates of IHD and overall mortality were found in those men expending 2000 kcal·week^{-1} in these activities. An energy expenditure greater than this was not associated with any further protective effect from IHD. Data on men at high risk for IHD followed in MRFIT[21,22] are consistent with these findings. An optimal reduction in the risk of IHD mortality was found in those men expending 1500 kcal·week^{-1} in predominantly light- and moderate-intensity LTPA (e.g. walking and working around the house and yard for approximately 45 min·day^{-1}) when compared with age-matched sedentary men who performed these activities less than 30 min·day^{-1}. Again, there was no added benefit concerning risk reduction of IHD mortality with an energy output (i.e., 90 min·day^{-1} of similar LTPA) above this threshold.

A similar dose–response relationship has recently been shown for levels of physical fitness and IHD mortality and total mortality.[28] Those men and women followed by Blair et al.[28] who were moderately fit (7 to 8 MET* capacity), based on maximal treadmill testing, had a substantially reduced risk of cardiovascular as well as all-cause mortality compared with the least-fit (less than or equal to 6 MET capacity) individuals. Higher levels of fitness were associated with relatively little additional reduction in risk of mortality. Data from the Lipid Research Clinics follow-up study in men[100] also demonstrated a substantially reduced risk of cardiovascular mortality in the moderately fit men (based on submaximal exercise heart rate) compared with those with the highest heart rate (least-fit men). However, in contrast to the highly fit men followed by Blair et al.,[28] those men with the lowest heart rate demonstrated a substantial additional reduction in risk of mortality. Likewise, in addition to demonstrating a reduced risk for cardiovascular mortality in those Norwegian men who were moderately fit (quartile 3) compared with the least-fit (quartile 1) based on maximal bicycle ergometry, Sandvik and co-workers[29] also reported a marked additional reduction in risk of cardiovascular mortality for the most fit (quartile 4) compared to those men with moderate levels of fitness (quartiles 2 and 3).

These observational studies suggest that there is a continuous (as opposed to a minimal threshold) relationship between increasing levels of physical activity or fitness and reduced risk of IHD mortality and total mortality. The relationship, however, does not appear to be linear, with the greatest rate of reduction in risk occurring between those individuals who are least active and those regularly performing moderate levels of physical activity.

Limited data exist regarding the systematic study of the dose–response relationship between physical activity or fitness and a variety of other adverse health outcomes. However, Haskell[213] recently reviewed data showing favorable changes in obesity, plasma HDL-C, plasma triglycerides, resting blood pressure, and insulin sensitivity with moderate levels of physical activity. Haskell emphasizes that although most health-related outcomes probably respond through the full continuum of exertion, some (i.e., resting blood pressure) may exhibit an "upper threshold" where greater amounts of exercise may be less effective than moderate levels.

It is important from the public health standpoint that high-intensity and/or large volumes of exercise do not appear to be required for sedentary people to gain some health benefit from increased levels of physical activity. This type of activity is perceived by most of the American population as requiring high exertion levels and is intimidating, contributing to adherence problems. Furthermore, the risk of negative health consequences (e.g., injuries to the muscles or joints and sudden cardiac death) is greater during high-intensity activity than during activities with a lower intensity. Blair et al.[6] emphasize that as little as 2 mi·day^{-1} of brisk walking performed most days of the week would result in the moderate level of fitness associated with reduced risk of total mortality in the Aerobics Center Longitudinal Study. A level of activity only slightly greater than this (2 to 3 mi of brisk walking 7 days·week^{-1}) would result in the 1500 to 2000 kcal·week^{-1} threshold of physical activity associated with optimal risk reduction for IHD mortality demonstrated in the MRFIT[21,22] and college alumni[12,19] cohorts, respectively. Furthermore, this level of energy expenditure is comparable with that used in the training studies reviewed by Haskell[213] previously referred to.

---

* MET = resting energy expenditure in the sitting position, approximately equal to 3.5 ml of oxygen per kg of body weight per minute.

The growing realization that moderately intense physical activity leads to important health benefits influenced to a large degree the content of the Healthy People 2000 objectives for the priority area, Improve Physical Fitness.[218] The core set of behavioral objectives (objective A to E) reflects this influence in that the objectives call attention to increasing moderately intense levels of various physical activities. For instance, the first objective (objective A) states "By 2000, the proportion of Americans who regularly participate in moderately intense physical activities such as walking for 3 or more times per week, 30 or more minutes per occasion should be increased from 50 percent to 60 percent."[218]

Surveys by the National Center for Health Statistics and the Behavioral Risk Factor Surveillance Systems indicate that less than 50% of the adult American population engages in exercise of any type on a regular basis (exercise of 20 minutes or longer duration, 3 or more days·week^{-1}).[218] These surveys also indicate that less than 10% of adults perform "Exercise which involves large muscle groups in dynamic movement for periods of 20 minutes or longer, 3 or more days per week, and which is performed at an intensity of 60 percent or greater of an individual's cardiorespiratory capacity," which is the level recommended by the 1990 objectives.[218] Objective B of the year 2000 objectives addresses this issue by recommending that "By 2000, the proportion of Americans who participate in vigorous physical activities that promote the development and maintenance of cardiorespiratory fitness, for 3 or more times per week, 30 or more minutes per occasion should increase from 22 percent to 34 percent." It is noteworthy that "vigorous" is defined as "50 percent or greater of maximal cardiorespiratory capacity," which is 10% lower than the intensity specified by the 1990 objectives.

In light of the potential health benefits to be gained by the performance of relatively moderate levels of activity of reasonable intensity, the current low level of participation in such activity is disappointing. The public health impact of a high prevalence of inactive and low-fit individuals should be appreciated. Recently, Blair et al.[6] reviewed the population-attributable risks of low activity and fitness determined from several sources. Risk estimates for all-cause mortality due to sedentary habits were higher than those found for the major risk factors of elevated cholesterol and hypertension.[217,219] Risk estimates for low levels of fitness determined from the Aerobics Center Longitudinal Study[28] were higher than or comparable with cigarette smoking, high fasting blood glucose, high body mass index, and a positive family history of IHD in addition to elevated cholesterol and hypertension. Clearly, inactivity in the adult American population is a major public health burden.

Although there is much to learn regarding the dose–response relationship between health-related physiological adaptations and physical activity, the public health message is clear: "Doing some physical activity is better than doing none at all" and "… to a degree more is better than less."[6] Blair et al.[6] go on to emphasize that the type of physical activity performed is not so important as the total energy expended. This sentiment is echoed by Haskell,[213] who states that the stimulus for many of the health-related changes "… is a sustained, repeated increase in metabolic rate and any way this can be achieved during physical activity is of benefit." Research efforts should continue to focus on the issue of dose–response relationship and on the development of effective population strategies to promote the adoption and maintenance of an active life-style.

ACKNOWLEDGMENTS

Dr. Leon is partially supported by the Henry L. Taylor Professorship in Exercise Science and Health Enhancement and NHLBI Grant 5R01-HL47323-05.

REFERENCES

1. Blackburn, H., Jacobs, D. R., Jr., Physical Activity and the Risk of Coronary Heart Disease, paper presented at the 5th World Congress on Cardiac Rehabilitation, Bordeaux, France, July 6, 1992 (in press).
2. U.S. Department of Health and Human Services, Physical Activity and Health. A Report of the Surgeon General, Pittsburgh, PA: Superintendant of Documents, 1196, 81–172.
3. Morris, J. N., Kagan, N., Pattison, D. C., Gardner, M. J., Raffle, P. A. B., Incidence and prediction of ischemic heart disease in London busmen, *Lancet*, 2, 533, 1966.
4. Morris, J. N., Clayton, D. G., Everitt, M. G., Semmence, A. M., Burgess, E. M., Exercise in leisure time: coronary attack and death rates, *Br. Med. J.*, 63, 325, 1990.
5. Taylor, H. L., Klepter, E., Keys, A., Parlin, W., Blackburn, H., Puchner, T., Death rates among physically active and sedentary employees in the railroad industry, *Am. J. Public Health*, 52, 1697, 1962.
6. Blair, S. N., Kohl, H.W., Gordon, N. F., Paffenbarger, R. S., Jr., How much physical activity is good for health?, *Annu. Rev. Public Health*, 13, 99, 1992.

7. Bouchard, C., Shepard, R. J., Stephens, T., Sutton, J., McPherson, B., Eds., *Exercise, Fitness and Health. A Consensus of Current Knowledge,* Human Kinetics, Champaign, IL, 1990.

8. Watson, R. R., Eisinger M., Eds., *Exercise and Disease,* Boca Raton, CRC Press, 1992.

9. Stamler, J., Established major coronary risk factors, in *Coronary Heart Disease Epidemiology: From Aetilogy To Public Health,* Marmot, M., Elliott, P., Eds., Oxford, Oxford Medical, 1992, 35–66.

10. Leon, A. S., Blackburn, H., Physical activity in the prevention of coronary heart disease: an update, in *Advances in Disease Prevention,* Vol. 1, Arnold, C. B., Kuller, L. H., Coreenlick, M. R., Eds., Springer Publishing Co., New York, 1981, 97–135.

11. Leon, A. S., Blackburn, H., The relationship of physical activity to coronary heart disease and life expectancy, *Ann. N.Y. Acad. Sci.,* 301, 561, 1977.

12. Paffenbarger, R. S., Jr., Hyde, R. T., Exercise in the prevention of coronary heart disease, *Prev. Med.,* 13, 3, 1984.

13. Powell, K. E., Thompson, P. D., Casperson, C. J., Kendrick, J. S., Physical activity and the incidence of coronary heart disease, *Annu. Rev. Public Health,* 8, 253, 1987.

14. Berlin, J. A., Colditz, G. A., A meta-analysis of physical activity in the prevention of coronary heart disease, *Am. J. Epidemiol.,* 132, 612, 1990.

15. Froelicher, V. F., Exercise, fitness and coronary heart disease, in *Exercise, Fitness, and Health: A Consensus of Current Knowledge,* Bouchard, C., Shepard, R. J., Stephens, T., Sutton, J. R., and McPherson, B. D., Eds., Human Kinetics, Champaign, IL, 1990, 429–450.

16. Leon, A. S., Physical activity and risk of ischemic heart disease — an update 1990, in *Sport for All,* Rothelma, O. J. A., Ed., Elsevier, Amsterdam, 1991, 251–264.

17. Haskell, W. L., Leon, A. S., Casperson, C. J., Froelicher, V. F., Hagberg, J. M., Harlan, W., Holloszy, J. O., Regensteiner, J. G., Thompson, P. D., Washburn, R. A., Wilson, P. W. F., Cardiovascular benefits and assessment of physical activity and physical fitness in adults, *Med. Sci. Sports Exercise,* 24, Suppl., S201, 1992.

18. Morris, J. N., Everitt, M. G., Pollard, R., Chave, S. P. W., Vigorous exercise in leisure-time: protection against coronary heart disease, *Lancet,* 2, 1207, 1980.

19. Paffenbarger, R. S., Jr., Wing, A. L., Hyde, R. T., A natural history of athleticism and cardiovascular health, *J. Am. Med. Assoc.,* 252, 491, 1984.

20. Slattery, M. L., Jacobs, D. R., Jr., Nichaman, M. Z., Leisure time physical activity and coronary heart disease death: the U.S. railroad study, *Circulation,* 29, 304, 1989.

21. Leon, A. S., Connett, J., Jacobs, D. R., Jr., Rauramaa, R., Leisure-time physical activity levels and risk of heart disease and death: the Multiple Risk Factor Intervention Trial, *J. Am. Med. Assoc.,* 258, 2388, 1987.

22. Leon, A. S. Connett, J., Physical activity and 10.5 year mortaility in the multiple risk factor intervention trial (MRFIT). *Int. J. Epidemiol.,* 20, 690, 1991.

23. Kannel, W. B., Sorlie, P., Some health benefits of physical activity: the Framingham Study, *Arch. Intern. Med.,* 139, 857, 1979.

24. Salonen, J. T., Slater, J. S., Tuomilehto, J., Rauramaa, R., Leisure time and occupational activity: risk of death from ischemic heart disease, *Am. J. Epidemiol.,* 127, 87, 1988.

25. Garcia-Palmier, M. R., Costas, R., Jr., Cruz-Vidal, M., Sorlie, P. D., Havlik, R. J., Increased physical activity: a protective factor against heart attacks in Puerto Rico, *Am. J. Cardiol.,* 50, 749, 1982.

26. Donahue, R. P., Abbott, R. D., Reed, D. M., Yano, K., Physical activity and coronary heart disease in middle-aged and elderly men: the Honolulu Heart Study, *Am. J. Public Health,* 78, 683, 1988.

27. Paffenbarger, R. S., Jr., Hyde, R. T., Wing, A. L., Lee, I. M., Jung, D. L., Kampert, J. B., The association of changes in physical-activity level and other life-style characteristics with mortality among men, *N. Engl. J. Med.,* 328, 538, 1993.

28. Blair, S. N., Kohl, H. W., III., Paffenbarger, R. S., Jr., Clark, D. G., Cooper, K. H., Gibbons, L. W., Physical fitness and all-causes mortality: a prospective study of healthy men and women, *J. Am. Med. Assoc.,* 262, 2395, 1989.

29. Sandvik, L., Eriksen, J., Thaulow, E., Erikssen, G., Mundal, R., Rodahl, K., Physical fitness as a predictor of mortality among healthy, middle-aged Norwegian men, *N. Engl. J. Med.,* 328, 533, 1993.

30. Leon, A. S., Jacobs, D. R., Jr., Debacker, G., Taylor, H. L., Relationship of physical characteristics and life habits to treadmill exercise performance, *Am. J. Epidemiol.,* 113, 653, 1981.

31. Gordon, D. J., Leon, A. S., Ekelund, L.-G., et al., Smoking, physical activity, and other predictors of endurance and heart rate response to exercise in asymptomatic hypercholesterolemic men: the Lipid Research Clinics Coronary Primary Prevention Trial, *Am. J. Epidemiol.,* 125, 587, 1987.

32. Bouchard, C., Genetic determinants of endurance performance, in *Endurance in Sports,* Shepard, R. J., Astrand, P. O., Eds., Blackwell Scientific, Oxford, 1992, 149–159.

33. O'Conner, G. T., Buring, J. E., Yusaf, S., et al., An overview of randomized trials of rehabilitation with exercise after myocardial infarction, *Circulation,* 80, 234, 1989.

34. Oldridge, N. B., Guyatt, G. H., Fischer, M. E., Rimm, A. A., Cardiac rehabilitation after myocardial infarction, *J. Am. Med. Assoc.,* 260, 945, 1988.

35. Kramsch, D. M., Aspen, A. J., Abramowitz, B. M., Kreimendahl, T., Hood, W. B., Jr., Reduction of coronary atherosclerosis by moderate conditioning exercise in monkeys on atherogenic diet, *N. Engl. J. Med.,* 305, 1483, 1981.

36. Ornish, D., Brown, S. E., Scherwitz, L. W., et al., Can life-style changes reverse coronary heart disease? *Lancet,* 336, 129, 1990.

37. Wood, P. D., Stefanick, M. L., Exercise, fitness and atherosclerosis, in *Exercise and Health: A Consensus of Current Knowledge*, Bouchard, C., Shepard, R. J., Stephens, T., Sutton, J. R., McPherson, B. D., Eds., Human Kinetics, Champaign, IL, 1990, 409–424.

38. Schroll, M., Hagerup, L. M., Risk factors of myocardial infarction and death in men aged 50 at entry. A ten-year prospective study from the Glostrup Population Studies, *Dan. Med. Bull.*, 24, 252, 1977.

39. Expert Panel: Report of the National Cholesterol Education Program Expert Panel on Detection, Evaluation, and Treatment of High Blood Cholesterol in Adults, *Arch. Intern. Med.*, 148, 36–39, 1988.

40. Pekkanen, J., Linn, S., Heiss, G., Suchindran, C. M., Leon, A., Rifkind, B. M., Tyroler, H. A., Ten-year mortality from cardiovascular disease in relation to cholesterol level among men with or without pre-existing cardiovascular disease, *N. Engl. J. Med.*, 322, 1700, 1990.

41. Frick, M. H., Elo, O., Haapa, K., Heinonen, O. P., et al. Helsinki Heart Study: primary-prevention trial with gemfibrozil in middle-aged men with dyslipidemia, *N. Engl. J. Med.*, 317, 1237, 1987.

42. Gordon, D. J., Knoke, J., Probstfield, J. L., Superko, R., Tyroler, H. A., High-density lipoprotein cholesterol and coronary heart disease in hypercholesterolemic men: the Lipid Research Clinics Coronary Primary Prevention Trial, *Circulation*, 74, 1217, 1986.

43. Miller, C. J., Miller, N. E., Plasma high-density lipoprotein concentrations and the development of ischemic heart disease, *Lancet*, 1, 16, 1975.

44. Gordon, T., Castelli, W. P., Hjortland, M. C., Kannel, W. B., Dawber, T. R., High density lipoprotein as a protective factor against coronary heart disease: the Framingham Study, *Am. J. Med.*, 62, 707, 1977.

45. Wallace, R. B., Anderson, R. A., Blood lipid, lipid-related measures, and the risk of atherosclerotic cardiovascular disease, *Epidemiol. Rev.*, 9, 95, 1987.

46. Lithell, M., Orlander, J., Shele, R., Changes in lipoprotein lipase activity and lipid stores in human skeletal muscle with prolonged heavy exercise, *Acta Physiol. Scand.*, 107, 257, 1979.

47. Hartung, G. H., Squires, W. G., Gotto, A. M., Effect of exercise training on plasma high-density lipoprotein cholesterol in coronary disease patients, *Am. Heart J.*, 101, 181, 1981.

48. Superko, H. R., Exercise training, serum lipids, and lipoprotein particles: is there a change threshold?, *Med. Sci. Sports Exercise*, 23, 677, 1991.

49. Leon, A. S., Physiological interaction between diet and exercise in the etiology and prevention of ischemic heart disease, *Ann. Clin. Res.*, 20, 114, 1988.

50. Leon, A. S., Exercise and risk of coronary heart disease, in *Exercise and Health*, Eckert, H. M., Montoye, J. H., Eds., Human Kinetics, Champaign, IL, 1984, 14-31.

51. Dyer, A. R., Persky, V., Stawler, J., et al., Heart rate as a prognostic factor for coronary heart disease and mortality: findings in three Chicago epidemiologic studies, *Am. J. Epidemiol.*, 112, 736, 1980.

52. Hickey, N. R., Mulcahy, G. J., Bourke, I., et al., Study of coronary risk factors related to physical activity in 15,171 men, *Br. Med. J.*, 3, 507, 1975.

53. Superko, H. R., Haskell, W. L., The role of exercise training in the therapy of hyperlipoproteinemia, *Clin. Cardiol.*, 5, 285, 1987.

54. Superko, H. R., Krauss, R. M., LDL and HDL particle subclass differences in CHD patients treated with selective and nonselective beta blocking medications, in *Proceedings of the 8th International Symposium on Atherosclerosis*, Rome, Italy, 1988, p. 908.

55. Wood, P. D., Haskell, W. L., Blair, S. N., et al., Increased exercise level and plasma lipoprotein concentrations: a one-year randomized controlled study in sedentary middle-aged men, *Metabolism*, 32, 31, 1983.

56. LaPorte, R., Brenes, G., Dearwater, S., HDL-cholesterol across a spectrum of physical activity from quadriplegia to marathon running, *Lancet*, 1, 1212, 1983.

57. Durstine, J. L., Pate, R. R., Sparling, P. B., Wilson, G. E., Senn, M. D., Bartoli, W. P., Lipid, lipoprotein, and iron status of elite women distance runners, *Int. J. Sports Med.*, 8, 119, 1987.

58. Martin, R. P., Haskel, W. L., Wood, P. D., Blood chemistry and lipid profiles of elite distance runners, *Ann. N.Y. Acad. Sci.*, 301, 386, 1977.

59. Williams, P. T., Krauss, R. M., Wood, P. D., Lingren, F. T., Giotas, C., Vranizan, K. M., Lipoprotein subfractions of runners and sedentary men, *Metabolism*, 35, 45, 1986.

60. Haskell, W. L., Taylor, H. L., Wood, P. D., Schrott, H., Heiss, G., Strenuous physical activity, treadmill exercise test response and plasma high density lipoprotein cholesterol. The Lipid Research Clinic Program Prevalence Study, *Circulation*, 62, Suppl. IV, 53, 1980.

61. Gordon, D. J., Probstfield, J. L., Rubenstein, C., et al., Coronary risk factors and exercise test performance in asymptomatic hypercholesterolemic men: application of proportional hazards analysis, *Am. J. Epidemiol.*, 120, 210, 1984.

62. Leon, A. S., Effects of exercise conditioning on physiologic precursors of coronary heart disease, *J. Cardiopulm. Rehabil.*, 11, 46, 1991.

63. Haskell, W. L., Durstine, L., Impact of exercise training on lipoprotein metabolism, in *Diabetes Mellitus*, Devlin, J., Horton, E.S., Vranic, M., Eds., Smith-Gordon, London, 205, 1992.

64. Tsopanakis, A. D., Sgouraki, E. P., Pavlov, K. N., Nadel, E. R., Bussolari, S. R., Lipids and lipoprotein profiles in 4-h endurance test on a recumbent cycloergometer, *Am. J. Clin. Nutr.*, 49, 980, 1989.

65. Gordon, N. F., Cooper, K. H., Controlling cholesterol levels through exercise, *Compr. Ther.*, 14, 52, 1988.

66. Holloszy, J. O., Skinner, J. S., Toro, G., Cureton, T. K., Effects of a six month program of endurance exercise on the serum lipids of middle-aged men, *Am. J. Cardiol.*, 14, 753, 1964.

67. Goldberg, L., Elliot, D. L., The effect of physical activity on lipid and lipoprotein levels, *Med. Clin. North Am.*, 69, 41, 1985.

68. Weintraub, M. S., Rosen, Y., Otto, R., Eisenberg, S., Broslov, J. L., Physical exercise conditioning in the absence of weight loss reduces fasting and post-prandial triglyceride-rich lipoprotein levels, *Circulation*, 79, 1007, 1989.

69. Haskel, W. L., The influence of exercise training on plasma lipids and lipoproteins in health and disease, *Acta Med. Scand.*, 11, Suppl. 7, 25, 1986.

70. Wood, P. D., Stefanick, M. L., Dreon, D. M., et al., Changes in plasma lipid and lipoproteins in overweight men during weight loss through dieting as compared with exercise, *N. Engl. J. Med.*, 319, 1173, 1988.

71. Sopko, G., Leon, A. S., Jacobs, D. R., Jr., et al., The effects of exercise and weight loss on plasma lipids in young obese men, *Metabolism*, 39, 227, 1985.

72. Santiago, M. C., Alexander, J. F., Stull, G. A., Serfass, R. C., Hayday, A. M., Leon, A. S., Physiological responses of sedentary women to a 20-week conditioning program of walking or jogging, *Scand. J. Sports Sci.*, 9, 33, 1987.

73. Santiago, M. C., Effects of a forty-week walking program of twelve miles per week on physical fitness, body composition, and blood lipids and lipoproteins in sedentary women. A thesis in partial fulfillment of the requirements for the Ph.D. degree. Minneapolis, University of Minnesota, 1990, 1–208.

74. Estelles, A., Tormo, G., Aznar, J., Espana, F., Tormo, V., Reduced fibrinolytic activity in coronary heart disease in basic conditions and after exercise, *Thromb. Res.*, 40, 373, 1985.

75. Rauramaa, R., Salonen, J. T., Seppanen, K., et al., Inhibition of platelet aggregability by moderate-intensity physical exercise: a randomized clinical trial in overweight men, *Circulation*, 74, 939, 1986.

76. Eichner, E., Coagulability and rheology: hematologic benefits from exercise, fish, and aspirin: implications for athletes and nonathletes, *Physician Sports Med.*, 14, 102, 1986.

77. Lee, G., Amsterdam, E. A., DeMara, A. M., Davis, G., LaFave, T., Mason, T. D., Effect of exercise on hemostatic mechanisms, in *Exercise in Cardiovascular Health and Disease*, Amsterdam, E. A., Wilmore, J. H., DeMara, A. N., Eds., Yorke Medical Books, New York, 1977, 122–136.

78. Rauramaa, R., Physical activity and prostanoids, *Acta Med. Scand. Suppl.*, 711, 37, 1986.

79. Stratton, J. R., Chandler, W. L., Schwartz, R. S., et al., Effects of physical conditioning of fibrinolytic variables and fibrinogen in young and old healthy adults, *Circulation*, 83, 1692, 1991.

80. Thompson, P., The benefits and risks of exercise training in patients with chronic coronary artery disease, *J. Am. Med. Assoc.*, 259, 1537, 1988.

81. Leon, A. S., Comparative cardiovascular adaptations to exercise in animals and man and its relevance to coronary heart disease, in *Comparative Pathophysiology of Circulatory Disorders*, Bloor, C. M., Ed., Plenum Publishing Corporation, New York, 1972, 143.

82. Froelicher, V., The effect of exercise on myocardial perfusion and function in patients with coronary heart disease, *Eur. Heart J.*, 98 (Suppl. G), 1, 1987.

83. Leon, A. S., Bloor, C. M., Effects of exercise and its cessation on the heart and its blood supply, *J. Appl. Physiol.*, 24, 485, 1968.

84. Leon, A. S., Bloor, C. M., The effect of complete and partial deconditioning on exercise-induced cardiovascular changes in the rat, *Adv. Cardiol.*, 18, 81, 1976.

85. Leon, A. S., Epidemiological aspects of physical activity and coronary heart disease, *Finn. Sports Exercise Med.*, 2, 10, 1983.

86. Rissanen, V., Occupational physical activity and coronary artery disease: a clinicopathologic appraisal, *Adv. Cardiol.*, 18, 113, 1976.

87. Pelliccia, A., Spataro, A., Granata, M., Biffi, A., Caselli, G., Alabiso, A., Coronary arteries in physiological hypertrophy: echocardiographic evidence of increased proximal size in elite athletes, *Int. J. Sports Med.*, 11, 120, 1990.

88. Eckstein, R. W., Effect of exercise and coronary artery narrowing on coronary collateral circulation, *Circ. Res.*, 22, 230, 1957.

89. Bloor, C. M., White, F. C., Sanders, T. M., Effects of exercise on collateral development in myocardial ischemia in pigs, *J. Appl. Physiol.*, 56, 656, 1984.

90. Schevre, J., Effects of physical training on myocardial vascularity and perfusion, *Circulation*, 66, 491, 1982.

91. Dawson, A. K., Leon, A. S., Taylor, H. L., Effect of submaximal exercise on vulnerability to fibrillation in the canine ventricle, *Circulation*, 60, 798, 1979.

92. Van Camp, S. P., Exercise-related sudden death: risks and cause, *Physician Sportsmed.*, 17, 97, 1988.

93. Siscovick, D. S., Weiss, N. S., Fletcher, R. H., Lasky, T., The incidence of primary cardiac arrest during vigorous exercise, *N. Engl. J. Med.*, 311, 874, 1984.

94. Jennings, G., Nelson, L., Nestel, P., et al., The effect of changes in physical activity on major cardiovascular risk factors, hemodynamics, sympathetic function, and glucose utilization in man: a controlled study of four levels of activity, *Circulation*, 73, 30, 1986.

95. Cousineau, D., Ferguson, R. J., De Champlin, J., Gauthier, P., Cote, P., Bourassaa, M., Catecholamines in coronary sinus during exercise in man, before and after training, *J. Appl. Physiol.*, 43, 801, 1977.

96. Noakes, T., Higginson, L., Opie, L., Physical training increases ventricular fibrillation thresholds of isolated rat hearts during normoxia, hypoxia, and regional ischemia, *Circulation*, 67, 25, 1983.

97. Posel, D., Noakes, T., Kantor, P., Lambert, M., Opie, L. H., Exercise training after experimental myocardial infarction increases the ventricular fibrillation threshold before and after the onset of reinfarction in the isolated rat heart, *Circulation*, 80, 138, 1989.

98. Scheuer, J., Bhan, A. K., Penpargkul, S., Malhotra, A., Effects of physical training and detraining on intrinsic cardiac control mechanisms, *Adv. Cardiol.*, 18, 19, 1976.

99. Weber, J.-R., Left ventricular hypertrophy. Its prime importance as a controllable risk factor, *Am. Heart J.*, 116, 272, 1988.

100. Ekelund, L., Haskell, W. L., Johnson, J. L., Whaley, F. S., Criqui, M. H., et al., Physical fitness as a predictor of cardiovascular mortality in asymptomatic North American men: the Lipid Research Clinics Mortality Follow-Up Study, *N. Engl. J. Med.*, 319, 1379, 1988.

101. Anonymous, Hypertension prevalence and the status of awareness, treatment and control in the United States: final report of the Subcommittee on Definition and Prevalence of the 1984 Joint National Committee, *Hypertension*, 7, 457, 1985.

102. Leon, A. S., Recent advances in the management of hypertension, *J. Cardiopulm. Rehabil.*, 11, 182, 1991.

103. Leon, A. S., Blackburn, H., Physical activity and hypertension, in *International Medical Reviews: Cardiology 1. Hypertension*, Sleight, P., Freis, E., Eds., Butterworths, London, 1982, 14–36.

104. Tipton, C. M., Exercise and resting blood pressure, in *Exercise and Health*, Eckert, H. M., Montoye, H. J., Eds., Human Kinetics, Champaign, IL, 1984, 32–41.

105. McHaiton, M., Palmer, R. M., Exercise and hypertension, *Med. Clin. North Am.*, 69, 57, 1985.

106. Hagberg, J. M., Exercise, fitness, and hypertension, in *Exercise, Fitness, and Health: A Consensus of Current Knowledge*, Bouchard, C., Shepard, R. J., Stephens, T., Sutton, J. R., McPherson, B. D., Eds., Human Kinetics, Champaign, IL, 1990, 455–467.

107. Paffenbarger, R. S., Jr., Wing, A. L., Hyde, R. T., Jung, D. L., Physical activity and incidence of hypertension in college alumni, *Am. J. Epidemiol.*, 117, 245, 1983.

108. Blair, S. N., Goodyear, N. N., Gibbons, L. W., Cooper, K. H., Physical fitness and incidence of hypertension in healthy normotensive men and women, *J. Am. Med. Assoc.*, 252, 487, 1984.

109. Fagard, R., Bielin, E., Hespel, P., Lijren, P., Staessen, J., Vanhees, L., Van Hoff, R., Amery, A., *Physical Exercise in Hypertension: Pathophysiology, Diagnosis, and Management*, Largah, J. H., Brenner, B.M. Eds., Raven Press, New York.

110. Jennings, G., Nielson, L., Nestel, P., Esler, M., Korner, P., Burton, D., Bazelman, J., The effects of changes in physical activity on major cardiovascular risk factors, hemodynamics, sympathetic function, and glucose utilization in man: a controlled study of four levels of activity, *Circulation*, 75, 30, 1986.

111. Reaven, G. M., Banting Lecture 1988: Role of insulin resistance in human disease, *Metabolism*, 37, 1595, 1988.

112. Hiatt, W. R., Regensteiner, J. G., Hargarten, M. E., Wolfel, E. E., Brass, E. P., Benefit of exercise conditioning for patients with peripheral arterial disease, *Circulation*, 81, 602, 1990.

113. Regensteiner, J. G., Steiner, J. F., Panzer, R. J., Hiatt, W. R., Evaluation of walking impairment by questionnaire in patients with peripheral arterial disease, *J. Vasc. Med. Biol.*, 2, 142, 1990.

114. Sternfeld, B., Cancer and the protective effect of physical activity: the epidemiological evidence, *Med. Sci. Sports Exercise*, 24, 1195, 1992.

115. Shephard, R. J., Physical activity and cancer, *Int. J. Sports Med.*, 11, 413, 1990.

116. Calabrese, L. H., Exercise, immunity, cancer, and infection, in *Exercise, Fitness, and Health: a Consensus of Current Knowledge*, Bouchard, C., Shepard, R. J., Stephens, T., Sutton, J. R., McPherson, B. D., Eds., Human Kinetics, Champaign, IL, 1990, 567–579.

117. Cordain, L., Lain, R. W., Benke, J. J., The effects of an aerobic running program on bowel transit time, *J. Sports Med. Phys. Fitness*, 26, 101, 1986.

118. Holdstock, D. J., Misiewicz, J. J., Smith, T., Rowlands, E. N., Propulsion (mass movements) in the human colon and its relationship to meals and somatic activity, *Gut*, 11, 91, 1970.

119. Bartram, H. P., Wynder, E. L., Physical activity and colon cancer risk? Physiological consideration, *Am. J. Gastroenterol.*, 84, 109, 1989.

120. Demers, L. M., Harrison, T. S., Halbert, D. R., Effect of prolonged exercise on plasma prostaglandin levels, *Prostaglandins Med.*, 6, 413, 1981.

121. Tutton, P. J. M., Barkla, D. H., Influence of prostaglandin analogues on epithelial cell proliferation and xenograph growth, *Br. J. Cancer*, 41, 47, 1980.

122. Thor, P., Konturek, J. W., Konturek, S. J., Role of prostaglandins in control of intestinal motility, *Am. J. Physiol.*, 248, G353, 1985.

123. Frisch, R. E., Wyshak, G., Albright, N. L., Lower lifetime occurrence of breast cancer and cancers of the reproductive system among former college athletes, *Am. J. Clin. Nutr.*, 45, 328, 1987.

124. Henderson, B. E., Ross, R. K., Pike, M. C., Toward the primary prevention of cancer, *Science*, 254, 1131, 1991.

125. Rudden, R. A., *Cancer Biology*, 2nd edition, Oxford University Press, New York, 1987.

126. Henderson, B. E., Ross, R. K., Pike, M. C., Casagrande, J. T., Endogenous hormones as a major factor in human cancer, *Cancer Res.*, 42, 3232, 1982.

127. Leon, A. S., Diabetes, in *Exercise Testing and Exercise Prescription for Special Cases*, Skinner, J., Ed., Lea and Febiger, Philadelphia, 1987, 115–134.

128. Petrides, P., Weiss, L., Loffler, G., Wieland, O. H., *Diabetes Mellitus: Theory and Management*, Urban and Schwarzenberg, Baltimore, 1978.

129. West, K. M., Epidemiology of diabetes and its vascular complications, Elsevier, New York, 1978.

130. Wilson, P. W., McGee, D. L., Kannel, W. B. Obesity, very low density lipoproteins, and glucose intolerance over fourteen years: the Framingham Study, *Am. J. Epidemiol.*, 114, 697, 1981.

131. Karan, J. H., Obesity and diabetes in humans, in *Diabetes Mellitus and Obesity*, Brodoff, B. N., Bleicher, S. J., Eds., Williams and Wilkins, Baltimore, 1982, 294–300.

132. Marble, A., Krall, L. P., Bradley, R. F., Christlieb, A. R., Soeldner, J. S., Eds., *Joslin's Diabetes Mellitus*, 12th ed., Lea and Febiger, Philadelphia, 1985.

133. Paffenbarger, R. S., Jr., Wing, A. L., Chronic disease in former college students. XII. Early precursors of adult-onset diabetes mellitus, *Am. J. Epidemiol.*, 97, 314, 1973.

134. Barrett-Conner, E., Epidemiology, obesity and non-insulin-dependent diabetes mellitus, *Epidemiol. Rev.*, 11, 172, 1989.

135. Vranic, M., Wasserman, D, Exercise, fitness, and diabetes, in *Exercise, Fitness and Health: A Consensus of Current Knowledge*, Bouchard, C., Shepard, R. J., Stephens, T., Sutton, J. R., McPherson, B. D. Eds., Human Kinetics, Champaign, IL, 1990, 467.

136. Bjorntorp, P., Fahlen, M., Grimby, G., et al., Carbohydrate and lipid metabolism in middle-aged, physically well-trained men, *Metabolism*, 21, 1037, 1972.

137. Horton, E. S., Exercise and physical training: effects on insulin sensitivity and glucose metabolism, *Diabetes Metab. Rev.*, 2, 1, 1986.

138. West, K. M., *Epidemiology of Diabetes and Its Vascular Complications*, Elsevier, New York, 1978.

139. Frisch, R. E., Wyshak, G., Albright, T. E., Albright, N. L., Schiff, I., Lower prevalence of diabetes in female former college athletes compared with nonathletes, *Diabetes*, 35, 1101, 1986.

140. Taylor, R., Ram, P., Zimmet, L. R., Rapar, L. R., Ringrose, H., Physical activity and prevalence of diabetes in Melanesian and Indian men in Fiji, *Diabetologia*, 27, 578, 1984.

141. Helmrich, S. P., Ragland, D. R., Leung, R. W., Paffenbarger, R. S., Physical activity and reduced occurrence of non-insulin-dependent diabetes mellitus, *N. Engl. J. Med.*, 325, 147, 1991.

142. Lipman, R. L., Raskin, P., Love, T., Triebwasser, L., LeCoq, F. R., Schure, J. J., Glucose intolerance during decreased physical activity in man, *Diabetes*, 21, 101, 1972.

143. Lipman, R. L., Schnure, J. J., Bradley, E. M., Le Cocq, F. R., *J. Lab. Clin. Med.*, 76, 221, 1970.

144. Leon, A. S., The role of exercise in the prevention and management of diabetes mellitus and blood lipid disorders, in *Exercise and the Heart in Health and Disease*, Shephard, R. J., Miller, H. S., Jr., Eds., Marcel Dekker, New York, 1992.

145. Vranic, M., Wassarman, D., Bukowiecki, L., *Diabetes Mellitus, Theory and Practice*, 4th ed., Rifkin, H., Ponte, D., Jr., Eds., Elsevier, New York, 1990, 198–219.

146. Akerblom, K. H., Koivukangas, T., Ikka, J., Experiences from a winter camp for teenage diabetics, *Acta Paediatr. Scand.*, 283, 50, 1980.

147. Campaigne, B. N., Gilliam, T. B., Spencer, M. L., Lampman, R. M., Schork, M. A., Effects of a physical activity program on metabolic control and cardiovascular fitness in children with insulin-dependent diabetes, *Diabetes Care*, 7, 57, 1984.

148. Landt, K. W., Campaigne, B. N., James, F. W., Sperling, M. A., Effects of exercise training on insulin sensitivity in adolescents with type I diabetes, *Diabetes Care*, 8, 461, 1985.

149. Walberg-Henriksson, H., Gunnarson, H., Henriksson, J., DeFronzo, R., Felig, P., Ostman, J., Wahren, J., Increased peripheral insulin sensitivity and muscle mitochondrial enzymes but unchanged blood glucose control in type I diabetics after exercise training, *Diabetes*, 31, 1044, 1982.

150. Yki-Jarvinen, H., DeFronzo, R., Koivisto, V. S., Normalization of insulin sensitivity in type 1 diabetic subjects by physical training during insulin pump therapy, *Diabetes Care*, 7, 520, 1984.

151. Walberg-Henrikkson, H., Gunnarson, H., Rossner, S., Wahren, J., Long-term training in female type I (insulin-dependent) diabetic patients: absence of significant effect on glycaemic control and lipoprotein levels, *Diabetologia*, 29, 53, 1986.

152. Goodyear, L. J., Hirshman, M. F., King, P. A., Horton, E. D., Thompson, C. M., Horton, E. S., Skeletal muscle plasma membrane glucose transport and glucose transporters after exercise, *J. Appl. Physiol.*, 68, 193, 1990.

153. Hirshman, M. F., Wardzala, L. J., Goodyear, L. J., Fuller, S. P., Horton, E. D., Horton, E. S., Exercise training increases the number of glucose transporters in rat adipose cells, *Am. J. Physiol.*, 257, E520, 1989.

154. Koivisto, V. A., et al., Insulin binding to monocytes in trained athletes. Changes in the resting state and after exercise, *Am. Soc. Clin. Invest.*, 64, 1011, 1979.

155. Koivisto, V. A., et al., Exercise and insulin: insulin binding, insulin mobilization, and counter-regulatory hormone secretion, *Fed. Proc.*, 39, 1481, 1980.

156. Pedersen, O., Beck-Nielsen, H., Heding, L., Increased insulin receptors after exercise in patients with insulin-dependent diabetes mellitus, *N. Engl. J. Med.*, 302, 886, 1980.

157. Soman, V. R., et al., Increased insulin sensitivity and insulin binding to monocytes after physical training, *N. Engl. J. Med.*, 301, 1200, 1979.
158. West, K. M., *Epidemiology of Diabetes and Its Vascular Lesions*, Elsevier-North Holland, New York, 1978, 1–579.
159. Truglia, J. A., Livingston, J. N., Lockwood, D. H., *Am. J. Med.*, 79(Suppl.), 13, 1985.
160. Despres, J.-P., Moorjani, S., Lupien, P. J., Tremblay, A., Nadeau, A., Bouchard, C., Regional distribution of body fat, plasma lipoproteins, and cardiovascular disease, *Atherosclerosis*, 10, 497, 1990.
161. Ohlson, L. O., Larsson, B., Swardsudd, K., Wilhelmsen, L., Bjortorp, P., Tibblin, G., The influence of body fat distribution on the incidence of diabetes mellitus. 13.5 years of follow-up of the participants in the study of men born in 1913, *Diabetes*, 34, 1055, 1985.
162. Despres, J.-P., Tremblay, A., Nadeau, A., Bouchard, C., Physical training and changes in regional adipose tissue distribution, *Acta Med. Scand.*, 723, 205, 1988.
163. Horton, E. S., Exercise and decreased risk of NIDDM, *N. Engl. J. Med.*, 325, 196, 1991.
164. Kuczmarski, R. J., Flegal, K. M., Campbell, S. M., Johnson, C. L., Increasing prevalence of overweight among U.S. adult. The National Health and Nutrition Surveys, 1960 to 1991, *JAMA*, 272, 205, 1994.
165. Leon, A. S., The role of physical activity in the prevention and management of obesity, in *Sports Medicine*, 2nd ed., Ryan, J. A., Allman, F. L., Jr., Eds., Academic Press, San Diego, 1989, 5943.
166. Anonymous, Hearing before the Senate Select Committee on Nutrition and Human Needs of the United States Senate Ninety-Fifth Congress First Session Feb. 1–2, 1977. Diet Related to Killer Disease, II. Part 2. Obesity, U.S. Government Printing Office, Washington, D.C., 1977, 1–246.
167. Bray, G. A., The energetics of obesity, *Med. Sci. Sports Exercise*, 15, 32, 1983.
168. Braitman, L. E., Aldin, E. V., Stanton, J. L., Obesity and caloric intake: the national health and nutrition examination survey of 1971–1975 (HANES I), *J. Chronic Dis.*, 38, 727, 1985.
169. Kromhout, D., Energy and macronutrient intake in lean and obese middle-aged men: the Zutphen Study, *Am. J. Clin. Nutr.*, 37, 295, 1983.
170. Folsom, A., Caspersen, C. J., Taylor, H. L., et al., Leisure time physical activity and its relationship to coronary risk factors in a population-based sample. The Minnesota Heart Survey, *Am. J. Epidemiol.*, 12, 570, 1985.
171. Keys, A., *Seven Countries. A Multivariate Analysis of Death and Coronary Heart Disease*, Harvard University Press, Cambridge, MA, 1980, 161–195.
172. Montoye, J. H., *Physical Activity and Health*, Prentice-Hall, Englewood Cliffs, NJ, 1975, 95.
173. Thompson, J. K., Javie, G. J., Lahey, B. B., Cureton, K. J., Exercise and obesity: etiology, physiology, and intervention, *Psychol. Bull.*, 91, 55, 1982.
174. Pollock, M. L., Wilmore, J. H., Fox, S. M., III., *Exercise in Health and Disease. Evaluation and Prescription for Prevention and Rehabilitation*. W.B. Saunders, Philadelphia, 1984, 97–130; 217–228.
175. Brownell, K. D., Stunkard, A. J., Albaum, J. M., Evaluation and modification of exercise patterns in the natural environment, *Am. J. Psychiatry*, 137, 1540, 1980.
176. Chiraco, A., Stunkard, A. J., Physical activity and human obesity, *N. Engl. J. Med.*, 263, 935, 1960.
177. Rand, C., Stunkard, A. J., Obesity and psychoanalysis, *Am. J. Psychiatry*, 135, 547, 1974.
178. Mayer, J., Roy, P., Mitka, K. P., Relation between caloric intake, body weight, and physical work studies in an industrial male population in West Bengal, *Am. J. Clin. Nutr.*, 4, 169, 1956.
179. Lincoln, J. E., Caloric intake, obesity and physical activity, *Am. J. Clin. Nutr.*, 25, 390, 1972.
180. Maxfield, M., Konishi, F., Pattern of food intake and physical activity in obesity, *J. Am. Diet Assoc.*, 49, 406, 1966.
181. Brownell, K. D., Stunkard, A. J., Physical activity in the development and control of obesity, in *Obesity*, Stunkard, A. J., Ed., W.B. Saunders, Philadelphia, 1980, 300–324.
182. Anonymous, American College of Sports Medicine position statement on proper and improper weight loss programs, *Med. Sci. Sports Exercise*, 15, 9, 1983.
183. Epstein, L. H., Wing, R. R., Aerobic exercise and weight, *Addict. Behav.*, 5, 371, 1980.
184. Martin, J. E., Dubbert, P. M., Exercise applications and promotion in behavioral medicine. Current status and future directions, *J. Consult. Clin. Psychol.*, 50, 1004, 1982.
185. Shaw, W. E., The dilemma of obesity. Current concepts of causes and management, *Postgrad. Med.*, 72, 121, 1982.
186. Vasselli, J. R., Cleary, M. P., Van Itallie, T. B., Modern concepts of obesity, *Nutr. Rev.*, 41, 361, 1983.
187. Hagan, R. D., Upton, S. J., Wong, L., Whittam, J., The effects of aerobic conditioning and/or caloric restriction in overweight men and women, *Med. Sci. Sports Exercise*, 18, 87, 1986.
188. Lewis, S., Haskell, W. L., Wood, P. D., Manoogian, N., Baily, J. E., Perera, M., Effects of physical activity on weight reduction in obese middle aged women, *Am. J. Clin. Nutr.*, 29, 151, 1976.
189. Pavlov, K., Steffee, W. P., Lerman, R. H., Burrows, B. A., Effects of dieting and exercise on lean body mass, oxygen uptake and strength, *Med. Sci. Sports Exercise*, 17, 466, 1985.
190. Zuti, W. B., Golding, L. A., Comparing diet and exercise as weight reduction tools, *Phys. Sportsmed.*, 4, 49, 1976.
191. Larrson, B., Svardsudd, K., Wesin, L., Wilhelmsen, L., Bjorntorp, P., Tibblin, G., Abdominal adipose tissue distribution, obesity and risk of cardiovascular disease and death: 13 year follow-up of participants in the study of men born in 1913, *Br. Med. J.*, 288, 1401, 1984.
192. Lapidus, L., Bengtsson, C., Larsson, B., Pennert, K., Rybo, E., Sjostrom, L., Distribution of adipose tissue and risk of cardiovascular disease and death: a 12-year follow-up of participants in the population study of women in Gothburg, Sweden, *Br. Med. J.*, 289, 1261, 1984.

193. Stokes, J., III., Garrison, R. J., Kannel, W. B., The independent contributions of various indices of obesity to the 22-year incidence of coronary heart disease. The Framingham Heart Study, in *Metabolic Complications of Human Obesities*, Vague, J., Bjorntorp, P., Guy-Grand, B., Rebuffe-Scrive, M., Vague, P., Eds., Elsevier Science, Amsterdam, 1985, 49–57.

194. Ducimetiere, P., Richard, J., Cambien, F., The pattern of subcutaneous fat distribution in middle-aged men and the risk of coronary heart disease. The Paris Prospective Study, *Int. J. Obesity*, 10, 229, 1986.

195. Donahue, R. P., Abbot, R. D., Bloom, E., Reed, D. M., Yano, K., Central obesity and coronary heart disease in men, *Lancet*, 1, 822, 1987.

196. Bjorntorp, P., "Portal" adipose tissue as a generator of risk factors for cardiovascular disease and diabetes, *Arteriosclerosis*, 10, 493, 1990.

197. Anonymous, Osteoporosis: consensus conference, *J. Am. Med. Assoc.*, 252, 799, 1984.

198. Cummings, S. R., Kelsey, J. L., Nevitt, M. C., O'Dowd, K. J., Epidemiology of osteoporosis and osteoporotic fractures, *Epidemiol. Rev.*, 7, 178, 1985.

199. Martin, A. D., Houston, C. S., Osteoporosis, calcium and physical activity, *Can. Med. Assoc. J.*, 136, 587, 1987.

200. Snow-Harter, C., Marcus, R., Exercise, bone mineral density, and osteoporosis, in *Exercise and Sport Sciences Reviews*, Vol. 19, Holloszy, J. O., Ed., Williams and Wilkins, Baltimore, 1991, 351–388.

201. Smith, E. L., Smith, K. A., Gilligan, C., Exercise, fitness, osteoarthritis, and osteoporosis, in *Exercise and Health: A Consensus of Current Knowledge*, Bouchard, C., Shepard, R. J., Stephen, T., Sutton, J. R., McPherson, B. D., Eds., Human Kinetics, Champaign, IL, 1990, 517–528.

202. Tipton, C. M., Vailas, A. C., Bone and connective tissue. Adaptations to physical activity, in *Exercise and health: A consensus of current knowledge*, Bouchard, C., Shepard, R. J., Stephen, T., Sutton, J. R., McPherson, B. D., Eds., Human Kinetics, Champaign, IL, 1990, 331–344.

203. Dietrick, J. E., Whedon, C. D., Shorr, E., Effects of immobilization upon various metabolic and physiologic functions of normal men, *Am. J. Med.*, 4, 3, 1948.

204. Donaldson, C. L., Hulley, S. B., Vogel, G. M., et al., Effect of prolonged bed rest on bone mineral, *Metabolism*, 19, 1071, 1970.

205. Mazess, R. B., Whedon, C. D., Immobilization and bone, *Calcif. Tissue Int.*, 35, 265, 1983.

206. Whedon, G. D., Disuse osteoporosis: physiological aspects, *Calcif. Tissue Int.*, 36, S146, 1984.

207. Abramson, A. S., Delagi, E. F., Influence of weight-bearing and muscle contraction on disuse osteoporosis, *Arch. Phys. Med. Rehabil.*, 42, 147, 1961.

208. Nilsson, B. E., Westlin, N. E., Bone density in athletes, *Clin. Orthop.*, 77, 179, 1971.

209. Dalen, N., Olsson, K. E., Bone mineral content and physical activity, *Acta Orthop. Scand.*, 45, 170, 1974.

210. Jones, H. H., Priest, J. D., Hayes, W. C., et al., Humeral hypertrophy in response to exercise, *J. Bone Joint Surg. Am. Vol.*, 59A, 204, 1977.

211. Aloia, J. F., Cohn, S. H., Bab, T., et al., Skeletal mass and body composition in marathon runners, *Metabolism*, 27, 1793, 1978.

212. Huddleson, A. L., Rockwell, D., Kulund, D. N., et al., Bone mass in lifetime tennis athletes, *J. Am. Med. Assoc.*, 244, 1107, 1980.

213. Haskell, W. L., Dose-response relationship of physical activity and disease risk factors, in *Sports for All*, Ojrtelama, P., Ed., Elsevier, Amsterdam, 1991.

214. Haskell, W. L., Physical activity and health: need to define the required stimulus, *Am. J. Cardiol.*, 55, 4D, 1985.

215. Bouchard, C., Shephard, R. J., Physical activity, fitness and health: the model and key concepts, in *Physical Activity, Fitness, and Health: A Consensus of Current Knowledge*, Bouchard, C., Shephard, R. J., Stephens, T., Sutton, J. R., McPherson, B. D., Eds., Human Kinetics, Champaign, IL, 1993.

216. Paffenbarger, R. S., Jr., Hale, W. E., Work activity and coronary heart mortality, *N. Engl. J. Med.*, 292, 545, 1975.

217. Paffenbarger, R. S., Jr., Hyde, R. T., Wing, A. L., Hsieh, C.-C, Physical activity, all-cause mortality, and longevity of college alumni, *N. Engl. J. Med.*, 314, 605, 1986.

218. Anonymous, *Healthy People 2000: National Health Promotion and Disease Prevention Objectives*, Department of Health and Human Services, Jones and Bartlett Publishers, Boston, 1992.

219. Hahn, R. A., Teutsch, S. M., Rothenberg, R. B., Marks, J. S., Excess deaths from nine chronic diseases in the United States, 1986, *J. Am. Med. Assoc.*, 264, 2654, 1990.

Index

A

ACC, 137–138, 149
Acetylcholine (ACh), 51, 58, 60, 102
Acidosis
  and exercise intensity, 227
  metabolic, 7, 158, 228–229
  and oxyhemuclobin dissociation, 33
  and stroke volume, 10
  and ventilation changes, 35, 39, 42
ACSM. *See* American College of Sports Medicine
Actin, 58–63, 65–67
Action potentials, 49–50
Adenosine
  and blood flow, 93
  and echocardiography, 209–212, 214–216
  and radionuclide exercise testing, 200
  responses to exercise, 7
  and vasodilation, 15, 101, 190
Adenosine diphosphate (ADP), 62–63
ADH release, 7
Adrenals and cardiovascular control, 16, 98
Adrenergic receptors, 14, 53
Advanced Cardiac Life Support, 129
Aerobic capacity, 11
Aerobic power, 73–74, 78–79
Afterload, 96, 208
Aging
  and basal metabolism, 78, 258
  and coronary artery disease, 149
  effects on body systems, 258
  and exercise, 85–86, 230–231, 239, 244, 247, 258–259
  and flexibility, 83
  and hormonal changes, 84
  and muscle changes, 81–83, 258
  and osteoporosis, 83–84
  and oxygen transport, 78–81
  and protein synthesis, 83
  theories of, 77–78
  and training response, 81–82
AIDS and exercise testing, 139

Air pollution and oxygen partial pressures, 32
Alanine, calorimetry data for, 5
Alcohol intake, 5, 140, 158–159, 285
Aldosterone, 7, 15
Altitudes, high, and blood oxygen, 42
Alveoli, 24, 27–31, 36
American College of Cardiology (ACC), 137–138, 149
American College of Sports Medicine (ACSM)
  and contraindications to testing, 139
  on exercise and hypertension, 246
  exercise testing protocols, 238, 273
  screening recommendations, 129, 238–239
  and testing termination criteria, 144
  and test interpretation, 135, 145–146
American Heart Association (AHA), 137–138, 141, 144–145, 149
Aminophylline, 190, 212–214
Ammonia, 187
Anaerobic capacity and gender differences, 74
Anaerobic glycolysis, 228
Anaerobic threshold (AT), 227–229, 231–232
Anemia, 32, 162, 164
Aneurysm, 139, 161, 246, 287
Anger and health behavior change, 267
Angina
  characteristics of, 144
  and coronary artery disease, 148–150, 239
  and drug stressors, 212
  and echocardiography, 155, 166, 218
  and exercise testing, 138–141, 151, 165
  and myocardial infarction, 196
  pain scale of, 141–142
Angiogram, radionuclide, 18, 194, 197, 216
Angioplasty, 196, 217
Angiotensin release, 14–15, 246, 287
Anterior wall infarction, 158
Anxiety
  about behavior changes, 264, 267
  and exercise, 248
  and exercise testing, 126, 128–129, 140, 145, 248
  inventory of, 268